The psychopharmacology of smoking

The psychopharmacology of smoking

G. L. MANGAN

Research Fellow, Department of Psychology, University of Auckland

J. F. GOLDING

Research Associate, The Medical School, University of Newcastle upon Tyne

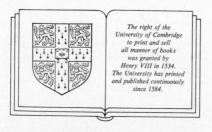

The right of the
University of Cambridge
to print and sell
all manner of books
was granted by
Henry VIII in 1534.
The University has printed
and published continuously
since 1584.

CAMBRIDGE UNIVERSITY PRESS

Cambridge

London New York New Rochelle

Melbourne Sydney

Published by the Press Syndicate of the University of Cambridge
The Pitt Building, Trumpington Street, Cambridge CB2 1RP
32 East 57th Street, New York, NY 10022, USA
296 Beaconsfield Parade, Middle Park, Melbourne 3206, Australia

First published 1984

Printed in Great Britain by
the Cambridge University Press, Cambridge

Library of Congress catalogue card number: 83-15275

British Library cataloguing in publication data
Mangan, G. L.
The psychopharmacology of smoking.
1. Tobacco – Physiological effect
I. Title II. Golding, J. F.
613.8′5   R1242.T6

ISBN 0 521 25806 5

Contents

Preface

It is probably true to say that the debate surrounding tobacco use has generated more heat than any other public health issue in recent years. The well-known reports of the Royal College of Physicians (1962, 1971, 1977) and the USA Surgeon General, and a number of subsequent epidemiological studies in many countries have confirmed a strong relationship between smoking cigarettes and increased morbidity and mortality rates. However, despite increasingly strong pressure from medical and health education authorities, these findings have made less impact on smoking prevalence rates than might be expected. Reasons for this are unclear, although a number of possibilities suggest themselves.

The first is the rationalisation, made by many smokers, that the health risks have been exaggerated. This is an aggressive defence which is difficult to shake, since it is surely a truism that correlational data of the sort reported in many of the 'critical' studies do not *demand* an assumption of causality. Nor, of course, do they disconfirm the hypothesis. It simply remains untested. But why should such a statement occasion, at times, such hostile reactions? Our own experience, and that of many workers in the field, suggests that some of the principals involved in what should be a serious scientific debate regard the issues as being moral rather than scientific ones. In a sometimes furious arena, we can detect distant echoes of that statement attributed to the president of the revolutionary tribunal which tried and convicted Lavoisier: 'La république n'a pas besoin de savants'.

Fortunately for science, however, facts are stubborn things. As Pavlov was fond of repeating, 'Mr Fact' is the final arbiter, and we follow where he leads. But what are the facts? If we accept that there is a substantial health risk from smoking, even though the exact nature and extent of this risk may not yet have been fully established, why then do individuals continue to smoke?

The most comfortable explanation is that individuals become addicted to nicotine, i.e., that they are 'hooked' and cannot 'kick' the habit. Arguing from this point of view, many advocate that our best efforts should be directed towards persuading young people not to start smoking. On the other hand, if we adopt a cost/benefit approach it could be argued that the confirmed smoker clearly sees more gain than disadvantage from smoking, this advantage maintaining the habit, especially since the gain is immediate whereas the disadvantage may occur some time in the smoker's future. But what is this advantage? If, for some individuals, it is substantial, and persuasive enough to outweigh the costs, can we, and should we, turn our attention to producing a 'safer' cigarette, i.e., one which maximises the benefits and minimises the costs for such individuals?

These are the questions which we address in the following pages. Inevitably, in view of the great proliferation of smoking research over the past twenty years, as evidenced, for example, in the Surgeon General's Reports, we have to select material. Where we place emphasis, and how we select studies for inclusion, will obviously reflect our personal judgement about what is representative and important, taking into account, of course, normally accepted criteria governing scientific investigation. The alternative is an unwieldy mass of information, difficult to digest and impossible to judge. We shall also attempt to point out the logical implications of such findings, again, we hope, with clarity and objectivity.

In view of the doubts sometimes expressed about the ethics of research funding from bodies which can be seen as having a vested interest in the research outcome, might we state that British-American Tobacco Company, whose support we enjoyed during the writing of this book, in no way whatsoever commented on our selection and perception of problem areas, or attempted to influence our judgement about any of the contentious issues examined.

The issues we discuss in the following chapters are as follows. In Part I we re-examine evidence for smoking–disease relationships, particularly in the light of some recent genetic studies, and describe theories about smoking. In Part II we review studies concerning the pharmacological and psychological effects of nicotine and smoking, and report a survey study of variables underlying recruitment to, and, with the older groups in the sample, maintenance of smoking amongst 2400 Oxfordshire school-children. This hitherto unpublished study was completed by one of the authors (GLM) during the tenure of a Social Science Research Council

Smoking Fellowship. We also review data relevant to an 'enhancement' model of smoking maintenance. In Part III we attempt to evaluate the various Health Education programmes and intervention and termination strategies essayed over the last twenty years. Finally, we raise the problem of the 'safer' cigarette, a contentious issue, since it seems to carry with it, inevitably, tacit acceptance of the fact that there are always going to be some individuals who smoke.

Gordon L. Mangan
John F. Golding
Department of Experimental Psychology,
University of Oxford

Abbreviations

ACh   acetylcholine
ACTH   adrenocorticotrophic hormone (corticotrophin)
Ad   adrenaline (epinephrine)
ADH   antidiuretic hormone (vasopressin)
CFF   critical flicker frequency, fusion
CNS   central nervous system
CNV   contingent negative variation
COHb   carboxyhaemoglobin
COLD   chronic obstructive lung disease
CRF   corticotrophin-releasing factor
CS   conditioned stimulus
CVS   cardiovascular system
Dz   dizygotic, twin
E   extraversion
ECG   electrocardiogram
EEG   electroencephalogram
EMG   electromyogram
EOG   electro-oculogram
EPQ   Eysenck Personality Questionnaire
GABA   *gamma*-aminobutyric acid

GSR   galvanic skin response (see SCR)
5-HT   5-hydroxytryptamine (serotonin)
i.p.   intraperitoneal, injection
i.v.   intravenous, injection
L   lie scale of EPQ
Mz   monozygotic, twin
N   neuroticism
NA   noradrenaline (norepinephrine)
NET   non-exposed twin
P   psychoticism scale of EPQ
SAE   spiral after-effect
s.c.   subcutaneous, injection
SCL   skin conductance level
SCN   thiocyanate
SCR   skin conductance response
SES   socioeconomic status
SFs   spontaneous fluctuation, in SCL
SS   self-stimulation, electrical
SSS   sensation-seeking scale
TPM   total particulate matter, in tobacco smoke
US   unconditioned stimulus

PART I

THE UNIVERSE OF DISCOURSE

Introduction

The ancestors of today's tobacco plant were undergoing evolution of their plant chemistry to produce alkaloids such as nicotine more than sixty-five million years ago. Alkaloids have no known function in plant metabolism, and it has been suggested that they are evolutionarily justified as a chemical deterrent against herbivores (Bever, 1970). Some authors (Swain, 1974; Gritz & Siegel, 1979) have noted that this evolutionary advance of plant chemistry coincided with the sudden extinction of the dominant animal life-form of that era – the dinosaurs. Perhaps these giant reptiles, unlike the birds and mammals which followed them, failed to evolve effective mechanisms with which to detect and/or detoxify alkaloids.

The effectiveness of alkaloids, and nicotine in particular, as a chemical defence against animals, can be judged from a contemporary account of the effects of a wild tobacco, *Nicotiana glauca* (African tobacco with a high nicotine content), on the ostrich. ' . . . the ostrich is particularly susceptible, the symptoms being staggering gait, spasmodic jerking of the head, dullness and stupor. Death occurs within a few hours . . . One seed is said to be certain death to a chick ostrich up to one month old' (Watt & Breyer-Brandwijk, 1962).

Although such experiences undoubtedly act as a deterrent for the would-be herbivore, the consumption of small quantities of toxic tobacco leaf is not lethal for many animals, and may even be reinforcing (Watt & Breyer-Brandwijk, 1962). Indeed, it has been suggested that humans learned much about plant-produced drugs through observing the effects of accidental self-administration by animals. Folklore abounds with accounts of the discovery of the various properties (which are due to the alkaloids they contain) of, for example, coffee (caffeine), qat leaves (cathine, cathedine, cathenine), coca (cocaine) and *Datura* (scopolamine and also atropine).

3

One typical story, told by an informant from the Huichol community of Bance de Calitice (Nayarit, Mexico), claims that tobacco was first used by birds which favoured the yellow flowers of the wild varieties (e.g., *N. rustica*). The tobacco enabled the birds to fly high and strong and to see great visions. Accordingly, early man copied such behaviours in attempting to communicate with gods and see visions. Of course, while high, verging on toxic, doses of nicotine may be hallucinogenic in their own right, it is possible that 'communication with gods' requires the addition of other alkaloids to a smoking mixture (consult Gritz & Siegel (1979) for review).

Nicotiana tabacum and *N. rustica* are plants indigenous to the Americas. Natives of the Americas had smoked and chewed these herbs for a variety of narcotic, stimulant, medicinal, social and religious reasons for a long time prior to the arrival of European explorers. Fig. 1 shows a stone carving of a Maya priest smoking a tube pipe. 'Tupa' or 'devil's tobacco' is the name by which the Mapuche Indians of Chile know the tall herb *Lobelia tupa*. The Mapuche smoked the leaves for their narcotic effect. The expressed juice was used to relieve toothache. In North America *L. inflata* was also chewed for its narcotic effects. The active principle, lobeline, is similar to nicotine in action.

Just as the natives of the Americas may have modelled animal drug-taking behaviour, so did the first Spaniards to set foot in the New World model the native predilection for tobacco smoke. De las Casas, the Bishop of Chiapas (located in present-day Mexico), who published the letters of Columbus, described the initial encounter with tobacco smoke. 'I know of Spaniards who imitate this custom, and when I reprimanded the savage practice, they answered that it was not in their power to refrain from indulging in the habit' (Lewin, 1931, p. 288).

Following the initial contact by Columbus and his men in 1492, tobacco was brought to Europe in the sixteenth century by explorers such as Sir Walter Raleigh, M. Jean Nicot (hence 'nicotine') and André Thevet. Although Jean Nicot and Sir Walter Raleigh are the individuals most often associated with the introduction of tobacco to Europe, the tobacco they introduced was the inferior *N. rustica* from North America, rather than its superior and eventually more successful Brazilian cousin *N. tabacum*, which was brought by Thevet to France in 1556. This issue of primacy of introduction seems to have been contested. It would appear from contemporary texts that Thevet objected strongly to Nicot's claim (Emboden, 1972).

It has been suggested that the first man to smoke in Europe was the Spaniard Rodrigo de Jerez, upon his return from the New World in 1493 (Barclays Bank, 1961). An approximate date for the introduction to

Fig. 1. Maya figure of an individual in the act of smoking. (After Corti, 1931.) Stone bas-relief in the Temple of the Foliated Cross, Palenque, Chiapas, Mexico. Middle Classic Period (AD 642–783 (Morley, 1947)): adjacent Temple dedication date glyphs give a Maya date equivalent to AD 692 (Anton, 1978). The figure has been variously described as 'Temple priest smoking' (Corti, 1931) or 'Maya rain god blowing smoke to the four winds' (Emboden, 1972).

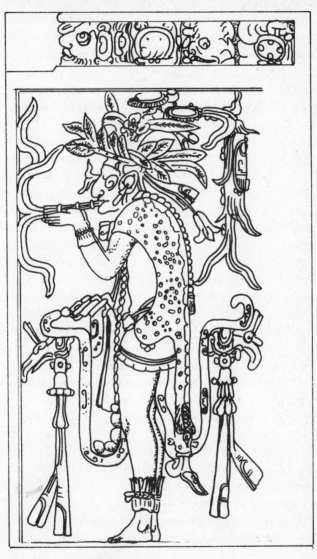

England is given by Edmund Howes (1631), who wrote that 'tobacco was first brought, and made known in England by Sir John Hawkins, about the yeare 1565 but not used by Englishmen in many yeares after, though at this day commonly used by most men, and many women' (Atkins, 1936).

Meanwhile, Portugese and Spanish sailors were introducing tobacco to the far corners of the world. The Portugese took the herb to West Africa, where its cultivation was begun; to India, where the first crop was grown in about 1605; and to Ceylon, Indonesia, China (today the world's largest producer and consumer of tobacco) and Japan. The Spaniards developed production in Central and South America and took tobacco to the Philippines (Barclays Bank, 1961). This spreading usage continues today in the underdeveloped countries of the world (Taha & Ball, 1980).

In this context, it is interesting to note that tobacco may replace an indigenous herb in popularity. For example, after the arrival of white men in Australia, tobacco became popular among the Aborigines. Formerly, leaves of the *Duboisia* species were used as a popular narcotic going under the name of 'pituri', the active principle of which is scopolamine. Scopolamine is primarily a depressant but has secondary activity as a hallucinogen. However, it was not long before these people became interested in 'white fellow pituri' (tobacco) (Emboden, 1972).

How rapidly the demand for tobacco grew can be gauged from the fact that by 1640 the annual export from Virginia and Maryland to England was over one million pounds weight, to service almost 7500 tobacco shops in London alone (Emboden, 1972). This was no doubt stimulated by the beliefs (then held) that tobacco had potent aphrodisiac powers, e.g., sailors told of the women of Nicaragua who smoked the weed and displayed an undreamed-of ardour (Emboden, 1972). In addition there were the widely touted medicinal benefits; tobacco was promoted as a remedy for many ailments, including 'sick kidnies' and 'naughty breath' (Buttes, 1599). In 1560 Nicot sent a gift of powdered tobacco leaves and seed to Catherine de Medici to be snuffed up the nose to relieve her headaches (Emboden, 1972). The prophylactic virtues of tobacco are underlined in the following entry from a dictionary published by Nicot with several other scholars in 1573. 'Nicotaine: a herb of marvellous virtue against all wounds, ulcers, face ulcers and similar things, which M. Jean Nicot, Ambassador to the King of Portugal, sent to France and from whom it has derived its name'. Tobacco was also thought to ward off other diseases, most notably the plague.

This rapid increase in tobacco usage was opposed from the outset, and anti-smoking measures were taken from the earliest times. The objections of non-smokers to the effects of smoking, which find a modern counterpart in objections to the suggested dangers of 'passive smoking', were aired by an Italian traveller in America, Girolamo Benzoni (1565). 'I have entered the house of an Indian who had taken this herb...and immediately perceiving the sharp fetid smell of this truly diabolical and stinking smoke, I was obliged to go away in haste, and seek some other place' (cited by Atkins, 1936). The Pope concurred with this view and outlawed all smoking in the Vatican under threat of excommunication in 1590. In 1604, James I, in his *A counterblaste to Tobacco*, described the habit thus: 'A custome lothsome to the eye, hatefull to the Nose, harmefull to the braine, dangerous to the Lungs, and in the blacke stinking fume thereof, neerest resembling the horrible Stigian smoke of the pit that is bottomelesse.'

Other countries took stronger measures. In Russia any person who smoked was exiled to Siberia after his nose and lips had been split wide open, and in Turkey the punishment was death (Duncan, 1951).

In England the official view (1604) was reinforced by imposition of an import duty of 6s 8d a pound on tobacco to limit the increasing imports '...by which great and immoderate takinge of Tabacco the Health of a great nomber of our People is impayred, and theire Bodies weakened and made unfit for labor...'

Charles I continued the restrictions on tobacco import and sale, and entertained a strong personal dislike to its use, one of the few attitudes that he held in common with his successor Oliver Cromwell who, sharing in the belief that to grow tobacco was to 'misuse and misemploy the soil', sent his troopers to trample down the crops (Tanner, 1912). However, despite the controversy both for and against 'the weed' aired by texts of that era, the use of tobacco increased.

The failure of these early anti-tobacco moves probably occurred for many reasons. It should be remembered that the introduction of tobacco was shortly followed by that of tea and coffee in the seventeenth century (Bianchini, Corbetta & Pistola, 1977), and this arguably may have directed some moralistic attention away from 'the weed'. The diversion is underlined in texts such as *The Women's Petition Against Coffee* (Anon., 1674), *The Character of a Coffee-House* (Eye and Ear Witness, 1665) and *Two Broad-Sides Against Tobacco* (Hancock, 1672), which include long polemics against coffee and alcohol. It can also be argued that the health risks claimed, e.g., by James I, could not be proven in the context of the shorter average life-span of that era, since we now know that the majority of smoking-related diseases occur at 40–50 years of age. We can cite evidence that the anti-smoking lobby of the early seventeenth century was fully aware of the difficulties of proving their case on health grounds alone. For example, possible objections to health arguments were anticipated by the anti-tobacco writer Philaretus (1602) in his chapter detailing the sixth reason for rejecting tobacco. 'But here may be objected, that if *Tabacco* were of that poysoned nature (as wee have affirmed) then no doubt, the Indians (who usually drinke it) should have long since bin poisoned therewith. But hitherto they have found no such hurt, but rather great commoditie and manifest benefit thereby.'

A crucial factor, of course, may have been the actual inhalation of the tobacco smoke, which was probably difficult, since manufacturers of that era had not yet mastered the secrets of tobacco maturing and blending to produce a less irritating smoke, a process which was eventually to lead to the popularisation of the cigarette in this century. Philaretus (1602, Sixth reason) commented that 'Fewe or none do take it downe the throates, and such as let it passe down, they mince it in such sort, and swallow it in so small quantitie, as that no great detriment can happen to them thereby.' However, all arguments, whether medical or moral (tobacco being a product of 'the devill'), crumbled before the very obvious pleasures given by smoking, and its more arguable medicinal and aphrodisiac properties. Finally, the increasing importance that tobacco was assuming in trade with the American colonies, and the lucrative tax consequences for the Exchequer, began to warm official opinion towards tobacco. The tobacco revenue was considerable; by the end of the seventeenth century tobacco was returning a greater revenue to the treasury than was any other product of the colonies (Brooks, 1953).

By the time of Charles II, tobacco had passed what may be termed its stage of persecution and was being cultivated all over Europe and Western Asia. For example, as early as 1615, a grower's guide entitled *An Advice How To Plant Tobacco In England; With the Danger of the Spanish Tobacco* had been published in England (C.T., 1615). Charles II prohibited its growth in England mainly to encourage commerce, although the difficulty in taxing home production may also have been an incentive. The subsequent history of tobacco to the mid-twentieth century mainly concerns the mode and prevalence of its usage, increasing sophistication of manufacture both in the blending of various tobacco strains and in curing, and its importance as regards commerce and tax revenue.

Historical and regional differences affected the mode of tobacco usage. Although pipe smoking had become general by the late seventeenth century, snuffing was particularly popular in Scotland and Ireland, the snuffing habit probably being copied from France, where Catherine de Medici had first set the fashion (Tanner, 1912). Snuffing appears to have reached its height of popularity in the eighteenth century, when the snuff box became the hallmark of elegance in the fashionable world. Snuffing has since declined to near negligible levels, snuffers currently representing less than 1 or 2% of the American adult population (Surgeon General, 1979, Ch. 14, p. 13). A similar growth and decline can be detected in the chewing of tobacco, which became most popular in the nineteenth century, when the spittoon was a common fixture, but subsequently declined. Today less than 6% of the adult population in the United States, and less still in the UK (in the new form of nicotine chewing-gum) indulge in the habit. The reasons for this initial upsurge in chewing are obscure except in certain instances, e.g., because of fire hazards in saw mills and British naval vessels. 'But whatever the reason, the fact remains that a large part of the population of the United States became ruminating animals' (Brooks, 1953). Chewing in itself may be reinforcing, of course, judging from the twentieth-century popularity of chewing-gum.

The century of the spittoon also saw the explosive growth in popularity of the cigar. Cigar smoking had always been popular with the Spanish, who no doubt copied the dominant (cigar) smoking behaviour of the American Indians indigenous to their colonies. By contrast, the Portugese indulged in both cigars and pipes, probably because the natives of Brazil used both, whereas the English and French, who came into contact with the North American Indians, tended to use the pipe, as did the original peoples of this region (Brooks, 1953, pp. 29 and 193). However, following the Iberian peninsular war, the cigar became popular in Britain. Similar Hispanic influences can be traced in the growth of popularity of the cigar in North America. The 'fat cigar' perhaps symbolised the violent expansion of industry and wealth in the nineteenth century. Meanwhile, in the mid-nineteenth century, the clay pipe evolved to the briar, cob and meerschaum pipes, similar to the forms of pipe seen today.

The late nineteenth and early twentieth centuries saw the cigarette become the most popular tobacco product. The origins of the cigarette can be traced to the Aztecs, who smoked tobacco-filled reeds a foot or so in length (approximately 30 cm in length). The Spanish conquerors experimented, made the refinement of using paper tubes – *papeletes* – and transmitted their use to other colonial possessions as well as to Portugal, Italy, the Levant, the Orient and South Russia. However, until the mid-nineteenth century the cigarette was never more than an oddity by comparison with the cigar. Women appear to have popularised early cigarette usage, the term 'cigarette' originating in France, where, in the 1840s, an English lady traveller reported that it had 'become la grande mode with certain French ladies' (Brooks, 1953). This feminine article quickly crossed the Atlantic to New York, where Dr Trall, in the mid-nineteenth century, commented: 'Some of the ladies…are aping the silly ways of some pseudo-accomplished foreigners, in smoking Tobacco through a weaker and more feminine article, which has been most delicately denominated cigarette.' The Crimean War introduced the cigarette to Britain via returning servicemen. However, the hand-rolled cigarette, filled with tobaccos from Turkey and the Near East, remained an exotic luxury by comparison with the pipe and cigar until the beginning of the twentieth century.

The first cigarette factory in England is believed to have been opened in 1856 in Walworth, London, by Robert Gloag, who served in the Crimea. His cigarettes were hand made and crude, with cane mouthpieces, and achieved little success. Cigarette popularity increased when Virginian

Fig. 2. (*a*) Historical trends in tobacco consumption for the UK. Consumption is in mean pounds weight of tobacco consumed per adult head of population (15+years of age) per year, i.e., not smokers only. Tobacco consumption is given for men and women, separately and combined. Tobacco in the form of cigarettes is shown separately. (Data from Lee, 1976.) (*b*) Trends in cigarette smoking in the UK for adult males and females (16+years of age). Consumption (top) and prevalence (bottom). (After Capell, 1978.) Continuations of these trends may be found in Cox, H. & Marks, L. (1983). *Health Trends*, **15**, 48–52.

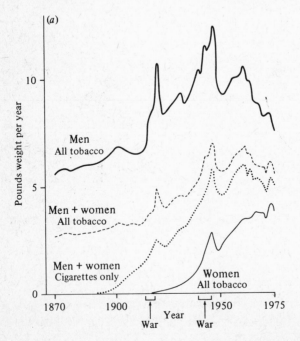

tobacco was used in the 1870s and 1880s, and when hand-rolled cigarettes were replaced by efficient machine-made cigarettes with fine-textured paper (Barclays Bank, 1961). Gritz & Siegel (1979) suggest a date as late as 1913 as the critical 'take-off' date for the cigarette, when Richard Joshua Reynolds blended a newly developed flue-cured (Virginia type) tobacco with air-cured (Burley) tobacco, resulting in an eminently inhalable mild cigarette. The pleasures of inhalation-style smoking, combined with modern manufacturing and sales techniques, rapidly led to the cigarette becoming the dominant mode of tobacco usage during the First World War.

Recent trends in tobacco consumption (in particular amongst women) and the prevalence of cigarette smoking are shown in Figs. 2a and 2b. Note that the dramatic rise in tobacco consumption by women is from a zero

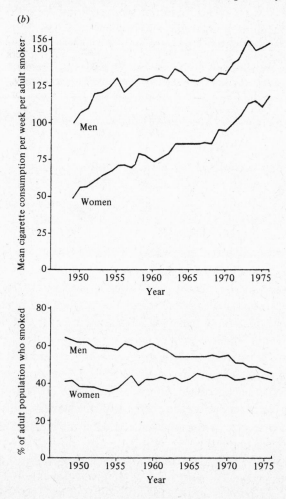

starting-point according to Tobacco Research Council data (Fig. 2*a*). This presumably reflects the paucity of early tobacco consumption data broken down by sex as there are certainly many early references to women smoking. Thomas Carlyle, for example, in *Reminiscences* (1881), recalled that Scottish peasant women smoked tobacco in short clay pipes during the latter part of the eighteenth century (1799) (Trevelyan, 1945; see Brooks, 1937, for extensive references).

Two aspects of the data shown in Figs. 2*a* and 2*b* are of particular interest. Firstly, there is a marked upsurge in smoking during time of war, which could be due to any one, or a combination, of several factors, of which perhaps the most plausible are easy access to, and cheapness of, cigarettes supplied to the armed services, and the postulated anxiety reducing effects of nicotine (see Chapter 2: Arousal modulation theory). The latter would be of obvious relevance in times of prolonged stress. A recent parallel is the increase in cigarette consumption and prevalence which occurred in Israel during and after the Yom Kippur War, which has been ascribed to tension and nervousness (Ben-Meir, 1977). However, availability and cost are probably limiting factors; during the Second World War tobacco consumption fell dramatically in Nazi Occupied Europe at the same time as consumption rose in Great Britain (Beese, 1972).

Secondly, there is recent evidence that while prevalence rates for males, although not for females, declined in the period 1950–75, consumption rates for both men and women rose quite steeply over this period. This could indicate that while a smaller section of the population was 'at risk' from smoking, for that section 'at risk', the health hazards may have increased appreciably, although the extent to which risk from increased consumption is counterbalanced by the increased popularity of lower nicotine/tar yield cigarettes is unknown.

From the graphs, a further inference is possible. If, as seems to be the case, prevalence curves for both males and females have flattened out, then probably, for the foreseeable future, there will be a hard core of smokers in the population, i.e., individuals who are untouched by anti-smoking campaigns aimed largely at persuading young people not to start smoking, or by intervention and termination strategies directed to the older, more committed smoker. Whether increased efforts along these lines will produce further down-turns in prevalence curves is problematical. This probably means that we need to re-examine some of the more important issues in the light of recent findings.

The first of these issues concerns relationships between smoking cigarettes and disease originally underlined in the Surgeon General's (1964) Report, and the Report of the Royal College of Physicians (1962). Some more recent studies suggest that these relationships may not be as simple and unequivocal as was first suggested, and that more research needs to be done to tease out the critical variables, and to establish their exact role in the aetiology of cause-specific morbidity and mortality.

As a case in point, one view attracting a good deal of attention, and commanding some empirical support, is the proposal that there is a genetic basis for smoking, and a genetic basis for certain cause-specific diseases such as lung cancer and heart disease. Given the high prevalence rates for smoking, a possible implication is that if certain individuals are predisposed to smoke, and if certain of these individuals are predisposed to contract diseases such as lung cancer and heart disease, such risks being increased by smoking, then the linked probabilities could artefactually boost the correlations typically reported between smoking and disease. The resolution of this issue is important, both in terms of removing any doubts in the smoker's mind about his personal health risk, which may lower his motivation to give up smoking, and also, in general public health terms, in assessing to what degree changes in other lifestyle variables such as diet, drinking and stressful activities may be important for the health of the population.

The second major issue concerns the reasons why individuals continue to smoke cigarettes given that major health risks are involved. A good deal of controversy has centred round this question, and a number of theories about smoking have been proposed. These can be conveniently divided into addiction and 'functional' theories. If we accept a simple addiction theory, we know why individuals continue to smoke. Such theories, however, having nothing to say about recruitment to smoking, i.e., the reasons why individuals started smoking in the first place, and we have to appeal to other explanatory concepts such as those proposed, for example, by social learning or social dysfunction theories of smoking to account for this.

Alternative, 'functional' theories have in common some version of cost/benefit analysis. Smoking damages health, that is the cost. But what is the compensating benefit? There is evidence to suggest that nicotine, as the primary reinforcer in smoking, contributes to both psychological comfort and performance enhancement. The implications of such findings for both intervention and termination strategies are obvious.

A number of secondary issues inevitably flow from the kinds of answers we propose to these major questions. For example, if we adopt a polydrug model, for which there is considerable support, i.e., the notion that nicotine, alcohol and minor tranquillisers are used, as available, and possibly in combination, as mood control agents, then what are the consequences of persuading individuals to stop smoking or drinking? Will the individual who stops smoking drink more, and vice-versa? If so, what are the likely health consequences? The possibility of 'displacement' or 'migration' of this sort becomes more plausible if we postulate some genetic component underlying drug use. This may be represented, at second order, by the excessive use of drugs by the stimulation-seeker, or by the highly anxious person, both stimulation-seeking and anxiety being personality dimensions which have genetic as well as environmental components.

1

The smoking/health debate

A question encountered at one time or another by most smokers is 'Why do you persist in smoking cigarettes when you know the health risks involved?' Usually, what is implied is a lack of will-power underlying this apparent inability to quit what is a socially distasteful, potentially dangerous habit.

A number of rejoinders are possible. One is the frequently advanced claim that the health risks have been exaggerated, a much-ado-about-nothing argument to counter what is regarded as the moralistic, almost religious fanaticism of a do-gooding section of the community which regards even the mildest form of self-indulgence as sinful. This argument still retains some force, at least superficially. Whether or not the health risk has been overly emphasised is still much debated. It is difficult, in this field, to find sober, measured judgements. Most of the early smoking/health studies were correlational studies, and surely it is axiomatic that while correlation may suggest, it certainly does not require, an assumption of causality. But neither is such an assumption necessarily untenable. The real problem is that the highly complex network of interrelated and interacting variables associated with smoking can only be identified in terms of cause–effect relationships by more powerful methodologies and statistical procedures than have usually been employed. This has been remedied to some extent in some more recent studies, such as those of Cederlof, Friberg & Lundman (1977), and it is to these that we will turn for more illuminating insights. The earlier studies may have exaggerated the risks which undoubtedly exist. On the other hand, the reduced risks suggested by more recent studies may be in part a function of changes in the product itself (lower tar content).

Thus, initially, we need to re-ask the question, one which is obviously critical in the debate, of just how substantial is the elevated mortality risk

15

from being a smoker, compared with being a member of some other group? As a background to this question we will first summarise findings concerning the toxicology of tobacco smoke itself.

The toxicology of tobacco smoke

The cigarette has been likened to a miniature chemical factory producing a complex mixture of gases and tar particles containing scores of organic compounds. In the gas phase the major constituents (by weight or volume) are nitrogen, oxygen and carbon dioxide, all present normally in the air. However, in the residual gases, apart from water vapour and the noble gases, carbon monoxide (CO) is present in significant concentrations (4% by volume approximately), together with smaller amounts of other gases including isoprene, acetaldehyde, acetone and hydrogen cyanide. In the particulate phase the major components are nicotine, in pharmacologically active concentrations, and tar. Tar is the sticky brown residual substance left after removing nicotine and moisture, and consists of a complex mixture of polynuclear aromatic hydrocarbons including benzopyrene, pyrene, catechol and N'-nitrosonornicotine (for detailed chemical breakdowns see Surgeon General, 1979, Chs. 14 and 15, and Table 1).

Attention has focused on nicotine, CO (for cardiovascular disease) and tar (for cancer) as the components of smoke that represent health hazards.

Nicotine is a powerful sympathomimetic agent which produces widespread effects on the cardiovascular system (see Chapter 3). There is no strong evidence that smoking dosages of nicotine lead to acute adverse effects in normal healthy smokers. For example, it is difficult to explain why pipe smokers, who show serum cotinine levels (cotinine is the principal metabolite of nicotine) equal to those of cigarette smokers, should show little, if any, excess risk from coronary heart disease (Wald, Idle & Boreham, 1981). However, it is possible that nicotine can aggravate existing cardiovascular disease such as ischaemic heart disease (by increasing cardiac output but not coronary blood flow), and peripheral vascular disease, such as Raynaud's syndrome (through peripheral vasoconstriction), and can also be a factor in aortic rupture and cerebral aneurysms (through acute rises in blood pressure) (Surgeon General, 1979). Additionally, nicotine from maternal smoking may contribute to foetal hypoxia via uterine vasoconstriction (Manning & Feyerabend, 1976).

Carbon monoxide is only absorbed from tobacco smoke if it is inhaled. It has the property of combining with haemoglobin to form carboxy-haemoglobin (COHb). Owing to the much greater affinity of CO, as opposed to oxygen, for haemoglobin, the COHb complex dissociates much

Table 1. *Gas and particulate phase components of cigarette smoke.* (*Adapted from Surgeon General, 1979*)

Gas phase components[a]	μg/cigarette
Carbon monoxide	13400
Carbon dioxide	50600
Ammonia	80
Hydrogen cyanide (hydrocyanic acid)	240
Isoprene (2-me-1,3-butadiene)	582
Acetaldehyde	770
Acrolein (2-propenal)	84
Toluene	108
N-Nitrosodimethylamine	0.08
N-Nitrosomethylethylamine	0.03
Hydrazine	0.03
Nitromethane	0.5
Nitroethane	1.1
Nitrobenzene	25
Acetone	578
Benzene	67

Particulate phase components[a]	μg/cigarette
Tar (minus nicotine, minus H_2O)	26100
Nicotine	1800
Phenol	86.4
o-Cresol	20.4
m- and p-Cresol	49.5
2,4-Dimethylphenol	9.0
p-Ethylphenol	18.2
β-Naphthylamine	0.028
N′-nitrosonornicotine	0.14
Carbazole	1.0
N-Methylcarbazole	0.23
Indole	14
N-Methylindole	0.42
Benz(a)anthracene	0.044
Benzo(a)pyrene	0.025
Fluorene	0.42
Fluoranthene	0.26
Chrysene	0.04
Dichloro diphenyl dichloroethane (DDD)	1.75
Dichloro diphenyl trichloroethane (DDT)	0.77
4,4′-Dichlorostilbene	1.73

[a] These values are for cigarettes without a filter tip. Changes in cigarette tobacco and construction as well as different ways of puffing will change deliveries, see the text for details.

less readily and more slowly than does the oxyhaemoglobin complex. Consequently, the CO from inhaled cigarette smoke effectively reduces the oxygen-carrying capacity of the blood, reductions of up to 15% being possible after a day's heavy smoking. Although the body of the smoker makes compensatory changes, such as increasing the total haemoglobin (as also seen amongst people living at high altitude), under certain circumstances, e.g., myocardial disease and pregnancy, it is probable that CO has deleterious effects both on its own account and also in combination with the acute effects of nicotine (Surgeon General, 1979). Although the position is far from clear, and the causal mechanisms far from certain, many authors believe CO to be a greater hazard than nicotine. The Surgeon General (1979) concludes that CO in particular has been identified as a possible critical factor in coronary heart disease, atherosclerosis and sudden death, chronic respiratory disease and foetal growth retardation.

Unlike the doubts concerning the relative and absolute contributions of nicotine and CO as causative and aggravating agents for cardiovascular disease, the position of tar as a cancer agent is clear. Extensive animal experiments have demonstrated the role of the various individual tar components as cancer-initiating, cancer-promoting and cancer-accelerating agents. Moreover, in generalising from animal models to humans, careful studies reveal that the carcinogenic role of cigarette smoke is causal and direct (although, as we note later, (pp. 30ff), there is evidence, from twin studies, of genetic disposition to cancer). The simple observation that (generally non-inhaling) cigar and pipe smokers show elevated rates for cancers of the upper aerodigestive tract rather than for lung cancer, which is seen in (generally inhaling) cigarette smokers, is most compelling (see Surgeon General, 1979, for individual studies).

The tobacco industry has made attempts to reduce cigarette yields of these various toxic substances while preserving the taste and flavour. Over the period 1934–79, for cigarettes manufactured in the UK, the average tar yield decreased by 49%, the nicotine yield by 31% and the CO yield by 11% (Wald, Doll & Copeland, 1981). This has been achieved firstly by changes in the tobacco itself (through selection of particular genetic strains of tobacco plant and changes in fertiliser use, in the time and manner of harvesting, in leaf storage and curing, and in processing techniques including tobacco sheet reconstitution) and secondly by changes in the construction of the cigarette (changes in the packing density and moisture content of the cut tobacco, in cigarette length, in paper porosity and ventilation characteristics and in the filtration efficiency of the butt) (for detailed studies see Surgeon General, 1979, Ch. 14; and Gori, 1977). The reductions in tar and nicotine yields have been achieved mainly by reducing the levels in the tobacco itself and the addition of filter tips. Lowering the CO yield proved more difficult. CO is produced both by incomplete oxidation of tobacco constituents in the high temperature zone of the glowing tip and by decarboxylation processes in the lower temperature pyrolysis and distillation zones behind the glowing tip. Since CO is a small molecule (a gas) it cannot be readily trapped in the filter tip, as can tar and nicotine. Consequently, attention has turned towards alternative cigarette construction methods in order to change the burning temperature of tobacco, the burning rate and the rates at which CO diffuses out of the side of the cigarette. Smoke dilution through perforated filters also offers some control of the delivery of CO and other offending constituents of cigarette smoke.

However, the way in which the cigarette is smoked affects the tar, nicotine and CO deliveries (see Chapter 3: Regulation of nicotine intake). If, as we argue later, smokers desire some optimum dose of nicotine from their cigarettes, then they will simply compensate by puffing harder and smoking more low tar/nicotine delivery cigarettes, thus obviating any health advantages of these 'safer' cigarettes (see Chapter 2: Simple addiction models). Such observations have led Russell (1980) to strongly champion the case for medium-nicotine, low-tar, low-CO cigarettes or alternative forms of tobacco use such as snuffing (see Chapter 3: Pharmaco-kinetics, Absorption; and Chapter 5: Drug therapy).

Smoking and morbidity/mortality

There are various ways of examining the risks associated with being a cigarette smoker. The usual index is the mortality ratio, i.e., the ratio of the death rate of smokers to that of a group of non-smokers who are comparable in age, sex, race, social class and so on. Using this index, hyper-mortality ratios for cigarette smokers (ratios greater than 1.0 denoting increased risk for smokers) range from 1.25 (Japanese males) to as high as 1.83 (USA males) or nearly 2.0 (Swedish males) (Surgeon General, 1979, Ch. 2, p. 15; Cederlof *et al.*, 1977). Mortality for smokers versus non-smokers peaks for the early (35- to 44-year-old) and mid (45- to 55-year-old) middle-age groups (mortality ratio 2.0 for USA males), and then declines in later age (1.3 for 65- to 74-year-old USA males). This decline with age does not, however, imply a decreasing effect of cigarette smoking on health, but rather a process of 'natural selection', the more susceptible smokers having already been 'weeded-out' (Surgeon General, 1979, Ch. 2, p. 17).

Sex differences are also apparent in mortality ratios, female smokers being at lower risk than males smoking equivalent amounts (Doll, Gray,

Hafner & Peto, 1980). These ratios are, of course, affected by a number of variables, for example consumption and the age of recruitment to smoking; the longer and more frequently a person smokes, the greater is the risk. The mode of consumption also affects mortality, the smoking of higher tar/nicotine cigarettes representing a greater risk than cigar or pipe smoking. The latter carry a risk which leads to a mortality ratio not much above 1.1; some studies have even reported a slight advantage, for example Rogot (1974) reports a mortality ratio of 0.93. This is probably due to the fact that cigar and pipe smokers tend to inhale less than cigarette smokers rather than to the fact that cigar and pipe smoke is less toxic than cigarette smoke. Of interest here is the observation that cigarette smokers who claim (by self-report) to inhale only slightly, show lower mortality ratios than 'deep-inhalers', although in view of the notorious unreliability of self-report, we should treat such data with reserve.

Of relevance also is the finding that ex-smokers show overall mortality ratios which decline as a function of increase in the number of years 'off' cigarettes. After 15 years, these mortality ratios are similar to those of individuals who have never smoked, although such savings are reduced if the smoker quits because of illness rather than for other reasons. The finding that ex-smokers' mortality ratios decline as a function of the length of time since quitting smoking has, however, been criticised on the grounds that the group of smokers who give up may be self-selected for a relative preponderance of individuals with low risk factors in the first place, particularly with regard to cardiovascular disease (i.e., type of constitution, diet and level of alcohol consumption) (Seltzer, 1980; see also later in this chapter). However, in the case of pulmonary morbidity (i.e., still-living subjects), careful studies of non-smokers, smokers and ex-smokers indicate that quitting smoking protects against the accelerated loss of pulmonary function seen over the years in those who do not quit (Bosse, Sparrow, Rose & Weiss, 1981), and one recent study indicates that some recovery of bronchial epithelium is possible (biopsy specimens were examined for mucous-cell hyperplasia and squamous-cell metaplasia) (Bertram & Rogers, 1981).

In terms of the actual number of deaths, the major contributors to cause-specific mortality amongst cigarette smokers are, in order of decreasing importance, coronary heart disease, lung cancer, chronic obstructive lung disease (COLD) and cancer of the larynx (Surgeon General, 1979). In addition, pipe and cigar smoking are associated with elevated mortality ratios for cancer of the upper aerodigestive tract, including cancer of the oral cavity, the larynx and the oesophagus. Lung cancer is not so evident amongst pipe smokers, perhaps reflecting the fact that pipe smokers do not inhale as much as cigarette smokers. Note, however, that the highest *mortality ratios*, by contrast with *death rates*, are represented by lung cancer, COLD and cancer of the larynx, in that order. This is because coronary heart disease, as a cause of death in the population at large, far outweighs death from lung cancer and COLD. This point can be appreciated more fully if we examine the number of deaths, as opposed to mortality ratios, in typical breakdowns of cause-specific mortality associated with cigarette smoking, such as those reported by Doll & Peto (1976) and Rogot & Murray (1980). These are reproduced in Tables 2a and 2b. We might also note national differences in death rates, some quite obvious, as, for example, between developed and underdeveloped countries. Within the industrialised world, however, one of the most important differences is that bronchitis, as a sub-set of COLD, is highest of all in Great Britain.

Quite apart from mortality, the morbidity data (disease amongst still-living people) suggest that both male and female current cigarette smokers tend to report more conditions such as chronic bronchitis and chronic emphysema, sinusitis, peptic ulcer disease and heart disease than persons who have never smoked. As in the case of mortality, here a dose–response gradient is also apparent: the more cigarettes smoked a day, the greater is the prevalence of these symptoms (Surgeon General, 1979, Ch. 1, p. 12).

From Tables 2a and 2b, it is apparent that the primary cause of death, cardiovascular disease, can be broken down into fatal and non-fatal myocardial infarction (in simple terms, heart attacks), ischaemic heart disease, arteriosclerotic peripheral vascular disease, and aneurysm of the aorta. We can also add to this list angina pectoris and cerebrovascular disease, manifested as stroke, although the Surgeon General (1979) notes that, as yet, epidemiological data on the association between cigarette smoking and angina pectoris and cerebrovascular disease are not conclusive.

Subsidiary findings are reported in terms of morbidity, with both nicotine and CO aggravating exercise-induced angina. It is clear that women who smoke and use oral contraceptives are at a significantly elevated risk for fatal and non-fatal myocardial infarction. Also noteworthy is recent evidence indicating that smoking during pregnancy may cause slightly smaller babies, although whether this is due to cigarette-associated malnourishment of the mother as opposed to direct (e.g., CO-aggravated hypoxia) action on the foetus is debatable (D'Souza, Black & Richards, 1981).

Table 2a. *Death rates in smokers and non-smokers. (From Doll & Peto, 1976)*

Cause of death	No. of deaths	Non-smokers	Current or ex-smokers	Ex-smokers	Current smokers, any tobacco	Current smokers, any tobacco (g/day)			X^{2a}	
						1–14	15–24	≥25	Non-smokers v. others	Trend
Cancer										
Lung	441	10	83	43	104	52	106	224	41.98	197.04
Oesophagus	65	3	12	5	16	12	13	30	3.94	14.94
Other respiratory sites	46	1	9	4	11	6	9	27	3.31	21.68
Stomach	163	23	28	21	32	28	38	32	–	–
Colon	195	27	34	34	34	35	33	31	–	–
Rectum	78	6	14	14	14	10	14	27	2.81	10.76
Pancreas	92	14	16	12	18	14	18	27	–	3.98
Prostate	186	39	30	31	30	28	31	38	–	–
Kidney	46	3	8	9	8	8	9	9	–	–
Bladder	80	9	14	11	16	16	16	12	–	–
Marrow and reticuloendothelial system	152	33	24	26	24	27	22	19	–	(3.51)
Unknown site	64	12	11	9	12	10	13	14	–	–
Other site	151	25	26	29	24	19	24	35	–	–
Respiratory disease										
Respiratory tuberculosis	57	3	11	11	10	8	7	21	3.83	10.51
Asthma	40	4	7	12	5	5	7	0	–	–
Pneumonia	345	54	59	62	57	47	62	91	–	6.94
Chronic bronchitis and emphysema	254	3	48	44	50	38	50	88	25.58	47.23
Other respiratory disease	121	16	21	24	19	20	14	26	–	–

Ischaemic heart disease	3191	413	554	533	565	501	598	677	22.59	53.56
Myocardial degeneration	615	67	108	98	116	111	111	160	9.58	13.92
Hypertension	239	37	41	41	41	33	43	58	–	4.67
Arteriosclerosis	117	21	20	17	21	17	21	46	–	4.85
Aortic aneurysm (non-syphilitic)	121	5	22	16	26	18	28	45	8.40	25.60
Venous thromboembolism	48	9	8	8	8	8	5	14	–	–
Cerebral thrombosis	616	86	106	105	107	92	123	131	–	9.54
Other cerebrovascular disease	692	107	118	122	115	112	114	128	–	–
Other cardiovascular disease	267	53	44	49	41	37	42	52	–	–
Other diseases										
Parkinsonism	51	14	8	13	5	8	1	4	–	(9.10)
Peptic ulcer	79	8	14	12	15	10	20	23	–	8.26
Cirrhosis of liver, alcoholism	80	7	14	10	16	10	10	40	–	22.53
Hernia	16	0	3	2	4	3	4	7	–	4.16
Other digestive disease	144	20	25	27	24	18	33	26	–	3.25
Nephritis	79	10	14	10	16	15	14	21	–	–
Other genitourinary disease	136	19	23	24	23	22	24	26	–	–
Other disease	391	59	67	73	64	65	58	73	–	–
Violence										
Suicide	173	21	31	27	32	30	28	46	–	6.26
Poisoning	74	9	13	6	16	12	14	26	–	6.86
Trauma	240	46	39	36	41	47	25	56	–	–
All causes	10072	1317	1748	1652	1802	1581	1829	2452	68.47	244.16
(No. of deaths)		(940)	(9132)	(3114)	(6018)	(2707)	(1986)	(1325)		

[a] Figures are given whenever the value was greater than 2.71 ($p < 0.1$); figures in parentheses indicate a decreasing trend from non-smokers to heavy smokers; others indicate an increasing trend.

Table 2b. *Observed deaths (O), expected deaths (E) and mortality ratios (O ÷ E) for pure cigarette smokers, pure cigar smokers and pure pipe smokers for selected causes of death, USA veterans study, 1954–69. (From Rogot & Murray, 1980)*

Cause of death[a]	Pure cigarette smokers			Pure cigar smokers			Pure pipe smokers		
	Observed deaths	Expected deaths	O ÷ E[b]	Observed deaths	Expected deaths	O ÷ E[b]	Observed deaths	Expected deaths	O ÷ E[b]
All causes	15091	8112	1.86	2653	2302	1.15	1545	1432	1.08
Cardiovascular diseases	8920	5257	1.70	1681	1522	1.10	984	948	1.04
Cancers, all sites	3138	1401	2.24	510	386	1.32	307	237	1.29
Coronary heart disease	5740	3414	1.68	1077	965	1.12	606	596	1.02
Stroke	1172	796	1.47	267	249	1.07	157	159	0.99
Influenza and pneumonia	200	96	2.08	28	34	0.82	22	23	0.97
Aortic aneurysm	359	68	5.28	38	19	2.04	24	12	2.07
Respiratory diseases	879	185	4.75	51	61	c	57	39	1.44
Bronchitis and emphysema	568	43	13.13	10	14	0.84	22	9	2.53
Lung cancer	1095	91	12.06	41	25	1.66	32	15	2.14

[a] For 'Cause of death', 'All causes' refers to all deaths observed, most, but not all, of which can be classified under the general categories of 'Cardiovascular diseases', 'Cancers, all sites' and 'Respiratory diseases'. In addition, a number of more specific categories of major interest, which can be subsumed under the above, are also given, e.g., the category 'Lung cancer' is one of the categories subsumed under 'Cancers, all sites'.

[b] Based on expected number to 2 decimal places.

[c] Ratio not shown for observed values of less than 20.

There remain a number of important causes of death which appear to be linked, in an as yet unknown fashion, with cigarette smoking, e.g., suicide, cirrhosis of the liver and poisonings. Also of interest, as regards the 'fine detail' of cause of death, is the repeated finding that smokers suffer significantly less from Parkinson's disease than do non-smokers. This negative association is not simply due to the inability to continue to smoke (because of motor dysfunction) since ex-smokers show similar reduced risks. While it should be remembered that Parkinson's disease is relatively infrequent as compared to cardiovascular disease, the negative association reported with cigarette smoking merits serious study (Rogot & Murray, 1980).

Another way of looking at smoking-associated risk is to study life expectancy, i.e., the number of years a cigarette smoker can expect to live beyond a particular age when compared to a non-smoker. A 30- to 40-year-old (USA) male smoking more than 40 cigarettes a day loses an estimated 8 years of life; if he smokes fewer than 10 cigarettes a day, he will lose around 4 years of life. These figures obviously drop off with older age groups, the equivalent figures being 5 years and 2 years respectively for the 60-year-old. This reflects both the process of 'natural selection', many smoking-related excess deaths having already occurred amongst 40- to 50-year-olds, and also the fact that the older person, overall, has fewer years left to live.

Expressed in these simple terms, the risks associated with smoking are substantial. However, we should be wary of superficial interpretation of such findings. In the first place, different modes of analysis can, at times, throw up quite different results. For example, if we sub-categorise groups and re-analyse the data, in certain instances different, sometimes reversed, relationships emerge. One example is presented in Table 3. For individuals who regard their lives as stressful (they answer 'yes' to questionnaire statements such as 'my position has involved too much responsibility'), mortality ratios are 1.3 for the total sample, but 1.6 for non-smokers and 1.2 for smokers; for those reporting financial worries, the figures are 1.4 for the total sample, 1.8 for non-smokers and 1.3 for smokers (Floderus, 1974). Thus, amongst individuals leading stressful lives, smokers have lower mortality ratios than non-smokers.

Again, other reported data raise questions which are difficult to answer if we assume a simple causal relationship between smoking and mortality. Consider, for example, the observation from some recent studies that the incidence of certain types of smoking-related disease, e.g., lung cancer, may be falling in smokers (Wald, 1978). The obvious explanation is that this is due to changes in both the quantity and the quality of tar delivered, although the evidence is not yet very convincing owing to the time lag between smoking and the onset of disease. Changes over the last few years in cigarette tar yield will probably not be reflected in mortality rates for some years to come. However, some preliminary evidence is available on this point. Auerbach, Hammond & Garfinkel (1979) report differences in pre-malignant changes in the bronchial epithelium of cigarette smokers that are consistent with the gradual reduction in tar delivery over the past thirty years (filter cigarettes seem to have had less impact on heart disease (Castelli *et al.*, 1981), perhaps because the role of CO has not been appreciated until recently).

Contrast this finding concerning the decreased incidence in lung cancer amongst smokers, however, with the reported increase in lung cancer in non-smokers (rates are, of course, much lower than for smokers (see Enstrom, 1979)). It has been suggested that this may be due to increased environmental pollution and passive inhalation of other people's tobacco smoke (BMJ Editorial, 1978; Surgeon General, 1979, Ch. 11; Hirayama, 1981). Of particular relevance is the fact that 'side-stream', as opposed to 'mainstream', cigarette smoke may contain different amounts of potentially

Table 3. *Mortality ratios in total group[a] and by smoking in 'factor-positive' versus 'factor-negative' individuals, and proportion of 'factor-positive' cases in total group;[b] old Swedish Twin Registry, A Series. (Condensed from Floderus, 1974; detailed in Cederlof et al., 1977)*

	Mortality ratios			Proportion of 'factor-positive' cases
Factor	Total group[a]	Non-smokers	Smokers	
Financially I have not achieved what I hoped for	1.4[s]	1.8[s]	1.3	0.23
My position has involved too much responsibility	1.3[s]	1.6	1.2	0.38
I have had a lot of difficulty in my marriage	1.4	3.5[s]	0.9	0.09
I have often been restless	1.4	1.8[s]	1.3	0.18
I have often had difficulties in falling asleep	1.6[s]	2.0[s]	1.4[s]	0.12
I have often felt somewhat uneasy in my work	1.7[s]	2.3	1.5	0.07

[a] Total group: non-smokers + smokers.
[b] The total group size is approximately 5000 individuals, the exact numbers for a particular factor depending on the non-response rate to a particular questionnaire item (for details see Floderus, 1974).
[s] Significant effect.

toxic chemicals (Stock, 1980). The health hazards of passive smoking have been underlined in a number of studies. Hirayama's (1981) study claims that the effects of passive smoking are 'about half to one-third of direct smoking in terms of mortality ratio or relative risk'. The children of cigarette smokers appear to have an elevated risk for respiratory diseases (Colley, 1974). Recent evidence suggests that even such simple measures as children's height and weight show small, but significant inverse relationships with the number of smokers in the home. Thus, it is argued, certain groups of non-smokers, for example the non-smoking husbands, wives and children of smokers, are at risk from increased exposure conditions because of close physical proximity.

Alternative explanations can be offered, of course, for the passive smoking data. Neglecting for the moment the fact that Hirayama's results have been criticised because of the dubious statistical procedures used (Correspondence, 1981), a genetic argument could account for his and Colley's results, insofar as smokers' children are concerned. Concerning the reduced height and weight of these children, alternative possibilities have been proposed in terms of restricted diet, both because of the proportion of the household budget required to support the habit, and because nicotine, a well-known appetite suppressant, may lead smoking parents to provide poorer meals (Berggreen, 1981). Additional indirect effects of smoking may occur on the foetuses of pregnant mothers. Evidence suggests that the birth weight of such infants is lower, and gestation and birth complications greater, even when relevant factors such as social class and maternal weight are allowed for (Surgeon General, 1979, Ch. 8; *Lancet*, 1979*a*). Foetal hypoxia caused by CO from cigarette smoke has been suggested as one possible mechanism for these effects.

But even if, for the sake of argument, we accept that increased exposure from passive smoking carries an elevated risk, this is relevant to the question of increased mortality amongst non-smokers only if we assume that there is a higher level of passive smoking today than in the past, which is highly improbable, to say the least, or that passive smoking interacts with the effects of other environmental pollutants to exert differential effects on smokers and non-smokers, for which there is no evidence whatsoever. It may be, of course, that there is a marked reduction in mortality amongst smokers due to lower tar delivery, which masks a relatively small increase due to pollution, this latter being reflected in increased mortality rates amongst non-smokers.

Finally, we might note that some reported changes in mortality rates over time, which have been assumed to be related (and superficially are so) to changes in smoking habits and in the tar/CO delivery of cigarettes, may be due to entirely unrelated, but as yet unrecognised, factors. For example, the 'savings' gained with regard to smoking-related deaths amongst British doctors as a consequence of giving up smoking during the years 1951–71 reported by Doll & Peto (1976) are not as substantial as originally supposed (see Lee, 1979). Although this group of doctors has substantially reduced hyper-mortality rates for lung cancer and heart disease, comparison with an equivalent social class I/II group not showing the same decline in smoking over this period reveals a similar though less

Table 4. *Lee's (1979) re-analysis of Doll & Peto's (1976) data concerning mortality in doctors, smokers versus non-smokers. (From Lee, 1979)*
(a) *Observed (O) and expected (E_1) numbers of deaths from various causes among doctors aged under 65 during 1949–53 and 1970–2. Age-standardised mortality ratios (SMR) calculated as (ratio of O to E_1) × 100*

Cause of death	1949–53			1970–2		
	O	E_1	SMR	O	E_1	SMR
Coronary heart disease	345	249	139	261	305	86
Stroke	106	76	140	44	54	81
Lung cancer	46	92	50	31	97	32
Other malignant tumours	131	165	79	106	128	83
Bronchitis	18	76	24	13	45	29
Cirrhosis of the liver	12	5	240	14	5	311
Suicide	61	27	226	55	16	335
Accidents, poisonings, etc.	42	61	69	60	47	128
All other causes	247	378	65	81	124	65
Total	1008	1129	89	665	821	81

(b) *Observed (O) and expected (E_1) numbers of deaths from each cause among all men in social classes I and II combined during 1949–53 and 1970–2. Age-standardised mortality ratios (SMR) taken as 100*

Cause of death	1949–53			1970–2		
	O	E_1	SMR	O	E_1	SMR
Coronary heart disease	21989	20077	110	20378	22874	89
Stroke	6607	6185	107	3440	4063	85
Lung cancer	5971	7318	82	4788	7294	66
Other malignant tumours	11576	12785	91	8397	9414	89
Bronchitis	3102	6232	50	1673	3451	48
Cirrhosis of the liver	580	360	161	455	332	137
Suicide	2342	1987	118	1093	1166	94
Accidents, poisonings, etc.	3304	4245	78	2680	3663	73
All other causes	21770	28385	77	6734	9237	73
Total	77241	87574	88	49638	61494	81

dramatic trend as far as heart disease is concerned. This may be due to other factors such as dietary fat about which doctors might be expected to be well informed. In any event, these 'savings' have to be set against increased 'losses' from stress-related causes such as cirrhosis of the liver, suicide, accidents and poisonings compared with rates for equivalent social classes. It could be argued that these increases in stress-related deaths in doctors may be due, paradoxically, to actually giving up smoking, since there is evidence in the literature that smoking has a protective function

Table 4 (*cont.*)

(c) *Observed (O) numbers of deaths from each cause in 1970–2 and expected (E$_2$) numbers had standardised mortality ratios remained at 1949–53 values. 'Savings' represent negative values of O − E$_2$ and 'losses' positive values of O − E$_2$*

Cause of death	O	E$_2$	Saving	Loss
Coronary heart disease	261	423	162	–
Stroke	44	75	31	–
Lung cancer	31	49	18	–
Other malignant tumours	106	102	–	4
Bronchitis	13	11	–	2
Cirrhosis of the liver	14	12	–	2
Suicide	55	36	–	19
Accidents, poisonings etc.	60	32	–	28
All other causes	81	81	–	–
Total[a]	665	821	211	55

(d) *Observed (O) numbers of deaths from each cause in doctors during 1970–2 and expected (E$_3$) numbers had doctors shown same improvement in standardised mortality ratios as men in social classes I and II as a whole. 'Savings' and 'losses' calculated as in (c)*

Cause of death	O	E$_3$	Saving	Loss
Coronary heart disease	261	344	83	–
Stroke	44	60	16	–
Lung cancer	31	39	8	–
Other malignant tumours	106	100	–	6
Bronchitis	13	10	–	3
Cirrhosis of the liver	14	10	–	4
Suicide	55	29	–	26
Accidents, poisonings, etc.	60	30	–	30
All other causes	81	77	–	4
Total[b]	665	699	107	73

[a] Difference = 156 net saving.
[b] Difference = 34 net saving.

vis-à-vis stress. We refer the reader back to the mortality figures cited for stressed smokers versus stressed non-smokers. Lee's (1979) figures are shown in Table 4.

Although Lee's re-analysis has drawn some criticism, it appears to be basically sound (see Lee, 1980, for criticisms and reply). However, caution should be exercised in extrapolating from the re-analysis of the British doctors' data to the general population because doctors as a group may be exposed to relatively higher levels of stress.

Thus, even from what appear to be relatively straightforward studies, there are sometimes serious difficulties of interpretation. We have mentioned the most serious underlying problem, i.e., weak methodology and inappropriate statistical procedures. There are, however, a few more recent (mostly genetic) studies which meet more rigorous scientific criteria, and it is on these that we choose to place most weight.

Genetic studies

The genetic approach to smoking focuses on two interrelated issues: the degree of genetic disposition to smoking and the degree of genetic disposition to smoking-related diseases, although in some of the relevant studies problem areas have not been differentiated so that analyses are not addressed specifically to one or the other problem.

A body of largely non-medical professional opinion (mainly that of geneticists and statisticians) has proposed a genetic hypothesis which suggests that independent or possibly linked mechanisms account for both smoking (recruitment to, and persistence of, the habit, and consumption rates) and its associated disease (Fisher, 1959; Berkson, 1962; Burch, 1976). A variant of this is constitutional theory, which suggests that the smoking-disease relationship is due primarily to factors, loosely described as 'personality' and 'life-style', which themselves may have strong genetic underpinnings, and which carry second-order dispositions to both smoke cigarettes and contract certain diseases (Eysenck, 1980).

Of course, intermediate positions are possible. For example, it could be argued that while tar may cause lung cancer, and nicotine and CO may cause cardiovascular disease, this is more likely in cases where the individual is peculiarly vulnerable to such insults, i.e., cigarette smoking causes elevated disease rates in individuals who are genetically more susceptible (see, e.g., Hopkins & Evans, 1980). Again, it might be that other factors, which themselves are under genetic control, are strongly implicated in the aetiology of certain diseases when in interaction with smoking, but that their influence has been masked in the smoking/health debate.

Mixed or interactive models of this sort can be very complex, suggesting, in some cases, a subtle underlying causal nexus. For example, let us assume a genetic predisposition to alcohol use, for which there is some support (see, e.g., Strickenberger, 1968). Consider also the evidence that pre-loading smokers with alcohol increases tobacco use (Griffiths, Bigelow & Liebson, 1976), perhaps because it prevents the disruptive effects of alcohol on performance while preserving the pleasant tranquillising effects on emotion (Myrsten & Andersson, 1978). However, it is well established that excessive alcohol consumption itself causes disease, as well as being a 'promoter', with cigarette smoking, of cancer of the oesophagus (Surgeon General, 1979, Ch. 13, p. 25). The mechanisms underlying this synergistic alcohol/smoking action are uncertain, though it may be that alcohol acts as a solvent for carcinogenic hydrocarbons in tobacco smoke, or alters microsomal enzymes in the mucosal cells, or, again, causes nutritional deficiencies which weaken the individual's resistance to certain diseases (Surgeon General, 1979, Ch. 5, p. 44).

Failure to document and allow for such risk factors by multivariate analysis may obscure and even confound relationships between smoking and disease entities. Interactions and interrelationships can be intricate, and may exaggerate risk factors to an unknown extent. Taking the case of cigarettes and alcohol, for example, the net risk appears to be larger than the sum of the individual risks (Surgeon General, 1979).

A crucial question is that of the degree of genetic predisposition to diseases which have been regarded as smoking-related (cause-specific). A second question, that of the genetic disposition to smoking, is discussed in the next chapter.

As far as lung cancer is concerned, information is meagre. Only a few studies have been reported, as Doll (1974) and Burch (1976) have remarked, but these seem to point to a reasonably firm conclusion. Tokuhata (1963, 1964) and Tokuhata & Lilienfeld (1963a, b), in a comparison of first-degree relatives of 270 lung cancer probands and first-degree relatives of 270 controls, report a ratio of 3.8:1 for deaths from lung cancer among non-smoking first-degree relatives of probands compared with non-smoking first-degree relatives of controls. The corresponding ratio amongst smoking first-degree relatives was 2.3:1, the combined probability being highly significant (p < 0.0006). This evidence indicates the existence of a genetic predisposing factor in the development of lung cancer. Of interest also is the fact that in these studies a significantly higher rate for all causes of death is reported in relatives of probands than in the relatives of controls. For all cancers, the difference is at the level p = 0.0006. It is important to view this work in the context of the first-order lung cancer/cigarette smoking relationship which has been frequently reported in the literature. The usual statistical relationship was also found in these studies: 93% of the lung cancer cases and only 59% of the controls were smokers, the difference being highly significant. The results of the Tokuhata studies, therefore, suggest strongly that certain genes predispose to lung cancer, a point underlined by Burch (1976).

Of interest in this connection is the study by Harvald & Hauge (1965). They report significant differences between monozygotic (Mz) and dizygotic (Dz) twins (see Appendix) in concordance rates for cancer at the same site, although for cancer rates at all sites there was no significant difference between the groups. There is evidence that, for some tumours in man there is a dominantly inherited form, which is characterised by 'high risk for specific kind of tumour; earlier age of occurrence of the tumour than is usual; and a multiplicity of primary tumours' (Knudson, 1978).

As far as coronary heart disease is concerned, evidence points in the same direction, namely, that the disease has a large genetic component (de Faire, 1974; Rose, 1977a). It has been suggested that serum cholesterol levels are implicated in ischaemic heart disease, and there is some evidence of a genetic component controlling such levels (Pikkarainen, Tukkunen & Kulonen, 1966).

Liljefors' (1970) clinical twin study, concerning the hereditary aspects of coronary heart disease is particularly important since initial results were supported by a seven-year follow-up study of surviving pairs (Liljefors, 1977). The differences between the Mz and Dz pairs were highly significant. Other familial studies, such as that of Thomas & Cohen (1955), have examined the familial occurrence of hypertension in coronary artery disease, and report a strong degree of association between hypertension and coronary disease. Thomas & Cohen (1955) report that the incidence of coronary artery disease was nearly four times as great amongst siblings of individuals with coronary artery disease than amongst siblings of persons without it. The data showed the highest incidence of coronary artery disease amongst offspring where both parents were affected, and the lowest incidence amongst offspring where both parents were unaffected. The suggestion of a genetic link is most compelling.

De Faire (1974) reports data, concerning coronary heart disease, on 205 survivors from 262 death-discordant twin pairs from the Swedish Twin Registry. The prevalence of myocardial infarction, angina pectoris and pathological Q-wave in the electrocardiogram (ECG) in the examined twins was 4/10 in the male Mz group whose partners had died from coronary heart disease against 4/25 in the Dz group. The prevalence was non-significantly lower in the group whose partners had died from other causes. If electrocardiographic signs of coronary heart disease were also included, nearly all Mz co-twins were affected. This high prevalence of coronary heart disease in the most genetically predisposed co-twins, that is, in the Mz co-twins whose partners had died from coronary heart disease, again strongly suggests a genetic component in coronary heart disease.

More recently, extensive data from a longitudinal twin study of smoking-related mortality and morbidity have been reported by Cederlof *et al.* (1977). These authors employed a number of additional techniques in an attempt to circumvent some of the problems usually encountered in classic twin study methodology. Three types of analysis were performed on data derived from the Swedish Twin Registry: 'A' Series analysis, 'B' Series analysis and non-exposed twin (NET) analysis.

A Series analyses compare, in a conventional manner, all individuals who are exposed (i.e., smokers) with all those who are not exposed (i.e., non-smokers) for a number of variables. These comparisons confirm, or disconfirm, that the generally found results vis-à-vis smoking and health are present in their twin data, and can be employed to generate expected prevalence rates for disease in smokers and non-smokers.

B Series and NET analyses focus on smoking-discordant pairs. In B Series analysis, prevalence rates for certain behaviours and disease entities are observed in smoking-discordant twin pairs, i.e., those twin pairs in which one partner smokes and the other partner is a non-smoker. The B series disease ratio is based on the disease prevalence rates for the smoking compared with the non-smoking co-twins. This B Series ratio (from smoking-discordant twins) can then be compared with the A Series ratio (from the rest of the sample: smoking- and non-smoking-concordant twins), for the relevant disease or behaviour under study. If the A Series ratio for heart disease, for example, is 2.0, this indicates that this disease is twice as prevalent amongst smokers than amongst non-smokers. This (A Series) ratio can then be compared with the (B Series) ratio between non-smoking and presently smoking co-twins in smoking-discordant pairs. Here a ratio of 1.0 would indicate that both partners are equally susceptible to heart disease. Thus, smoking could hardly be regarded as a 'cause' of heart disease. A genetic explanation seems more likely. On the other hand, a ratio of 2.0, which conforms with the expected ratio, would suggest that the higher incidence of heart disease in the smoking co-twin is due to some non-genetic effect, for which smoking is a strong (but not the only) causative candidate, this being the criterion for categorising groups. Intermediate values suggest an interaction between genetic and environmental effects.

In NET analysis, the disease, psychological and psychosocial characteristics of the non-smoking twin in smoking-discordant pairs are examined and compared with these characteristics in all non-smoking twins. Ratios above unity reflect the extent to which the non-smoking co-twin is different, in some fundamental way, from all non-smoking concordant twin pairs. For example, a NET ratio of 1.3 for heart disease indicates that the non-smoking co-twin is more susceptible to this disease than non-smoking twins in concordant pairs, indicating some extra susceptibility to heart disease in non-smoking co-twins whose twin partner smokes. This might well suggest some genetic predisposition to heart disease. On the other hand, NET ratios of around or below 1.0 indicate that the non-smoking co-twin is no more susceptible, or is less susceptible (respectively), to this disease than non-smoking twins in concordant pairs. Thus a NET ratio of 1.0 or less, in the context of a statistical association between smoking and heart disease (the latter having been revealed in many other epidemiological studies and also by the A Series analysis of Cederlof *et al.* (1977)), would strongly suggest that smoking is, in fact, implicated as one of the causal factors in this disease. A NET ratio of 1.0, of course, indicates no extra susceptibility to heart disease in non-smoking co-twins whose twin partners smoke, and thus suggests, by default, that the statistical association between smoking and heart disease is causal.

An important feature of the NET and B Series analyses is that, in comparing outcome (i.e., mortality) amongst smoking and non-smoking partners in smoking-discordant twin pairs, some control can be exercised over the possible confounding effects of certain psychological, behavioural and psychosocial variables. This type of control, of course, is not perfect, but appears to be particularly appropriate for variables such as alcohol consumption which are known to bear some relationship to mortality. In the case of alcohol consumption, for Mz twins, the smoker/non-smoker ratio observed in discordant pairs is 1.1, compared with an expected ratio of 1.5. This means that in smoking-discordant pairs, the non-smoker drinks (nearly) as much as the smoker, despite the expectation that his consumption, as a non-smoker, should be considerably lower. Equivalent ratios for excessive drinking are 1.5 as against 4.5. If, from these analyses, it appears that the non-smoker in smoking-discordant pairs drinks, uses drugs, is stressed, is disturbed, is more often divorced, and so on, to the same extent as his smoking co-twin, then probably we are referring to a lifestyle of which smoking has been selected as one marker. Possibly it is this lifestyle, or its consequences, which is related to overall mortality, rather than, or in addition to, any particular index such as smoking. This, in effect, would imply rejection of the environmental hypothesis that the entire association between morbidity or mortality and smoking is due wholly to the effects of smoking on body tissues.

A Series analyses of the old Swedish Twin Registry data, in which the twins were simply regarded as a group of unrelated individuals, confirmed the well-established picture of smoking as an indisputable risk factor for disease and premature death, results which did not deviate from those reported in the well-known USA and UK epidemiological studies of smokers and non-smokers. Prevalence rates were shown to be almost consistently dose-related. Gross mortality is strongly related to present smoking, the group smoking more than 10 cigarettes a day showing hyper-mortality ratios of about 2.0. This mortality rate, however, is also connected with other risk factors. For example, alcohol registration (Scandinavian definition) is associated with mortality in non-smokers as well as in smokers.

From the new Twin Registry data, Cederlof *et al.* (1977) were able to derive morbidity figures. They report clear relationships between smoking and symptoms such as cough and angina pectoris in both the Swedish and the USA registries. In the former, stomach disorders, impaired hearing, migraine, asthma, long-lasting illness and a disproportionate amount of sick leave all seem to be smoking related. Hyper-morbidity ratios of around 2.0 and 3.0 are recorded for some of these conditions. However, some high ratios were also found in the youngest age groups, and amongst individuals who smoked seven cigarettes or fewer a day. Back disorders have ratios of 2.9 amongst young males and 2.5 amongst young females. Stomach disorders in the youngest and lowest-smoking female groups show a hyper-morbidity ratio of 1.6. Cederlof *et al.* (1977) claim that as far as respiratory symptoms are concerned, it is not unreasonable to suggest that even a short exposure time (in all cases of the youngest age groups) would give rise to symptoms in susceptible individuals. However, it is more difficult to argue that there could be a causal association between smoking and symptoms such as back disorders. They suggest, therefore, that in the smoking groups there is an over-representation of individuals who are constitutionally different from non-smokers, or who pursue an unhealthy lifestyle.

As far as cause-specific mortality rates are concerned, these are increased for coronary heart disease, with relative risks of about 2.0 amongst smokers in general and 3.0 amongst males who are smoking more than 10 cigarettes a day. Lung cancer is also closely associated with the amount smoked, and mortality ratios are 5.0–6.0 in the lower (less than 10 cigarettes per day), and 13.0–25.0 in the higher (more than 10 cigarettes per day) smoking category amongst males.

In B Series analyses of mortality rates, one approach was to simply compare smoking-discordant twin pairs in which one partner did not smoke at all. The other approach (which increased the numbers in the sample), was to compare, in addition, those twins from smoking-concordant twin pairs who were smoking widely differing amounts of tobacco each day. Thus pooled high cigarette consumption and pooled low cigarette consumption groups with similar zygosity status could be assembled. These are referred to as the pooled groups.

For smokers versus non-smokers, discordant Dz pairs showed a hyper-mortality of 55 to 37 (ratio = 1.49) for males, and 52 to 43 (ratio = 1.21) for females. For the discordant Mz pairs, the figures were 15 to 10 (ratio = 1.5) and 22 to 18 (ratio = 1.22), respectively. For the pooled groups, there was an obvious hyper-mortality in the high-smoking group compared with the low-smoking group. For Dz pairs, figures were 82 to 54 (ratio = 1.52) for males and 60 to 44 (ratio = 1.36) for females, and for Mz pairs the figures were 27 to 24 (ratio = 1.13) for males and 26 to 22 (ratio = 1.18) for females. The ratios are significant only for the Dz pairs. Although excess mortality amongst smokers is only significant for the Dz groups, Cederlof *et al.* (1977) found no significant differences in direct comparison between the Dz and Mz groups. Therefore, this part of the data does not support a simple hereditary model of smoking-related mortality. However, as will be seen, more detailed analysis by cause-specific mortality/morbidity reveals important differences between respiratory diseases and coronary heart disease in terms of their causal or non-causal relationship with smoking.

As far as cause-specific deaths are concerned, the lung cancer figures reflected findings in the A Series analysis, although the number of cases reported is small. Because of the small numbers, and because of the importance of the problem, these authors also analysed data from the oldest cohort of twins (1886–1900) (Cederlof *et al.*, 1977). For all age groups combined, 12 cases of lung cancer are reported in the pooled high-smoking group of Dz pairs as against 2 cases in the pooled low-smoking group and 5 against 1 in the Mz pairs. For females, only 2 cases occurred, 1 in the Dz pooled high-smoking group, and 1 in the Mz pooled low-smoking group.

In the case of coronary heart disease, inspection of data from pooled high- and low-smoking groups revealed a distribution of deaths of 25 to 13 for male and 11 to 5 for female Dz twins, and of 10 to 8 for male and 3 to 1 for female Mz twins.

Cederlof *et al.* (1977), from the B Series analyses, report that for Dz pairs, as far as respiratory morbidity, total morbidity and death from specific causes including lung cancer and coronary heart disease are concerned, the more exposed partner in smoking-discordant pairs shows increased relative risk. The Mz picture agrees with this in several respects, particularly with regard to respiratory symptoms and lung cancer. For coronary heart disease, the situation is less clear-cut. The Dz ratio of 1.9 for males indicates a significantly higher mortality from coronary heart disease in smoking versus non-smoking co-twins in discordant pairs. The Mz ratio of 1.2, however, is not significant. Interestingly enough, where former smokers are excluded, the corresponding ratios are 2.6 and 1.0. Also of interest is the finding, which agrees with an earlier report of Friberg *et al.* (1973), that there is no evidence of hyper-mortality in the pooled high-smoking Mz group.

NET analyses of morbidity data show that symptoms such as cough, shortness of breath, stomach disorders, back disorders and migraine, as well as extensive periods of sick leave, occurred more often amongst Mz non-smokers with a currently smoking partner than amongst all the other non-smokers in the twin series (Cederlof *et al.*, 1977). For males, the ratios ranged from 1.3 to 1.9. Only with regard to stomach disorders were ratios reliably increased for Dz pairs. NET analyses of gross morbidity, mortality, coronary heart disease and cancer at all sites also indicate that non-smokers in smoking-discordant pairs have higher rates than other non-smokers.

In summarising a considerable amount of data, Cederlof *et al.* (1977) state that they are in no doubt about the causal link between smoking and the development of lung cancer, and comment that results from the Swedish Mz twin series speak strongly against a constitutional hypothesis such as that advanced by Fisher (1959). They also comment, however, that constitution may be important in the sense that certain individuals may be more susceptible, and suggest possible mechanisms. They note, for example, that the enzyme aryl hydrocarbon hydroxylase (AHH) may have a genetic basis, and may mediate an increased susceptibility to certain carcinogens found in tobacco smoke. A rather similar situation applies in the case of chronic bronchitis. Constitutional factors may have an importance equal to that of smoking in the development of the disease, a point reinforced by the recent Minnesota study of a small sample of Mz twins, reared apart, which examined pulmonary function in non-smoking concordant, smoking-discordant and smoking-concordant Mz twins (Hankins, Drage, Zamel & Kronenberg, 1982). Diet may modify susceptibility to lung disease. Thus, Shekelle *et al.* (1981) report epidemiological data suggesting that a diet relatively rich in *beta*-carotene may reduce the risk of lung cancer, even among smokers.

The role of smoking in the pathogenesis of coronary heart disease, however, is unclear. This is a multi-factorial disease in which several risk factors play an important role, perhaps interactively. The Swedish B Series data do not identify smoking as the most important aetiological factor.

Nor do Lundman's (1966) twin data. He reports no greater prevalence rates amongst smokers than amongst non-smokers in smoking-discordant pairs. Indirect evidence on this point is also offered by Liljefors (1970). In this study, smokers did not predominate amongst deceased partners, as compared with non-deceased partners, in twin pairs discordant for coronary heart disease. The possibility that genetic factors may play a part in the development of the disease is indicated in de Faire's (1974) study, which reports that surviving partners of deceased twins who had died from coronary heart disease more often had the signs and symptoms of the disease.

In a recent longitudinal study, Friedman, Siegelaub, Dales & Seltzer (1979) demonstrated that current smokers who later quit to become ex-smokers show physiological characteristics at baseline indicative of significantly lower coronary heart disease risk than smokers destined to continue. Seltzer (1980) argues that these results, in combination with those reported by Rose & Hamilton (1978), suggest that 'there is no established proof that cigarette smoking is causally related to coronary heart disease' (Seltzer, 1980). Rose & Hamilton (1978) report that in the case of middle-aged smokers at high risk for cardiorespiratory diseases who were randomly assigned to 'intervention' (58% quit at 3 years) and 'normal-care' groups (14% quit at 3 years) with regard to cigarette smoking cessation, there were no significant differences in mortality rates after almost 8 years follow-up.

The bulk of medical opinion would doubtless disagree with Seltzer. Nonetheless, there is still no unequivocal evidence of a causal link between smoking and cardiovascular disease. Unlike the case of lung cancer, where the potent carcinogen present in tobacco tar is delivered to the site of action, the postulated culprit in cardiovascular disease, nicotine and/or CO, has not yet been proved guilty. Another difficulty is that cigarette smoking is only one of the three (possible) major independent risk factors for cardiovascular disease, the other two being cholesterol level and blood pressure (Surgeon General, 1979, Ch. 4, p. 21). In addition, it seems highly likely that a number of other risk factors, in various combinations, interact with smoking to produce elevated cardiovascular mortality. Stress, alcohol consumption, irregular meals and lack of exercise suggest themselves as prime candidates (Liljefors, 1970; Cederlof et al. 1977; CHD Report, 1983). In some instances, smoking may even exert a 'cancelling' effect. For example, chronic smoking appears to be associated with slight hypotension (Surgeon General, 1979, Ch. 4, p. 64; Lundman, 1966), whereas the acute effects of smoking tend to produce hypertension (see Chapter 3: The cardiovascular system). Clearly, the aetiological picture is very complex.

The problem, however, is an important one, since cardiovascular disease is a far greater source of (assumed) smoking-related mortality than is lung cancer.

Summary

Epidemiological studies in many countries have consistently pointed to a strong association between smoking and mortality/morbidity, the most important cause-specific diseases being cardiovascular disease, lung cancer and, with some variation between countries, COLD (chronic obstructive lung disease). The toxic nature of some of the constituents of cigarette smoke, the positive relationship between the onset and course of disease and the degree of exposure to these toxic agents, and the established reduction in risk as a function of number of years elapsed since giving up smoking, are cited as strong evidence for a causal link between smoking and these disease entities.

However, alternative explanations have been offered for the correlations reported. These include the suggestion that the associations are due to linked genetic predispositions to contract certain diseases, and to take up smoking. Another suggestion is that smoking is one of the constellation of behaviours which characterises certain personalities which themselves may predispose to, or even cause, the diseases under study in their own right. We examine these approaches in some detail in Chapter 2 (Theories about smoking).

From the large-scale epidemiological and the better-controlled laboratory studies, it seems clear that the smoking/lung cancer link is causal. Clearly, tar is a potent carcinogenic agent and is delivered directly to the site of action. This is not to deny, of course, that there may be some genetic predisposition to lung cancer in certain individuals. If so, predisposed individuals who smoke accept a double jeopardy.

As far as cardiovascular disease is concerned, however, the relationship is more blurred. Possible mechanisms involving CO or nicotine, for example, have not yet been clearly implicated. In addition, the influence of other factors, e.g., genetic predisposition, diet, stress and excessive alcohol use, undoubtedly play a part, both in their own right, and in interaction with smoking.

2

Theories about smoking

Given that the health risks from smoking cigarettes may be substantial, particularly in the case of certain cause-specific diseases such as lung cancer, we might well ask 'Why do people persist in smoking?'

In the search for aetiological factors underlying smoking, we encounter a number of methodological and theoretical problems:

(1) We have to distinguish initially between recruitment to, and persistence of the smoking habit, each of which may be determined by different mechanisms. For example, addiction models have little to say about aetiology vis-à-vis recruitment. It may be that the individual is recruited to smoking for a variety of psychosocial reasons, for example by peer group pressure or the desire to adopt adult status, and that the habit is then maintained by addiction. Addiction theory, therefore, is only incidentally concerned with factors underlying recruitment, except insofar as this may have relevance to techniques of intervention and termination of the smoking habit.

On the other hand, the genetic argument proposes that recruitment to, and persistence of the habit, and consumption levels (any or all of these) are governed by genetic dispositions, perhaps through the genetic underpinning of personality, which itself is related to smoking. A second-order variant of the genetic argument is arousal modulation theory, which proposes that nicotine is one of a group of mood control agents (alcohol and coffee are others) that the individual uses to modulate his psychological state in accordance with his genetically fixed optimal arousal level, i.e., the arousal level which promotes optimal psychological comfort and performance enhancement.

(2) Part of the difficulty in classifying theories about smoking arises from the fact that, to an extent, all theories of smoking are pleasure-seeking/reward theories. With the possible exception of genetic theories,

41

analysis of the nature of the rewards inherent in smoking inevitably leads on to one or other of the theoretical models described below. From this point of view, the main difference between the theories lies in the assumed nature of, and hence in the emphasis given to, both the social and pharmacological rewards of smoking. It is here that some of the problems emerge in clearest form. For example, consider the view proposed by addiction theory that smokers gain their reward from relief of nicotine withdrawal symptoms and compare this with the view proposed by arousal modulation theory that smokers enjoy primary reward from nicotine, which is employed as a psychological tool to maintain arousal level at a hypothetical optimum. The difference between these views reflects the as yet unresolved debate in the animal learning literature as to whether relief from punishment is equivalent to reward, and is mediated by similar mechanisms (Gray, 1971). The exact nature of the pharmacological reinforcement involved in smoking is thus problematical.

(3) As far as genetic determinants are concerned, twin methodology, from which heritability estimates are derived, presents some vexing problems (Cederloff *et al.*, 1977; Eysenck & Kamin, 1981). One of the general problems encountered in twin studies is that Mz twins share the same genes, and all twins share similar social histories provided they are not separated. Thus, if there are any familial/environmental influences initiating or affecting the behaviour under study, they are more likely to affect Mz twins most similarly, Dz twins to a slightly lesser extent and non-twin siblings, who obviously are of a different age but share the same genetic endowment as Dz twins, to a much lesser extent. One influence that is likely to be important is that of peers, and this has been shown in a number of studies (see Chapter 4: Recruitment to smoking; Chapter 5: Influences on adolescent smoking through exemplars) to be considerable with regard to initiation of the smoking habit.

Of course, the greater similarity in social-familial/age-group influences for twins as opposed to siblings does not imply that Mz and Dz twins are subject to entirely similar social influences. Mz twins tend to be treated as more alike by parents than do Dz twins; for example, they are more likely to be dressed alike and to have friends in common. There are grounds for assuming, however, that one twin of the pair takes a 'leading' role, even *in utero*; on the other hand, it could be argued that Mz twins identify with, i.e., partake of, a 'joint personality' to a greater extent than do Dz twins and to a significantly greater extent than do siblings. When we are dealing with highly 'voluntary' behaviours such as smoking, which, initially, may be guided by imitation or a desire to achieve adult status, concordance rates are likely to be distorted by such factors.

The alternative to the observation of non-separated twins involves the study of age of initiation, persistence and consumption rates of Mz twins reared apart; this perhaps will give us the only true values for concordance rates. For obvious reasons, data of this sort are extremely difficult to obtain, and only one or two studies have been reported in the literature. Indeed, in such cases, the smoking data are usually almost incidental. The main thrust of these investigations concerns psychiatric disorder, since often the reason for adoption in the first case is some psychiatric breakdown in the mother (Heston, 1966). However, in view of this dearth of separated-twin studies, data derived from conventional twin studies, and studies of adopted children, have undoubted value, although adoptee data reported in some studies (e.g., Eysenck, 1980) may have greater relevance to other problems in this area such as familial influences on smoking behaviour.

Unfortunately, the problems outlined above have seldom been recognised, and have certainly not been disentangled in smoking research, and this presents great difficulties for the reviewer. All we can do, therefore, is to consider the various theories as they are described in the literature while reminding the reader that some of these are relevant to only some aspects of the smoking habit, and that in few cases has the problem of the nature of reward as far as smoking is concerned been satisfactorily resolved.

Over the past twenty years, a variety of methodological and substantive bias has generated a broad spectrum of theories about reasons for smoking, which, for convenience, can be categorised as genetic, central nervous system (CNS), psychobiological and social learning theories.

Genetic theories
A genetic basis for smoking

Irrespective of evidence as to whether or not certain genes predispose to the type of disease implicated in the smoking/disease controversy, what evidence is there that certain genes predispose to smoking, a claim asserted by Burch (1976)?

In approaching this issue, a word of caution seems timely. While it is possible to make heritability estimates for physiological and psycho-physiological measures of human individual differences such as skin colour, size, blood group and electroencephalographic (EEG) parameters, it is conceded that estimates are much more difficult for more conceptual measures such as Intelligence Quotient (IQ) (see Eysenck & Kamin, 1981). This is both because the concepts are more nebulous and because of the greater importance assumed by the environment, and its interactions, in the development of human intellectual capacity.

How much more pertinent is this observation when we are considering highly 'voluntary' behaviours such as smoking cigarettes? Common sense dictates that it is highly unlikely that such behaviours can have a direct genetic component. Facile statements about direct genetic determination of smoking seem absurd. It is rather analogous to claiming that 'the wearing of trousers is strongly genetically determined'. Sex status is, of course, so determined, and in those societies in which men wear trousers and women skirts, wearing trousers is, in fact, a second-order or indirect marker of a genetically determined attribute, i.e., sex.

We choose to regard smoking in a similar light. No-one would seriously suggest that the gene pool has changed over the past fifty years, which would have to be the case to account for the increased smoking prevalence (and, for that matter, the wearing of trousers) amongst women over this period of time on a genetic basis. However, it may be that genetics are indirectly involved, a point we shall recapitulate when describing addiction and arousal modulation theories of smoking.

With this caveat in mind, we shall briefly review evidence for a genetic theory of smoking. For convenience, non-separated and separated twin studies will be considered independently.

Non-separated twins. The first evidence for a genetic basis for smoking habits derived from twin studies comes from the study made by Fisher (1958*b*). Of 51 Mz pairs examined, Fisher states that 33 pairs were wholly alike qualitatively, 6 pairs were classed alike and 12 pairs showed distinct differences, in their smoking habits. Of 31 Dz pairs examined, only 11 pairs were classed as wholly alike and 16 of the pairs were distinctly different. Thus, the difference between the Mz and the Dz pairs, in terms of 'distinct' differences in smoking habits, was that only 24% of Mz pairs were distinctly different compared with 51% of Dz pairs. Fisher concludes that the genotype exercises a considerable influence on smoking, and on the particular habit of smoking adopted. A similar outcome is reported by Fisher (1958*b*) in an analysis of female twins from the sample studied in somewhat greater detail by Shields (1962). In evaluating the findings of these studies, of course, the possibility of mutual influence cannot be excluded.

A similar result is reported by Todd & Mason (1959). Their data support the inheritance of the smoking habit. Division of respondents into smokers and non-smokers produced 43 concordant Mz pairs out of 52, while only 19 of the total of 32 Dz pairs were concordant. Concordance data are also reported by Friberg, Kaij, Dencker & Jonsson (1959), who investigated the smoking habits of Swedish pairs. Groups of 59 Mz and 59 Dz pairs, matched for age and sex, were selected for study. Their results indicate that

Mz twins resemble one another significantly more than do Dz twins for overall characteristics of the smoking habit. Roughly similar results have been reported by Conterio & Chiarelli (1962) in an investigation of Italian twins. They studied 77 pairs of male twins, all over 20 years of age, 34 pairs being classed as Mz and 43 pairs as Dz. Concordance for smoking versus non-smoking was significantly different between the two groups of twins, Mz pairs showing a greater resemblance than Dz twins. In a subsidiary analysis, classification by quantity of smoked products revealed the greatest difference in concordance between the two types of twins, with 26 of the 34 Mz pairs being concordant compared with 14 of the 43 Dz pairs ($X^2 = 12.92$; $p < 0.001$).

A number of Scandinavian studies are of interest. Raaschou-Nielsen (1960) recorded the smoking habits of 894 twin pairs. She categorised smokers into four groups: non-smokers, occasional smokers, former smokers, and combined regular + heavy smokers. Concordant pairs were defined as all those pairs in which members fall into identical groups. The results are shown in Table 5. It is obvious that Mz twins are, on the average, significantly more similar than Dz twins.

A study of Finnish twins has been reported by Partanen, Bruun & Markkanen (1966). Of 198 male Mz twin pairs, 75.3% were concordant with respect to smoking/non-smoking. The corresponding figures for Dz twins were 65.5% of the 640 pairs studied, the difference between Mz and Dz twins being highly significant.

Similar data are reported by Friberg, Kaij, Dencker & Jonsson (1959), Cederlof (1966) and Cederlof et al. (1977). Significantly elevated coincidence

Table 5. *Smoking habits in Mz and Dz twins.*
(*From Raaschou-Nielsen, 1960*)

| | Percentage concordant[a] | |
	Male	Female
Dz/Total	39.4	55.7
(n)	(223)	(328)
Mz/Total	57.2	69.4
(n)	(147)	(196)

[a] All same sex twins, pooled 1870–1910 birth cohorts. Percentage concordance based on four categories: non-smokers, light smokers, ex-smokers, regular + heavy smokers. Concordance rates are much higher if the simpler categorisation of smokers versus non-smokers is employed.

ratios for observed over expected rates of smoking versus not smoking for both Mz and Dz twins are reported in the old Swedish Twin Registry (Cederlof, 1966). This finding is supported by data from the new Swedish Twin Registry for both male and female Mz and Dz twins with the single exception of Dz female twins from the 1946–55 birth cohort (Cederlof *et al.*, 1977). Coincidence ratios for smoking are higher for Mz than for Dz twins. This is tested by the Mz/Dz quotients of the coincidence ratios, which are significant, thus indicating either a genetic component or a strong environmental pressure for conformity in smoking (Table 6).

Extensive data on this issue have been reported by Eysenck & Eaves (Eysenck, 1980), who used 1261 twin pairs from the Maudsley Twin Registry as subjects. These authors have addressed different issues from those considered in the studies already discussed, and employed different methodological and statistical techniques. They dealt separately with the issues of differentiating smokers from non-smokers, and, amongst the former, with different aspects of the smoking habit: age of onset, persistence and reported daily average consumption. In addition, they have advanced beyond simple concordance and the application of conventional or quantitative genetics to a more rigorous analysis of the causes of variation.

Eysenck & Eaves claim that the unidimensional, multi-factorial model of quantitative genetics is perfectly adequate to distinguish those who have

Table 6. *Heredity of smoking; coincidence ratios and quotients between Mz and Dz ratios by sex, age and zygosity; new Swedish Twin Registry.* (*From Cederlof et al., 1977*)

Cohort	Coincidence ratios observed/expected		Quotients Mz/Dz
	Mz	Dz	
Males			
1926–45	1.46[s]	1.20[s]	1.22[s]
1946–55	1.68[s]	1.26[s]	1.33[s]
1956–58	4.00[s]	2.67[s]	1.50[s]
Total	1.61[s]	1.32[s]	1.22[s]
Females			
1926–45	1.71[s]	1.41[s]	1.21[s]
1946–55	1.65[s]	1.33	1.24
1956–58	2.78[s]	2.18[s]	1.28[s]
Total	1.76[s]	1.44[s]	1.22[s]

[s] Significant effect.

never smoked from those who persistently smoke, and that those who began smoking, but subsequently gave up, are between the extremes of non-smoking and persistent smoking on the scale of genetic predisposition. They claim that this predisposition is inherited rather than cultural, since the inclusion of a family environmental effect in the model for twin similarity has little effect on the values reported. They also report, however, that in dealing with age of onset of smoking and reported average daily consumption of cigarettes, the situation is somewhat more complex. They suggest that there are genetic differences which affect both these variables, but that these are expressed in addition to other non-genetic family effects. They were unable to resolve the additive genetic effects and the family environmental effects with complete certainty. They comment that non-smokers are differentiated genetically from smokers along quite a distinct dimension from that which discriminates the different degrees of cigarette consumption amongst smokers.

In an overall study of smoking/drinking and personality, Eysenck & Eaves used not only the data from this twin sample but also family and adoption data, the adopted families, the normal pedigrees and the twins totalling 2469 individuals. Correlations between relatives for age of onset of smoking and for average reported consumption threw up some interesting results (Table 7). For age of onset (Eysenck, 1980, p. 242), the correlation for Dz twins was not significantly less than for Mz twins, which suggests that the effects of the family environment may be acting along

Table 7. *Pooled correlations between relatives for smoking.* (*From Eysenck, 1980*)

Relationship	n (d.f.)[a]	Age of onset	Average consumption
Mz twin	310	0.403	0.521
Dz twin	217	0.304	0.303
Sibling	406	0.139	0.108
Spouse	150	0.195	0.117
Parent/offspring	533	0.103	0.205
Grandparent/grandchild	45	−0.109	0.080
Avuncular	302	0.176	0.073
First cousin	101	0.176	0.096
Foster parent/foster child	218	−0.018	−0.016
Foster child/natural child	27 ⎫ 40	0.018 ⎫ 0.181	−0.097 ⎫ 0.047
Foster child/foster child	13 ⎭	0.483 ⎭	0.333 ⎭

[a] The number of pairs (n) for each group is reported here in terms of degrees of freedom (d.f.). Add approximately 10 pairs to each group to form an estimate of the n pairs in each group. (See Eysenck, 1980, pp. 238–42 for further details.)

with genetic effects in determining the age at which smoking commences. For average cigarette consumption, the difference in twin correlations was much more marked (p < 0.01). This confirmed the earlier finding that a genetic rather than a purely environmental explanation was more likely.

Table 7 discloses a number of other interesting findings. One, for example, is that the correlation between siblings is substantially lower than that between Dz twins, particularly in the case of average consumption. This suggests that twins are something of a special case, perhaps because of the exceptional similarity in their environments, or because of the interaction of genetic differences with age. Another comparison of interest is that between correlation of parents with their natural children and of parents with their foster children. The difference for age of onset is very slight, suggesting no hereditary influences on this aspect of smoking. For average daily cigarette consumption, the foster parent/foster child correlation is close to zero, suggesting little environmental influence or connection between the consumption of cigarettes in parents and in offspring. However, the correlation of 0.205 between natural parent and offspring is significantly different from zero and also significantly exceeds the foster parent/foster child correlation for cigarette consumption. This suggests that hereditary factors play some part in the continuance of the habit. All these data fit into the picture of the trait which is partly heritable, but for which unique environmental experiences play a major role in the determination of variation.

Eysenck & Eaves (Eysenck, 1980) state that their data make them question the simple-minded exploitation of the twin design and its conventional genetic interpretation in relation to smoking. They suggest that the similarity of twins for age of onset and consumption of tobacco is probably not purely genetic, a point which is particularly crucial if we are tempted to assert that the increased risk of non-smoking partners of smoking twins is due to genetic communality of smoking and disease (which is a possible inference from the Cederlof *et al.* (1977) NET Series analyses). Eysenck & Eaves suggest that the methods which have been employed in the conventional pursuit of smoking genotype do not seriously examine the possibility that part of the similarity of twins is a reflection of environmental similarities. From their data concerning age of onset and average consumption of cigarettes, it is likely that about 20% of the measured variation in these traits can be attributed to peer effects, for which twins are alike. In the case of age of onset, this amounts to half the total variation between Mz twin pairs, and is thus on a par with the estimated contribution of inherited factors. They suggest that if this is true for the smoking habit itself, then they cannot discount the possibility that, on the basis of available twin data alone, environmental factors, as well as common genetic factors, may account for some of the increased incidence of certain diseases in the non-smoking partners of smoking twins.

Overall, the Eysenck & Eaves evidence suggests a small but significant contribution of genetic factors to characteristics of the smoking habit. From the twin data, the most striking contribution is that which differentiates non-smokers from persistent smokers. Genetic contribution for age of onset and consumption is substantially less. About half the similarity between twins for the smoking habit is attributable to non-genetic effects such as environmental influences.

Separated twins. The most compelling source of evidence, as we have commented previously, is studies of separated twins. Unfortunately, these are rare.

One of the earliest studies was reported by Fisher (1958*b*). He reports smoking concordance rates for 27 female Mz twin pairs reared apart which are not statistically different from rates for Mz twins reared together. The latter, of course, are significantly higher than concordance rates for Dz twins reared together.

Juel-Nielsen (1960) reports that smoking concordance rates for 12 pairs of Mz twins reared apart were no different from those observed for the Mz twins reared together in the Raaschou-Nielsen (1960) series.

Shields (1962) reports somewhat more extensive data. Pooling over sexes, his sample consisted of 42 pairs of Mz twins separated from birth, 42 pairs of unseparated Mz twins, and 20 pairs of unseparated Dz twins. The question asked was 'How many cigarettes do you smoke a day?'. Responses were classified into the following categories: non-smokers, and

Table 8. *Concordance in the smoking habits of twins. Figures are the number of twin pairs with similar cigarette consumption (percentages given in parentheses). (From Shields, 1962)*

| | Twin type | | |
| | Mz | | |
Rating of similarity	Separated	Unseparated	Dz
Closely similar	28 (67)	21 (50)	7 (35)
Fairly similar	8 (19)	13 (31)	7 (35)
Dissimilar	6 (14)	8 (19)	6 (30)
Total number of pairs	42	42	20

smokers of 1–5 cigarettes per day, 6–10 cigarettes per day, 11–16 cigarettes per day and 16+ cigarettes per day. Pairs in which both twins fell into the same category were classified as closely similar, those which fell into neighbouring categories as fairly similar, and those which were less alike as dissimilar. Details are shown in Table 8. Clearly, both the separated and unseparated Mz twins showed significantly higher concordance rates than the Dz twins. Over and above this, however, the separated twins showed higher concordance rates, although not significantly so, than the unseparated twins, suggesting that family environment is not important in the determination of smoking.

Finally, we can refer to some very limited data, derived from the continuing University of Minnesota twin study of separated twins, which has been described by Holden (1980). Although cases were few in number, a considerable amount of detailed information was collected for each pair, and some of it is of interest in the present connection. The most interesting observation is that 'one of the greatest areas of discordance for twins was smoking. Of the nine pairs, there were four in which one twin smoked, and the other did not'.

A review of the major twin studies of smoking is given in Table 9.

Despite the general criticisms which can be directed at twin study methodology, and some conflicting results (e.g., the last-mentioned study), data from both the separated and unseparated twin studies suggest overall that there is some genetic basis for smoking behaviour.

Genetic basis for personality and behavioural traits which have been shown to be related to smoking

Personality traits. A considerable amount of evidence that is relevant to the question of the genetic basis of personality traits is now available (see Eysenck, 1980; Mangan, 1982*b*), and the reader is referred to these sources for fuller detail. Here we shall briefly summarise the main findings, limiting our observations to those personality dimensions which have been shown to be related to smoking.

There is now substantial agreement that variations in temperament and personality can be described in terms of Eysenck's personality factors, extraversion (E), neuroticism (N), psychoticism (P) and lie score (L) (see Appendix: Extraversion). A number of conjoint factor analyses (e.g., Vagg & Hammond, 1976) have clearly indicated that the primary factor structures suggested by other personality theorists such as Cattell and Guilford (see Vagg & Hammond, 1976 and Mangan, 1982*b* for extensive references) do not account for variation additional to that taken up by Eysenck's second-order factors. In addition, the Cattell and Guilford factors appear to be inherently unstable, and, arguably, redundant.

Vandenberg (1967), in a review of 15 studies, reports a significant genetic contribution to extraversion, and a number of subsequent studies have offered strong support for this (Eysenck, 1967; Gottesman, 1968; Jinks & Fulker, 1970; Eaves & Eysenck, 1975; Horn, Plomin & Rosenman, 1976; Eaves & Young, 1981). Eaves & Young (1981) report that shared family environment has no detectable role in generating the similarities in personality observed between relatives, but that measured differences in these dimensions are attributable about equally to random environmental and genetic factors, which, however, are not constant throughout life.

As far as neuroticism is concerned, the evidence appears to be less conclusive (Vandenberg, 1967; Mittler, 1971). Nonetheless, a number of studies report a strong genetic component in N (Gottesman, 1963; Jinks & Fulker, 1970; Shields, 1973; Eaves & Eysenck, 1975; Eaves & Young, 1981, e.g.).

It is only recently that data concerning the genetic contribution to Eysenck's third factor, psychoticism, or P, has become available. Eaves (1973) claims that P has heritability of 46%, while Eysenck & Eysenck (1976) cite an additive heritability figure of 81%. This figure is similar to that reported by Gottesman & Shields (1966a, b) for schizophrenia, which, according to Eysenck's definition of P, lies in the same dimension. Eaves & Eysenck (1977) report, from a sample of 544 twin pairs, that environmental differences between families account for 51% of the variation of P. However, the greater part (77%) of such environmental variation is due to random effects which are unlikely to be controllable.

Eaves & Eysenck, in a number of studies (1975, 1976, 1977), suggest a very simple basis for determination of differences in E, N and P. Gene action seems relatively straightforward, with little evidence of assortative mating. As noted above, however, they comment that a good deal of what passes for environmental variation is simply the result of error, for example errors in measurement. Such random variation can account for a substantial portion – around 75% in the case of P – of so-called environmental variation.

Over and above error variance of this sort, however, it has been suggested that environmental effects are largely confined to unique experiences of individual twins rather than to shared environmental effects common to both members of the pair. Loehlin & Nichols (1976), for example, claim that environments for twins are no more alike than those of two members of the population pairs at random.

Personality and smoking. Considerable data describing significant differences between groups of heavy and light smokers, and between groups of ex-smokers and non-smokers, in a number of personality and behavioural

Table 9. *Studies postulating the genetic determination of smoking behaviour*

Author(s)	Country of twin origin	No. of sample twin pairs[a,b]	Mz twins reared apart?	Results[c]
Cederlof, Floderus & Friberg (1970)	Sweden	3656 Mz, 6850 Dz	No	Smoking concordance: observations that discordant Mz twins were difficult to find
Cederlof, Friberg & Lundman (1977)	Sweden	5025 Mz, 7873 Dz	No	Smoking coincidence ratios: observed/expected, significant Mz/Dz quotients for these ratios – Mz more concordant than Dz
Conterio & Chiarelli (1962)	Italy	34 Mz, 43 Dz	No	X^2 smoking concordance: Mz significantly more concordant than Dz
Eysenck (1980)	England	316 Mz, 229 Dz, 1359 individuals from families and fostered individuals	No (fostering)	Correlation (complex family models for assessing significance levels). Smoking concordance for Mz greater than for Dz greater than for family relatives
Fisher (1958a)	Germany	51 Mz, 31 Dz	No	No formal statistics. Smoking concordance greater for Mz than Dz
Fisher (1958b)	England	89 Mz, 18 Dz, 27 Mz reared apart	Yes	No formal statistics. Smoking concordance for Mz reared apart similar to Mz reared together and greater than Dz
Friberg, Kaij, Dencker & Jonsson (1959)	Sweden	59 Mz, 59 Dz	No	X^2 smoking concordance: Mz significantly more concordant than Dz

Study	Country	Mz reared apart	Sample	Comments
				No formal statistics. Smoking concordance for Mz reared apart similar to that for Mz reared together in Raaschou-Nielsen (1960) and cited in that study
Partanen, Bruun & Markkanen (1966)	Finland	No	198 Mz, 640 Dz	X^2 smoking concordance: Mz significantly more concordant than Dz
Raaschou-Nielsen (1960)	Denmark	No	343 Mz, 551 Dz	X^2 smoking concordance: Mz more concordant than Dz, significant only for females
Shields (1962)	England	Yes	42 Mz, 20 Dz, 42 Mz reared apart	No formal statistics. Smoking concordance for Mz reared apart similar to that for Mz reared together and greater than that for Dz
Todd & Mason (1959)	Germany	No	52 Mz, 32 Dz	No formal statistics. Smoking concordance for Mz greater than for Dz

[a] Twin pairs reared together unless otherwise stated.
[b] Dz twins are both of the same sex except for Eysenck (1980).
[c] Where 'no formal statistics', results are almost invariably significant when formally analysed (see Eysenck (1980) for analyses).

traits have been reported. Useful summaries have been prepared by Matarazzo & Saslow (1960) and Smith (1970). Although there is a good deal of redundancy and overlap between the traits identified, largely because many of the trait descriptions, e.g., 'independent', 'energetic' and 'agreeable', are difficult to operationalise, there is general agreement on a number of points, which are discussed below.

Of relevance also is Smith's (1970) comment that even the most reliable personality predictors of smoking such as extraversion account for only 3–5% of the variance in measures of smoking, and that even the best univariate personality assessment can discriminate smokers from non-smokers in only about 60% of cases. On the other hand, he claims that his own multivariate studies were successful in discriminating such groups in 68–76% of cases, a similar discrimination efficiency (80%) being reported by Golding, Harpur & Brent-Smith (1983). (However, since smokers still comprise a comparatively large segment of the population, random allocation of individuals to such groups will give considerable 'discrimination' by chance. This should be taken into account when judging the 'discriminability' of personality dimensions vis-à-vis smoking status.)

A number of studies, mainly univariate, have underlined the relationship between extraversion and cigarette smoking (e.g., Matarazzo & Saslow, 1960; Cattell & Krug, 1976). Smith (1970), from an extensive review, reports that 22 of the 24 studies cited disclosed that smokers are more extraverted than non-smokers, a relationship which was generalised over different populations. This has been supported in many subsequent studies (e.g., Coan, 1973; Cederlof *et al.*, 1977), and in longitudinal studies (Reynolds & Nichols, 1976; Cherry & Kiernan, 1978). Russell (1971) has proposed that a number of variables cluster with extraversion in describing smokers, who are greater risk takers, more impulsive, more prone to divorce and to changing jobs, more interested in sex, and more likely to drink coffee, tea and alcohol than non-smokers. On the other hand, McCrae, Costa & Bosse (1978) found no evidence in their study of an extensive sample of American adult males that smokers are more extraverted than non-smokers, judging from scores on Cattell's 16 Personality Factors (PF) and a shortened form of the Eysenck Personality Inventory (EPI). Weeks (1979), Golding (1980) and Golding *et al.* (1983) have reported a similar lack of relationship between E and smoking.

More recently, Eysenck & Eysenck (1975) have developed a P scale, orthogonal to E, N and L, which incorporates some of the original 'impulsivity' sub-factor items of extraversion, together with 'risk-taking', 'tough-minded' and 'paranoia' items. It is possible that this new P scale may now be more predictive of smoking (Eysenck, 1980; Golding *et al.*, 1983) than the new E scale of the Eysenck Personality Questionnaire (EPQ), which has been somewhat narrowed in scope, and is biased towards measuring 'sociability', although some elements of an impulsivity sub-factor still remain. More work needs to be done, however, before this assertion can be made with full confidence.

There is some evidence that smokers rate high on anxiety (McArthur, Waldron & Dickinson, 1958; Lilienfeld, 1959; Matarazzo & Saslow, 1960; Straits & Sechrest, 1963; Thomas & Ross, 1968; Walker, Nicolay, Kluczny & Rudel, 1969). All these authors also note that smokers consume more alcohol and coffee than do non-smokers. Thomas (1973) reports that mean values on these variables for smokers who ultimately stopped are intermediate between those of continuing smokers and non-smokers. She suggests that these results fit well with Tomkins' (1966) model for smoking behaviour, which describes three types of smokers: the positive affect smoker, who smokes for enjoyment, the negative affect smoker, who smokes to alleviate distress, and the addictive smoker, for whom lack of a cigarette becomes an important source of distress. Presumably the anxious smoker is the negative affect smoker. This is also the view taken by McKennell (1970), who suggests that 'nervous irritation', which, as a reason for smoking, starts early, characterises Tomkins' negative affect and addictive smoker.

Smith (1970) reports that half of the 50 studies in his review show smokers to have slightly poorer 'mental health' than non-smokers, mental health referring rather loosely to anxiety or nervousness. Floderus (1974) and Cederlof *et al.* (1977) also report higher neuroticism scores in smokers, as did the first Surgeon General's Report (1964). McCrae *et al.* (1978) report that current heavy smokers, as a sub-group, score significantly higher than non-smokers on neuroticism and anxiety, as does Rae (1975) in his study. On the other hand, Eysenck (1963, 1973, 1980) reports that there is no evidence that smokers are more neurotic than non-smokers.

It is possible, of course, that there may be sex differences in the relationship between smoking and neuroticism. Waters (1971) reports a non-significant correlation between smoking habits and neuroticism for men, but a small, significant correlation for women. Clausen (1968), as part of the Oakland Growth Study, reports scores on psychoneurotic symptoms for boys and girls who later grew up to be smokers. Males showed a generally negative association between amount smoked during adulthood and their adolescent neuroticism scores. Females, on the other hand, showed a positive association. Thomas (1973), in a detailed study of smoking and habits of nervous tension amongst male medical students of

Johns Hopkins University, using stepwise discriminant function analysis, found that anxiety was significantly related to heavier smoking.

By far the most comprehensive study of smoking and personality is that reported by Eysenck (1980), which we have already referred to when discussing the contribution of genetic factors to characteristics of the smoking habit. In advancing his 'constitutional' model of smoking, Eysenck has reported discriminant function analysis of relationships between persistence in smoking, age of onset and consumption rates and the four EPQ scales, P, E, N and L. These data are reproduced in Table 10, and from the table it is clear that the most significant discriminators between phenotypic categories into which smokers and non-smokers sort themselves are high P and low L. These dimensions, according to Eysenck, reflect socialisation and social desirability respectively. This finding applied across the sexes and across the three response categories age of onset, persistence and average consumption.

Eysenck then attempts to establish whether these personality variables also discriminate between different grades of the smoking habit amongst smokers. Again the pattern of weights for the four personality variables is similar to that reported in the previous analysis (Table 10), although the differences here are somewhat less significant. This suggests that the measured personality traits contribute more to the determination of whether people begin to smoke at all (recruitment) than to the level of indulgence once the habit has been started (maintenance).

In attempting to assess the causal basis of these phenotypic associations, Eysenck (1980) reports analyses of twin and family and adoption data. As far as the twin data are concerned, he reports that the contribution of genetic factors to the association between smoking and personality is more significant for females than for males; the principal relationship reported is identical to that obtained from the discriminant function analyses of the phenotypic associations. A personality profile of the 'early onset/persistent heavy smoker' as being high on the P scale and low on the L scale is strongly suggested by the genetic analysis, especially in the case of the female twins. However, when we allow for the large genetic correlation (-0.51) between these two personality scales, and for the fact that genetic factors explain only 57% of the phenotypic variation of persistence in smoking, then only about 7% of such variation is predictable in principle from genetic variation in these two components of personality. Similar calculations yield comparable figures for the other components of the smoking habit (Eysenck, 1980, p. 305).

Overall, a significant phenotypic relationship between questionnaire measures of personality and aspects of the smoking habit is disclosed.

Table 10. *Personality and smoking: discriminant function analysis. (From Eysenck, 1980)*

Response	Sex	Coefficients				Correlation	χ^2	d.f.[a]	P (%)
		P	E	N	L				
Age of onset	Males	−0.62	+0.12	−0.23	0.58	0.233	63.70	24	< 0.1
	Females	−0.60	−0.24	−0.29	0.56	0.278	149.44	24	< 0.1
Average consumption	Males	−0.80	−0.05	−0.31	0.25	0.170	37.86	28	10.0
	Females	−0.68	−0.35	−0.39	0.31	0.250	133.38	28	< 0.1
Persistence	Males	−0.60	−0.07	−0.43	0.46	0.216	38.40	8	< 0.1
	Females	−0.57	−0.37	−0.36	0.49	0.266	134.48	8	< 0.1

[a] Degrees of freedom.

Smoking is associated with higher scores on the P scale and lower scores on the L scale. However, Eysenck & Eaves (Eysenck, 1980) comment that it is difficult to discriminate between genetic and environmental explanations of the familial components of the correlation. From their results, it is clear that the greater part of the variation in smoking cannot be predicted from personality measures. Thus, 'we are forced into virtual agnosticism about the relative contributions of heredity and environment to the inter-relations of smoking and personality' (Eysenck, 1980).

In addition to the studies already reviewed, there are a number of reports in the literature concerning the relationship of personality variables such as the internal/external locus of control and augmenting/reducing behaviour (see Appendix), to smoking behaviour.

As far as internal/external control is concerned, Smith's (1970) review indicates that only five studies of the relationship of this variable to smoking have been reported. Four of these show smokers to be more under the control of an external locus. Two more recent studies, by Berman (1973) and Hjelle & Clouser (1970), are divided in their support.

The relationship of augmenting/reducing behaviour to smoking behaviour presents a very confusing picture. Knott (1979a) accepts the original suggestion of Petrie (1967) that extraverts tend to be reducers, and introverts augmenters, a view internally consistent with the observation that reducers are more tolerant of pain, since it is well established that extraverts have greater pain tolerance than introverts (Eysenck, 1967). However, more recent evidence (Soskis & Shagass, 1974) calls this into question. Using evoked potential tests of augmenting/reducing behaviour they report that augmenters were more extraverted and reducers more introverted. Neuroticism (N) yielded no consistent relationships. Soskis & Shagass note this conflict of evidence, but point out that other studies, such as that of Buchsbaum (1971), also throw doubt on the notion that reducers are extraverted rather than introverted. We should also point out that in line with commonly held views on the arousal characteristics of extraverts and introverts, the low-aroused extravert might be expected to seek stimulation, i.e., to augment, and the highly reactive introvert to reduce. Of relevance here is more recent evidence which suggests that the augmenting/reducing phenomenon may not be a totally stable characteristic but may vary with concomitant changes in autonomic arousal (Birchall & Claridge, 1979).

Knott (1979a), however, reports that the low-arousal smoker is more introverted than extraverted, more stable and more augmenting, the latter attribute being predictable from the general theory outlined above. This result receives some limited support from the findings of Barnes &

Fishlinsky (1976) concerning augmenting/reducing. Much the same comment can be made about Knott's complementary finding that the high-arousal smoker is more extraverted, more neurotic and more reducing. Note also that Bartol's (1975) results favour the rather unexpected linking of extraversion with high-arousal or stress smoking, and introversion with low-arousal smoking, i.e. smoking to enhance arousal in boring or monotonous conditions.

Despite some conflict of evidence, therefore, it appears likely that there is a systematic relationship between smoking and certain aspects of personality. The major studies and reviews in this field, those of the Surgeon General (1979), Cederlof *et al.* (1977), Warburton & Wesnes (1978) and Eysenck (1980), conclude that there is reason to believe that smokers are, to a degree, more extraverted (reflected in sociability, risk-taking, aggression, divorce, job-changing, sex, e.g.) and more neurotic (i.e., unstable) than non-smokers. However, there have been some failures of prediction. No doubt that this may be due in part to the fact that smokers are a heterogeneous group. In particular, women smokers seem to show a better 'fit' with the concept that the heavier smoker is more neurotic (Warburton & Wesnes, 1978). Additionally, the relationship between extraversion (E) and smoking may be contaminated by the fact that both cigarette smoking and E are associated with other drug use: coffee, tea and alcohol. In fact, the association between smoking and other psychoactive drug use is one of the most consistently reported pieces of evidence. It may be more than coincidental that in the Weeks (1979) study, which failed to demonstrate significantly higher E in smokers, smoker and non-smoker groups had been matched for alcohol consumption.

Behavioural traits and characteristics. Here we are concerned with a number of behavioural and psychosocial attributes which appear to have genetic underpinnings, and which seem to be associated with smoking as opposed to the 'purer' concepts of personality discussed in the previous section.

In his review of the relationship of antisocial tendencies to smoking, Smith (1970) reports that 20 of 32 analyses show that smokers exhibit antisocial tendencies such as belligerence, psychopathic deviance, misconduct, defiance and disagreeableness to a greater extent than non-smokers. Subsequent studies have supported these findings (Lebovits & Ostfeld, 1971; Nesbitt, 1973; Reynolds & Nichols, 1976). Matarazzo & Saslow (1960) and Weatherley (1965), however, consider that admission of antisocial tendencies by smokers may indicate response bias, in that they are more willing to admit negative attributes, although in fact they may not differ from non-smokers in these respects. Eysenck's (1980) finding that smoking is associated with high P and low L scores is very much in line with this, since this profile would suggest both possession of, and willingness to admit to, antisocial tendencies.

Cederlof *et al.* (1977), from their A Series analyses, report a clear-cut association between drinking, particularly excessive drinking, and smoking. A distinct dose gradient was apparent, even in the youngest age group. Subjects who smoked more than 16 cigarettes a day drank excessive amounts of alcohol 3–10 times more often than did non-smokers. Roughly similar results are reported for drug consumption, particularly for prescription-free analgesics, sleeping pills and oral contraceptives. Smokers used sleeping pills and tranquillisers 3–5 times more frequently than did non-smokers. As in the case of alcohol consumption, there was little evidence of sex differences in the appropriate categories. Similar associations have been reported by Cummins, Shaper, Walker & Wale (1981) and Golding *et al.* (1983).

There was also evidence of psychosocial discord in heavy smokers. They scored higher on instability (similar to N), and reported sleeping difficulties and stress about twice as frequently as non-smokers. Divorce was about four times as common. Smokers showed more frequent changes of employer, lower levels of physical activity and more often drank five or more cups of coffee per day. Extraversion was moderately, but significantly, higher in smoking groups. As before, these trends applied to both men and women. Where appropriate, they also applied to the youngest age groups, boys and girls in the age range 15–17 years. For example, drinking was around five times more common amongst smokers and the use of oral contraceptives by the girl smokers was nine times more common than by non-smokers. These findings are strongly reinforced by Cederlof *et al.*'s B Series and NET analyses, summaries of which are presented in Table 11.

In the B Series analyses, ratios for many items were much lower than expected, particularly for Mz pairs. For example, in the case of alcohol consumption, the Mz ratio was 1.1, compared with the expected ratio of 1.5; the figures for excessive drinking were 1.5, as against the expected 4.5. This means that in discordant (for smoking) Mz pairs, the non-smoking twin drank almost as much as his smoking co-twin. A similar, but less dramatic effect applies in the case of drug use. Less good control is indicated for sleeping pills and tranquillisers, with ratios of 1.9 and 1.8 as against expected ratios of 2.3 and 1.9 respectively. In the NET analyses, where drinking and drug use prevalence rates for the non-smoking partner in smoking-discordant pairs are compared with rates for all non-smoking twins, excessive drinking was 2.6 times more prevalent, and the use of sleeping pills 1.2 times more prevalent, in the former group.

The B Series analyses also indicate that although ratios for concordant smokers versus concordant non-smokers for indices of psychosocial discord were generally well above one, ratios in smoking-discordant pairs were significantly reduced in the case of instability, sleeping difficulties and irregularity of meals in the case of Dz twins, and instability, divorce, change of employer and low physical activity for Mz twins. This means that the non-smoking partner in smoking-discordant pairs was significantly more alike to his smoking co-twin on these variables than were non-smoking concordant twins as compared with smoking concordant twins, or, for that matter, for smokers versus non-smokers in the population at large.

These findings are generally supported in NET analyses. Ratios were significantly elevated for Mz twins for instability, extraversion, divorce, low physical activity and coffee drinking; for Dz pairs, the relevant variables were instability, sleeping difficulties, stress, change of employer and irregularity of meals. These results indicate that the non-smoking partner in smoking-discordant pairs was more alike to his smoking co-twin on these psychosocial variables than concordant non-smoking twins, or indeed non-smokers in the population at large, these effects being more strongly represented in Mz than in Dz pairs.

There is a good deal of evidence to suggest that smokers score higher than non-smokers on aggressiveness (Thomas, 1960, 1973; Smith, 1970). Smith (1970) reports that from 19 studies reviewed, an aggressive personality dimension was stronger in smokers in 27 of the 32 analyses provided. Thomas (1973) has also observed that heavy smokers have higher 'chronic anger' scores, and that smoking prevents an increase in self-rated feelings of aggressiveness observed when non-smokers and deprived smokers perform stressful and monotonous tasks (Heimstra, 1973). Similarly, when smokers are deprived of cigarettes, they not only score higher on an inventory of questions concerning feelings of aggression, but also display more aggression on an 'aggression machine', by which they administer 'shocks' to other people (Schechter & Rand, 1974). This finding was essentially replicated in an analogous experiment which demonstrated that smoking reduced aggression as measured by a reduction in monetary punishments or aversive white noise punishments thought to be (but in reality actually not) delivered to another subject (Cherek, 1981).

These findings are congruent with evidence that nicotine reduces aggressiveness in animals as measured, for example, by predatory biting attack in the cat (Berntson, Beattie & Walker, 1976), post-shock biting attack in the squirrel monkey (Hutchinson & Emley, 1973) and social aggressiveness in rats (Silverman, 1971). There is some evidence that the mechanism of this nicotine-induced reduction in aggressiveness involves the activation of the (inhibitory) part of the mutually inhibitory nicotinic–

Table 11. *Summary of psychosocial variables related to smoking in the new Swedish Twin Registry. B series: Mz and Dz smoker/non-smoker prevalence ratios in smoking-discordant twins, and smoker/non-smoker prevalence ratios in concordant smoker/non-smoker prevalence ratios in concordant twins for comparison on the relevant items. NET (non-exposed twin): ratios of observed/expected prevalence rates amongst the non-smoking partners, grouped by smoking status of co-twin. (Adapted from Cederlof et al., 1977)*

| | B Series[a] | | | NET[b] | | | | | | | | |
| | Con-cordant smokers/ non-smokers in con-cordant non-smokers | Smokers/ non-smokers in discordant groups | | Non-smokers | | Present cigarette smokers | | All present smokers | | Former smokers | |
Variable		Dz	Mz	Dz	Mz	Dz	Mz	Dz	Mz	Dz	Mz
Elementary school only	1.24	1.03	0.96[s]	0.98	1.00	1.04	1.04	1.03	1.04	0.90	0.95
Employed	1.06	1.09	1.10	0.98	1.01	1.07[s]	0.96	1.07[s]	0.97	1.09[s]	1.06
Alcohol drinking[c] (born 1926–58)	1.48	1.22[s]	1.09[s]	0.93	0.93	1.25[s]	1.32[s]	1.23[s]	1.36[s]	1.15[s]	1.45[s]
(born 1901–25)	2.05	1.26[s]	1.22[s]								
Excessive drinking[c] (born 1926–58)	4.49	1.74[s]	1.49[s]	0.66	0.80	2.00[s]	2.81[s]	2.05[s]	3.48[s]	1.19	2.28[s]
(born 1901–25)	6.53	2.08[s]	1.72[s]								
Tonics and vitamins	1.01	0.92	0.94	0.99	1.01	1.00	0.97	0.99	0.96	1.11[s]	1.06
Prescription-free analgesics	1.28	1.04[s]	1.17	0.98	1.00	1.02	0.98	1.01	1.02	0.95	1.16
Sleeping pills	2.34	1.36[s]	1.85	0.84	0.70	1.37[s]	1.42	1.33[s]	1.75[s]	1.02	1.03
Tranquillisers	1.87	1.60	1.77	1.02	0.95	0.99	1.06	1.01	1.16	1.02	0.94
	2.21	1.19[s]	0.98[s]								

sleeping difficulties	1.77	1.39[s]	1.29	0.96	0.98	1.15[s]	1.39	1.12[s]	1.24	0.92
Stress	1.36	1.19	1.02	0.93	0.91	1.11	1.25	1.15[s]	1.19	1.04
Divorced	2.70	1.85	1.25[s]	0.87	0.79	1.11	2.03[s]	1.18	1.82[s]	0.91
Change of employer ≥ 3 times	1.40	1.15	0.81[s]	0.91	0.94	1.22[s]	0.99	1.25[s]	1.13	1.13
Low physical activity	1.64	1.57	1.20[s]	1.02	0.90	0.96	1.15	1.04	1.23[s]	0.79
Cooked food ≤ once a day	1.32	0.96[s]	1.17	0.97	1.01	1.18[s]	1.06	1.14[s]	1.03	0.98
Coffee ≥ 5 cups a day	1.75	1.90	1.44	1.01	0.97	0.96	1.01	0.98	1.18[s]	1.08

[a] Based on Tables 6.2B, 6.3B, 6.4B, 6.5B in Cederlof et al. (1977).
[b] Based on Tables 6.8, 6.10, 6.12, 6.14 in Cederlof et al. (1977).
[c] Combined years for 'NET' analysis.
[s] Significant effect.

muscarinic system controlling aggression (Berntson, Beattie & Walker, 1976). However, there are indications that other transmitters, e.g., nor-adrenaline (NA), 5-hydroxytryptamine (5-HT) and *gamma*-aminobutyric acid (GABA), may also be involved (Mandel *et al.*, 1978).

From both these sources, therefore, there seem grounds for suggesting that reduction in aggression in smokers with high chronic anger scores may be an important motivational factor for smoking. In this respect, nicotine may be acting similarly to other tranquillisers (Hutchinson & Emley, 1973).

With younger age groups also, a persistent theme is one of a relationship between smoking and deviancy or delinquency. For example, Clarke, Eyles & Evans (1972) report higher smoking rates amongst delinquent boys at all age levels. Backhouse & James (1969) and Brill, Crumpton & Grayson (1971) report significant correlations between smoking and drinking, and Backhouse & James (1969) report correlations between these and drug-taking. Bynner (1969) reports that young smokers show greater anticipation of, and higher desire for, adulthood than their non-smoking counterparts, and that they tend to be more delinquent and rebellious to authority at home and at school, although there was no evidence of greater feelings of inferiority, frustration or tension in this study. Bewley, Day & Ide (1974) suggest that these differences are linked with early recruitment rather than with smoking persistence since such differences are not found among adult smokers.

Although it is difficult to define a concept of delinquency as such, it seems reasonable, for present purposes, to regard it simply as formal social rule-breaking deviance (see Foggitt, 1974), of which smoking in adolescents could be an instance. Foggitt (1974) reports that the best predictor of rule-breaking deviance is the level of social dysfunction, as assessed by Robins' (1966) criteria, a listing of pathological social behaviours character-istic of the clinically diagnosed 'psychopath'.

At first glance, the fact that smokers are more 'antisocial' than non-smokers seems at variance with the well-established observation that smokers are more extraverted than non-smokers (McArthur *et al.*, 1958; Matarazzo & Saslow, 1960; Eysenck, 1963, 1973; Thomas, Fargo & Enslein, 1970). Thomas (1973), in attempting to resolve this impasse, suggests that these two findings, taken together, imply that smokers interact with others more readily than do non-smokers, but that in so doing they often encounter frustrations that arouse feelings of anger and rebelliousness. In this setting, smokers use cigarettes as a means of alleviating distress. Thus, according to Thomas, adolescents who are outgoing and desire social acceptance are often aware of anxiety and anger in situations of stress, and heavy smoking stems in part from the inner need to cope with negative affect. As these adolescents are drawn into situations and gain acceptance, their coffee and alcohol consumption tend to rise. This latter observation derives some support from McKennell's (1970) report (that a 'social smoking' factor loads items such as 'smokes when drinking tea or coffee', 'smokes when drinking alcohol', 'smokes in company' and 'smokes at a party'), which suggests the strong social implications of smoking and drinking coffee and alcohol.

A more persuasive explanation, however, derives from Eysenck's (1957) proposal that in high E/high N individuals, existing antisocial tendencies, which are due to lack of social–moral control as a consequence of poor early conditioning, are multiplied by N to produce psychopathic behaviour. Thus, it is the extreme neurotic extravert who is antisocial, by comparison with the socially mobile, stable, moderately extraverted individual. Both types smoke and use other psychoactive drugs. However, consumption rates, and motivations underlying these behaviours, will differ. As far as the stable extravert is concerned, we obviously need to look for other than antisocial factors in his psychological and/or biological makeup which would account for his greater consumption of cigarettes, coffee and alcohol. This leads on to a consideration of theories which are more properly described as psychobiological.

Central nervous system theories

The best examples of CNS theories of smoking are the pharmacological or 'drug' models, which are usually subsumed under the rubric 'addiction'.

Simple addiction models

The notion that the rate of cigarette consumption is maintained by nicotine addiction enjoys a wide acceptance (Frith, 1971 a; Schachter, 1975, 1978). Physiological addiction models, such as those proposed by Schachter (1978), postulate that certain CNS receptors, probably located in the medial forebrain bundle, become addicted to nicotine, i.e., they signal punishment when the nicotine level at these sites falls below a critical level. From this point of view, we might regard the desire to smoke as a consequence of nicotine 'hunger' in the classical drive sense, the purpose of smoking being to maintain nicotine homeostasis, just as regular heroin injections maintain opiate homeostasis at the CNS opiate receptors. The two main lines of evidence supporting an addiction model are 'withdrawal effects' following cessation of smoking and variations in smoking rate following experimental manipulation of nicotine levels in the smoker.

The notion that drug use is maintained by relief of withdrawal symptoms has considerable historical appeal. For example, we can cite De Quincey (1821, p. 114). 'The reader is aware that opium had long ceased to found its empire on spells of pleasure: it was solely by the tortures connected with the attempt to abdure it that it kept its hold'. Despite the fact that behavioural effects are commonly reported to follow the cessation of smoking, especially in heavy smokers (Ryan, 1973; Schachter *et al.*, 1977), in addition to psychophysiological effects (Knapp, Bliss & Wells, 1963; Ulett & Itil, 1969; Hall, Rappaport, Hopkins & Griffin, 1973; Knott & Venables, 1977), there is no evidence of withdrawal effects that are in any way comparable with those reported by subjects going 'cold turkey' in heroin addiction, or by alcoholics 'drying out' (see Table 12 for a review of such studies). From an addiction viewpoint, it is also difficult to account for the fact that some smokers can abstain for a day or more with little consciously experienced craving.

Even if significant withdrawal effects were to be demonstrated, however, it is debatable whether this would constitute direct support for an addiction hypothesis as far as the total population of smokers is concerned. While such an effect may be a 'rebound' phenomenon, suggesting that nicotine tolerance has occurred, particularly in long-term, heavy smokers, it is equally plausible that these effects may signal a return by some subjects to a more 'normal' constitutional level of functioning.

This possibility is strongly suggested by Brown's (1973) data, which compare the EEG characteristics of groups of heavy and light smokers, ex-smokers and non-smokers, and show that smokers and ex-smokers share some EEG characteristics not seen in non-smokers. Indeed, those findings may be cited as indirect evidence for an arousal modulation theory of smoking maintenance.

Longitudinal studies indicate that the teenager who eventually becomes a smoker is more emotionally labile than the future non-smoker (Cherry & Kiernan, 1978), and one can suggest that for these individuals cigarette smoking may have value as a 'psychological tool' in order to regulate mood. This view of smoker/non-smoker differences gains further credence in the light of evidence for a fair degree of genetic predisposition for smoking and other psychoactive drug use such as alcohol and coffee consumption (Strickenberger, 1968; also see this chapter: A genetic basis for smoking).

More convincing empirical support comes from studies in which nicotine levels in the smoker are artificially manipulated, and the effects on smoking rate assessed. The studies may be roughly divided into those concerned with the internal manipulation of nicotine delivery and those where the manipulation was done externally (see Tables 13 and 14).

The effects of manipulating nicotine levels on smoking behaviour. Direct pharmacological control of the nicotine supply to postulated mid-brain receptors has been obtained by intravenous or oral administration of nicotine or lobeline (Lucchesi, Schuster & Emley, 1967), or of nicotine receptor antagonists such as mecamylamine, which readily pass the blood–brain barrier (Stolerman, Goldfarb, Fink & Jarvik, 1973*b*), or through varying nicotine excretion rates by manipulating urinary pH (Schachter *et al.*, 1977). These studies claim to demonstrate that the smoker will adjust his smoking rate in the appropriate direction.

Perhaps the most interesting theory is that of Schachter (1975). He suggests that the control mechanism involved is the urinary pH level, which determines the rate of nicotine excretion by the kidneys. The crux of his argument is as follows. Nicotine is excreted more rapidly by the kidneys when the urine is acid since reabsorption of nicotine from the urine is then greatly reduced (see Chapter 3: Pharmacokinetics). If we assume that the nicotine receptors maintain a standard level of demand, then greater ingestion of nicotine is required under acid conditions, e.g., when the subject is stressed, and consequently the smoking rate will increase. Conversely, when the urine is alkaline, e.g., when the subject is relaxed, he will tend to smoke less.

Thus, Schachter (1975, 1978) reports that ingestion of sodium bicarbonate, which raises the urinary pH level, leads to decreased rates of smoking, and that ingestion of ammonium chloride or vitamin C tablets, which lowers the pH level, is followed by an increased desire to smoke. He claims to have shown, therefore, that both the nicotine level in the CNS and the rate of nicotine elimination are the critical factors maintaining cigarette smoking.

However, some of Schachter's interpretation of his results, and the derived theory, are not wholly convincing. Since it is generally agreed that about 80% of active nicotine is degraded into inactive metabolites in the liver (Goodman & Gilman, 1971), the urinary secretion rate can, at best, affect only 20% of active nicotine, a point also reinforced by the observations of Feyerabend & Russell (1978), which call into question the practical significance of this proposed mechanism (see Chapter 3: Pharmacokinetics).

Generally speaking, observed changes in smoking rates following such pharmacological interventions have been relatively small. A number of factors, however, could have depreciated the effects of treatment. For example, after oral ingestion of nicotine or lobeline, since there is considerable degradation of nicotine by the liver before the active molecule can reach the brain, nicotine dosage levels intended to mimic smoking may

Table 12. *Studies on the psychological and psychophysiological effects of smoking deprivation*

Author(s)	Country	Total no. of subjects	Breakdown of subjects[a]	Age	Sex	No. of cigarettes per day	Period of deprivation
Psychological studies							
1 Heimstra (1973)	USA	496	181 (NS) 166 (NDS) 149 (DS)	'Students'	M+F	> 20	16 min–6 h
2 Mausner (1970)	USA	111	64 (DS) 47 (NDS)	30–69	–	≈ 36	1–6 months
3 Pertschuk, Pomerleau, Adkins & Hirsh (1979)	USA	21	16 (DS) OC[b]	40±12.5	M+F	34.7±11.6	4 months
4 Ryan (1973)	USA	1385	941 (NS) 47 (DS @ 7 months)	> 14	M+F	–	1–7 months
5 Schechter & Rand (1974)	Australia	26	14 (NS) 12 (DS) OC[b]	18–24	M+F	'Habitual'	> 1½ h
6 Shiffman (1979)	USA	40	40 (DS) OC[b]	–	–	Mean ≈ 20 light and heavy	13 days
Psychophysiological studies							
7 Ek et al. (1977)	Sweden (Army)	129	19 (NS) 85 (NDS) 25 (DS)	20–24	M	5–15	4½ h
8 Frankenhaeuser, Myrsten, Post & Johansson (1971)	Sweden	12	6 (NDS) 6 (DS)	20–26	M	5–15	≈ 2 h
9 Friedman, Goldberg, Horvarth & Meares (1974a)	Australia	10	10 (DS) OC[b]	20–25	M	> 20	12 h
10 Hall et al. (1973)	USA	9	9 (DS) OC[b]	23–50	M+F	15–60	36 h
	USA	7	7 (DS)	–		40–60	5 days

				21 (NDS) 22 (DS)				3 days–1 week
13	Knott & Venables (1977)	England	40	10 (NS) 13 (NDS) 17 (DS)	19–23	M	≈ 20	13–15 h
14	Knott & Venables (1978)	England	30	10 (NS) 10 (NDS) 10 (DS)	20–30	M	> 10 mean = 18.3	15–18 h
15	Murphree & Schultz (1968)	USA	11	11 (DS) OC[b]	–	–	'moderate to heavy'	6 h
16	Myrsten, Post, Frankenhaeuser & Johansson (1972)	Sweden	6	6 (DS) OC[b]	20–26	M	10–15	2 h
17	Myrsten, Elgerot & Edgren (1977)	Sweden	27	14 (NDS) 13 (DS) OC[b]	21–55	M+F	21	5 days
18	Nesbitt (1973)	USA	60	30 (NS) 30 (DS) OC[b]	18–26	M	> 20	15 min
19	Schachter et al. (Exp. 1 & 5) (1977)	USA	59	59 (DS) OC[b]	20–52	M+F	> 10	–
20	Ulett & Itil (1969)	USA	8	8 (DS) OC[b]	16–21	M	> 20	24 h
21	Vogel, Broverman & Klaiber (1977)	USA	104	59 (NS) 45 (DS) OC[b]	18–55	M+F	10–40	> 3 h

[a] NS, non-smokers; NDS, non-deprived smokers; DS, deprived smokers; OC, own control.
[b] Deprived smokers were also observed when not deprived of smoking.

Table 12. (*cont.*)

	Technique	Results	Limitations/comments
1	Groups of students tested on driving simulator, reaction time, visual detection, tracking and during stressful film. Mood ratings (MACL)	Anxiety, aggression, fatigue, etc. increased during deprivation	—
2	Interview and mood self-report of patients with respiratory symptoms quitting smoking	Increased nervousness, irritability, weight gain commonly reported even after 6 months	Self-selection
3	Group subjects attending smoking clinic. Symptoms and subjective mood ratings	Little evidence for significant mood changes. Evidence for a significant weight increase although this also occurred for the subjects who failed to quit smoking	Self-selection
4	Public health campaign, mailed questionnaires	Increased irritability, depression, bad temper, laziness, mannerisms, appetite and weight gain both in short-term and for long-term (more than 7 months)	High drop-out rate
5	Aggression machine to give 'shocks', self-report aggression/hostility inventory	Increase in aggression for deprived smokers	Short period of deprivation
6	Daily mood and physical symptoms ratings on subjects quitting smoking	Both physical and mood symptoms (e.g. nervousness, drowsiness, etc.) rapidly decrease after 4 days but may start to reappear after 13 days	—
7	High stress versus low stress films, paced smoking, venous blood samples, urine analysis, subjective mood ratings	Some evidence for high adrenaline excretion in abstainers during stress. Little evidence for NDS versus NS differences. Complicated results on other physiological and mood indices	Short period of deprivation
8	Reaction time, pulse rate, urinary catecholamine analysis, subjective mood ratings	Deprivation versus smoking, increased reaction time, reduced adrenaline excretion and pulse rate, no significant effects on mood	Short period of deprivation. Small n
9	Visual and auditory evoked potentials, mood checklist	Visual evoked potentials decreased, auditory evoked potentials increased, anxiety increased during deprivation. Smoking reverses these effects	—
10	Visual evoked potentials, battery of subjective mood rating scales	Deprivation causes reduction in evoked potentials especially to weak stimuli: no significant effect on mood ratings	—
11	Sleep monitoring for 9–11 nights, EEG, EOG, EMG,	Deprivation causes a moderate increase in the amount of	Small n of heavy smokers

	Measures	Findings	Comments
13	EEG 'alpha' measurement	Deprivation causes lower dominant EEG alpha frequencies. Smoking reverses this and brings smokers back to non-smoker EEG frequencies	—
14	Visual evoked potentials	Hypersensitivity shown by deprived smokers: faster latency, larger amplitudes, especially to low intensity flash stimuli	—
15	EEG, cardiovascular and subjective mood (IPAT) measured	Deprivation causes reduction in pulse rate and blood pressure. EEG 'change' caused by resumption of smoking. No anxiety change	Very short report
16	Cardiovascular, urinary catecholamines, hand steadiness, reaction time, subjective mood rating measures	Deprivation causes decreased pulse rate and blood pressure, improved hand steadiness, increased reaction time and boredom, irritability and distractability. Smoking reverses this	Small n. Short period of deprivation
17	Cardiovascular, skin temperature, urinary analyses; hand steadiness, cognitive performance tests; mood questionnaire	Deprivation causes decreased pulse rate and adrenaline, noradrenaline excretion; skin temperature increase, improved hand steadiness, small differences on cognitive tests, increased irritation, sleeping difficulties, anxiety, tension, depression, etc.	—
18	Electric shock endurance, pulse rate and emotionality ratings. Both smokers and non-smokers smoke cigarettes	Endurance of electric shock decreased by deprivation and increased by smoking, in parallel to emotionality. This smoking effect does not occur for non-smokers	Short period of deprivation
19	Deprivation postulated to be induced by low nicotine delivery cigarettes or by urinary pH manipulation. Mood self-report	Some evidence that 'deprived' smokers show increased weight, aggression, tension	Extent of deprivation is uncertain
20	Cardiovascular, EEG, mood ratings	Deprivation causes slower pulse rate, increased systolic blood pressure, increased slow frequency EEG, subjective dysphoria. Reversed by smoking two cigarettes	Small n
21	EEG driving response: photic driving	Deprivation causes increased EEG driving response, smoking reverses these effects towards non-smoker levels	Short period of deprivation

[c] REM sleep, rapid eye movement sleep.

Table 13. *Studies of the effects of nicotine manipulations on smoking behaviour. I: Direct pharmacological manipulations of nicotine*

Author(s)	Country	No. of subjects	Technique	Results	Limitations/comments
Jarvik, Glick & Nakamura (1970)	USA	17	Ingestion of nicotine tartrate capsules (10 mg, 5 per day) versus placebo	8% (approx.) reduction in smoking rate with nicotine capsules versus placebo	It is probable that most of the nicotine was degraded in the liver before reaching general circulation
Johnston (1942)	England	1	Self-injection (s.c.) of 1.3 mg nicotine 3 or 4 times a day	Self-injection of nicotine began to be preferred to cigarette smoking after a course of 80 injections. Feelings of deprivation when this was discontinued	Single-case study
Kozlowski, Jarvik & Gritz (1975)	USA	56	Nicotine 'pre-loads' administered via nicotine cigarette (1.3 mg v. 0.3 mg v. lettuce leaf cigarette, 0 mg) and/or nicotine chewing gum (4 mg v. 1 mg)	High nicotine 'pre-load' via cigarette followed by significantly longer latencies to lighting next cigarette; high nicotine gum 'pre-loads' followed by significantly less puffing on subsequent cigarettes	–
Kumar, Cooke, Lader & Russell (1978)	England	12	Multiple 'bolus' (i.v.) injections of nicotine at rates designed to mimic nicotine absorption during normal smoking: 'shots' of 0 mg (water) v. 0.07 mg nicotine bitartrate in ten 5-s pulses	Puffing rates on cigarettes remained unaffected over the 40-min experimental (injection) periods, although alternatively given nicotine pre-loads via inhalation cigarette smoking postponed and significantly reduced subsequent puffing	Relative failures of i.v. nicotine to suppress smoking may be due to venous dispersion of nicotine, failure to provide the 'correct' dose, or indicate relative

& Emley (1967)			i.v. infusion of nicotine bitartrate (0 mg v. 1 mg v. 2 mg v. 4 mg per h) over 6-h sessions for 15 days. Nicotine dosages designed to provide nicotine at rates equivalent to smoking	Cigarette consumption significantly reduced by 30% (approx.) and residual butt weight increased by 15% (approx.) during the high nicotine versus saline infusion	reinforcing' characteristics of smoking
Russell, Wilson, Feyerabend & Cole (1976)	England	43	Nicotine chewing gum (2 mg, 10 per day) versus placebo gum for 2 days each with ad lib. smoking, followed by 1 week of each gum during an attempt to quit smoking	A small (10% approx.) but significant decrease in smoking rate and COHb with nicotine versus placebo chewing gum during ad lib. smoking. The effect of chewing gum itself versus baseline smoking was much greater than this nicotine effect (30% approx. reduction in cigarette consumption)	Authors suggest that 4-mg strength nicotine chewing gum could give better results
Stolerman, Goldfarb, Fink & Jarvik (1973b)	USA	52	Ingestion of central and peripheral nicotine antagonist (mecamylamine), peripheral antagonist (pentolinium) or placebo	Central but not peripheral nicotine antagonists, versus placebo, significantly increased cigarette smoking and puffing rates by 30% (approx.)	Smoking may increase with mecamylamine to overcome side effects of drug-induced drowsiness, poor concentration, etc.
Schachter et al. (1977)	USA	13	Daily ingestion of acidifying agents designed to decrease urinary pH (Vitamin C, Acidulin v. placebo) and postulated to increase excretion rate of nicotine	Significant increase (approx. 20%) in smoking rates under acidified versus placebo condition. Alkaline agents (such as bicarbonate) produced opposite effect, that of decreasing smoking rate, especially during stress-induced acidification of urine	Nicotine degradation in the liver is more important than excretion. See also Feyerabend & Russell (1978)

have been radically underestimated by experimenters. Again, with regard to cigarette smoking, nicotine may have to arrive at the CNS receptors in a concentrated bolus form (see Appendix), which suggests that the method of pulsed microinjections into the carotid artery to mimic the in vivo effects of cigarette smoking should be used. However, this procedure might be regarded as risky and not ethically justifiable. While Kumar, Cooke, Lader & Russell (1978) report minimal effects on smoking of discrete, rapid, intravenous nicotine injections at a rate designed to mimic in vivo 'boli', this may in part be a function of bolus dispersion due to venous mixing.

The effects of manipulating nicotine delivery of cigarettes. Attempts to vary the smoking rate by manipulating the maximum possible nicotine delivery of a cigarette have produced conflicting results. While Frith (1971*a*) and Schachter (1978) report significant variations in the number of cigarettes smoked under these conditions, Mangan & Golding (1978), and Goldfarb, Jarvik & Glick (1970) report no such relationship. Stepney (1980), in a review of many of the published experiments utilising this technique, suggests that for a 50% decrease in nicotine delivery, on average, an increase in cigarette consumption of only 9% will be observed.

While it is difficult to interpret these data unequivocally, since in most cases taste and draw factors are not well controlled, they are not incompatible with the generally accepted finding that pharmacological maintenance of nicotine homeostatis is of doubtful value in smoking modification programmes. The latter suggests that nicotine homeostasis is not the only, or possibly even the critical, factor involved in smoking maintenance.

There is, however, some relevant evidence concerning smoking style. It has been reported that the puffing rate increases as the nicotine delivery of the cigarettes is reduced (Ashton & Watson, 1970; Frith, 1971*a*) (see Table 14). It may be that other aspects of smoking style, e.g., puff strength, are also critical in determining the amount of nicotine extracted from a cigarette. Some such explanation must be advanced to account for the recent observation of Ashton, Stepney & Thompson (1979) which is detailed in Table 14. The so-called 'self-titration' for nicotine in the face of experimental variations in cigarette nicotine delivery may be extremely efficient. Thus the use of filters to produce large variations in tar/nicotine delivery from cigarettes resulted in subjects showing only small differences on a number of physiological variables (Golding, 1980). Upon smoking the second pair of high- versus low-nicotine delivery cigarettes, these small differences were reduced still further, the major effect being that of tachyphylaxis, i.e., reduced physiological effect from smoking the second cigarette. Analysis of smoking style and butts indicated that the crucial compensating variables were puff strength and/or duration rather than increased puffing rates or depth of smoke inhalation with the low-delivery cigarettes (Golding, 1980) (see Table 14 for a review).

Another factor of general relevance in studies involving manipulation of nicotine delivery is that smoking quickly acquires secondary reinforcing properties. Nicotine is a potent drug; the latency between the conditioned stimulus (CS) (lighting up, lip contact, taste, inhalation) and the unconditioned stimulus (US) (arrival of nicotine at the appropriate CNS receptors) is 8–10 s, and the smoker has previously experienced many thousands of CS/US pairings. Such conditions are known to favour the formation of classically conditioned responses. Secondary reinforcement undoubtedly operates as a confounding variable when we attempt to measure the effects of manipulation of nicotine on smoking rates.

As for the presumed nature of the target receptors in the CNS, there is, of course, the possibility that nicotine may have direct 'pleasure-centre' stimulating properties, which is analogous to brain electrical self-stimulation reward. Some data suggest that specific nicotinic system stimulants (e.g., nicotine) facilitate self-stimulation in rats, whereas muscarinic stimulants such as arecoline decrease self-stimulation rates (Newman, 1972). Critical data are lacking, as is the case for the pharmacological mechanism for 'nicotine addiction' postulated by Jaffe & Kanzler (1979). They suggest that nicotine from cigarette smoking may cause the release of 'internal opiates' in addition to the well-known action of nicotine in causing adrenocorticotrophin release (Jaffe & Kanzler, 1979). This speculation is based upon the observation that *beta*-endorphin and adrenocorticotrophin are secreted concomitantly in the pituitary gland. The analogy between opiate addiction and 'addiction' to nicotine may thus be closer than previously thought (see also Chapter 3: Specific reinforcing mechanisms, The brain).

Opponent-process theory

Opponent-process theory (Solomon, 1977; Surgeon General, 1979, Ch. 16, p. 9) attempts to combine various behavioural and physiological observations concerning smoking, and to relate these in a dynamic time-bound fashion to conditioning theory. Briefly, the theory states that:
  (i) the initial effects of smoking are pleasurable (A process), but this is followed by a more sustained, dysphoric, unpleasant period (B process);
  (ii) hedonic tone is determined by the algebraic summation of the pleasurable A state and the dysphoric B state at any given point in time;

Table 14. *Studies of the effects of nicotine manipulations on smoking behaviour. II: Manipulation of standard nicotine delivery of cigarette[a]*

Author(s)	Country	No. of subjects	Technique	Results	Limitations/comments[b]
Ando & Yanagita (1981)	Japan	14	1.9-mg, 0.3-mg and 0-mg (special nicotine-free tobacco from grafts) nicotine delivery cigarettes 'smoked' by monkeys	Low nicotine and nicotine-free cigarettes led to decreased 'smoking' behaviour.	Only 2 monkeys engaged in 'voluntary' smoking
Ashton & Watson (1970)	England	36	2.1-mg and 1.0-mg nicotine delivery cigarette during driving simulator task and resting	Significantly more puffing on the low-nicotine cigarette	–
Ashton, Stepney & Thompson (1979)	England	12	11-week study of smoking 1.84-mg, 1.4-mg and 0.6-mg nicotine delivery cigarettes	Slight changes in smoking and puffing rates. However, plasma and urine nicotine and COHb analyses indicated that smokers were maintaining their COHb and nicotine within a range of ±10% (approx.) in the face of expected experimental variations of +40%	–

Reference	Country	N	Method	Findings	Comments
			nicotine delivery smoked over 3 days. Puff pressure/volume observed on last cigarettes smoked of each type	for high-nicotine cigarettes. Puff pressure and volume were maximum for middle-nicotine cigarettes	
Goldfarb, Gritz, Jarvik & Stolerman (1976)	USA	35	Tar and nicotine deliveries varied independently: total range for all types of cigarettes, smoked over 3-week period, was tar, 0.29–19.0 mg, and nicotine, 0.26–1.4 mg	Urine nicotine analyses indicated compensation for variation in nicotine but not tar deliveries. Rated 'strength' of cigarette related to nicotine but not tar. No significant change in number of cigarettes smoked as a function of variation in delivery	Demonstrates importance of nicotine as opposed to tar. Self-titration probably occurs through 'smoking-style' rather than gross cigarette consumption
Goldfarb, Jarvik & Glick (1970)	USA	15	Lettuce cigarettes of 0 mg, and with added nicotine, 1.26 mg or 2.25 mg, smoked for 1 week each	No evidence for changes in consumption with variation in nicotine	Taste/smell of lettuce cigarettes may have been unpleasant
Golding (1980)	England	10	Ventilated holder used to vary nicotine delivery from 0.36 mg to 1.8 mg. Two cigarettes of each type per subject	Subjects appeared to self-titrate by taking more puffs and inhaling more deeply on the low-delivery cigarettes. However, increased puff pressure was probably the most critical variable. SCL, EEG, ECG responses to both cigarettes very similar	Demonstrates how rapidly 'self-titration' can occur

Table 14. (*cont.*)

Author(s)	Country	No. of subjects	Technique	Results	Limitations/comments
Herning, Jones, Bachman & Mines (1981)	USA	24	Single cigarettes of 0.4 mg, 1.2 mg, 2.5 mg nicotine delivery smoked after 10 h of deprivation	Puffing rate, puff number and puff duration did not significantly differ between cigarettes. However, puff volume significantly increased for the low nicotine cigarette. Butt analysis, exhaled CO and heart rate rise indicated that self-titration occurred but was not complete for the low-nicotine cigarettes	Demonstrates how rapidly 'self-titration' can occur
Schulz & Seehofer (1978)	Germany	Large	Thousands of different cigarette butts collected from ash-trays, litter bins, etc., and analysed for nicotine. These compared to same brand under standard machine smoking	Evidence for significant self-titration. Emphasises both between-brand variations, and between- and within-subject variations	
Stepney (1980)	England	Total 427	Review of 16 published experiments (1945–78), ⌐⌐⌐⌐ ⌐⌐⌐⌐⌐⌐⌐ ⌐⌐⌐ ⌐⌐⌐⌐	A significantly positive relationship was found ⌐⌐⌐⌐⌐⌐⌐ ⌐⌐⌐⌐⌐⌐⌐⌐ ⌐⌐	Changes in gross cigarette consumption are not the most important variable

Study	Country	N	Description	Results	Conclusion
			relationship between variation of cigarette consumption and variation in nicotine delivery of cigarettes used	delivery (r = +0.59,[c] for 50% reduction in nicotine, cigarette consumption rose by only 10%)	Self-titration probably occurs by increased inhalation or increased puffing rate/puff intensity
Sutton, Russell, Feyerabend & Saloojee (1978)	England	10	Ventilated holders used to produce predicted reductions in nicotine delivery of (0%), 25%, 58%, switching between them over a 2-week period	Plasma nicotine and COHb measures indicated that a partially successful self-titration had occurred. No significant variation in numbers of cigarettes smoked	
Turner, Sillett & Ball (1974)	England	10	Cigarettes of < 0.3 mg, 0.8 mg and 1.4 mg nicotine delivery smoked over three 1-week periods	No significant variation in cigarette consumption. Butt length, butt nicotine and COHb indicated that partially successful self-titration had occurred, probably by alterations in puffing rate/intensity and inhalation	—

[a] Where cigarette nicotine deliveries are given these refer to standard machine-smoked deliveries; actual delivery for human smokers may of course be very different from this: hence the concept of 'self-titration' for nicotine.
[b] The best studies are those which have some indication of nicotine *absorption* by the subject, e.g., plasma nicotine, urinary nicotine/metabolites or (indirect) COHb, exhaled CO or some reliable physiological effect of nicotine, e.g., heart rate elevation.
[c] r is the correlation coefficient.

(iii) stimuli associated with a given state can elicit this state as a conditioned response after repeated pairings.

As regards the establishment of smoking, while there may be some unpleasant effects (such as coughing and nausea) on the first few occasions, these are offset by the pleasurable effects of nicotine, or by social reinforcers such as peer acceptance. As smoking becomes more habitual, however, the relief of withdrawal symptoms, as opposed to the directly pleasurable effects, begins to predominate.

Over a sufficient number of occasions, the pleasurable A state becomes more transient and the B state assumes greater significance. Consequently, the smoker gradually slips into addiction. However, if a sufficient period of abstinence elapses, the B process weakens through disuse and the A process recovers. Subsequent exposure to smoking restores the pleasurable A state at levels approximating those observable from the outset. This presumably accounts for the rapidity with which the ex-smoker can resume the habit.

Elaboration of the theory borrows heavily from operant and classical (Pavlovian) conditioning theory. Stimuli associated with the A state (e.g. the sighting of matches or a packet of cigarettes) become conditioned reinforcers (CS_As) as do stimuli associated with the B state (CS_Bs) (empty cigarette packets, no shops, 'no-smoking' signs, etc.). It is suggested that CS_As may promote smoking by eliciting a transient A state and that this is inevitably followed by elicitation of a more extended, conditioned B state.

There is as yet little formal supportive evidence for this theory, although there are some data concerning opiate addiction (O'Brien *et al.*, 1977), for which a similar theory has been postulated. Further evidence and theorising of relevance is presented by Siegel (1978), who suggests that at least some kinds of drug tolerance can be viewed as contra-adaptations, serving to protect the organism by reacting in a direction opposite to the normal drug effect.

Psychobiological theories
Orality/psychoanalytic theories
It is reported that Freud smoked up to 20 cigars a day, and, at times, was much concerned about the effects on his health. In 1894, when he was 38, he temporarily gave up smoking, but is reported to have been irritable and depressed when so deprived (Simeon & Ariel, 1978). Presumably his apparent inability to control the habit stimulated his interest in the dynamics underlying smoking, which is shown in some of his early works. We quote from *Infantile Sexuality: Auto-Eroticism* (Freud,

1901, p. 182): 'It is not every child who sucks in this way. It may be assumed that those children do so in whom there is a constitutional intensification of the erotogenic significance of the labial region. If that significance persists, these same children, when they are grown up, will become epicures in kissing, will be inclined to perverse kissing, or, if males, will have a powerful motive for drinking and smoking.' Note that by '...sucks in this way.', Freud means here sucking purely for the pleasure of stimulating the mucous membranes of the mouth and that it thus acquires a sexual, as opposed to merely a feeding, motive. It is perhaps ironic that Freud himself died of cancer of the jaw.

This is the starting-point for orality models of smoking behaviour, which have burgeoned over the past fifty years or so. These range from rather simple models based on phallic analogies with the actual shape of the cigar/cigarette to the much more general 'oral frustration' theory.

As recently described by Izard (1978), 'oral frustration' may be the source of behaviours in which anxiety, depression and even aggression predominate. If a lack of maternal affection, or hardness or coolness is present in the mother, then the child is likely to become a heavy and neurotic smoker, who, compared with the non-smoker, will demonstrate rebellion, impetuosity, 'looking for dangerous situations' and disdain for authority. This view has some congruence with one description of the smoker's personality described in the literature, namely, that of the risk-taking, aggressive, extraverted person (see this Chapter: personality variables, behavioural traits and characteristics). From an aetiological point of view, this also lines up with evidence, which we shall report later (in Chapter 4: Recruitment to Smoking) concerning the role of family dynamics and relationships, and delinquency/deviance in early smoking recruitment.

A somewhat less robust hypothesis is that 'nipple deprivation' in infancy is at the root of smoking. Here, however, the evidence is equivocal. Although relationships between early weaning, breast versus bottle feeding and thumbsucking have been demonstrated, no clear relationship has been reported with subsequent smoking (Salber, 1964). Of course, this is not to deny that deprivation of maternal warmth and love, perhaps as a consequence of too early weaning, may predispose a child to smoke. There is evidence from smoking/personality studies that insecurity and anxiety are in fact related to smoking. Data reported by Harlow & Harlow (1962) concerning maternal deprivation in young monkeys strongly suggest that warmth and tactile experience, i.e., 'contact comfort', are more crucial early determinants of emotional development than the supply of milk via the nipple.

Finally, one prediction we might make from orality theory is that smokers can be expected to indulge in many other types of 'oral' behaviours. There is some evidence, superficially, to support this. Although Smith (1970), in his review, found no evidence of such relationships, later studies (Cederlof *et al.*, 1977; adolescent study reported in Chapter 4: Recruitment to smoking) have thrown up impressive evidence that smokers drink more tea, coffee, and alcohol than do non-smokers. However, this finding lends itself to a different interpretation if we regard smoking as a marker for multiple drug use rather than as oral behaviour *per se*. Smokers tend to take more tranquilliser pills and proprietary medicines, as well as tea, coffee and alcohol (Cederlof *et al.*, 1977). The 'orality' component of pill-taking is obviously minimal. Similarly, smokers do not consume more milk and soft drinks (Straits & Sechrest, 1963; Larson & Silvette, 1968), as might be expected on the basis of an oral indulgence hypothesis.

In summary, however useful 'orality' theories might be in terms of theoretical starting-point and richness of concepts, in hard-nosed scientific terms these have tended to suffer the same fate as the better-known analytic theory of mental illness. They are difficult to test, and even where this has been possible, they have failed to survive strict experimental scrutiny.

Arousal modulation theory

What has sometimes been described as the hedonic theory of arousal postulates

(i) a homeostatic principle of an individually-specific optimal level of stimulation or arousal, a concept variously described in the literature as 'pacer stimulus' (Dember & Earl, 1957), 'optimal flux or arousal potential' (Berlyne, 1960);

(ii) a 'hedonic tone' concept, which can be traced to Wundt (1874) but is most explicitly stated by Berlyne (1971), that increase in arousal from low levels, and decrease in arousal from unpleasantly high levels, 'low' and 'high' being relative to the (assumed) optimal level, are seen as reinforcing events.

This is the rationale of the arousal modulation theory of smoking, which suggests that smoking is an activity which has the function of controlling arousal, i.e., the smoker smokes to increase arousal when bored or fatigued, and to reduce arousal when tense. When the smoker is neither under- nor over-aroused, smoking continues partly through habit and partly because it has become a positive reinforcer. On a somewhat broader scale, we might expect individuals who are typically under- or over-aroused, the latter possibly, though not necessarily, testing out as high on neuroticism (N), to use any readily available stimulant or depressant to maintain a homeostatic arousal level.

Some support for the 'low arousal leading to stimulation-seeking' argument comes from studies investigating behavioural correlates of the personality trait or motive of arousal seeking. As we have previously noted, Eysenck (1967) reports a correlation between smoking and extraversion, the extravert, because of high impulsivity and low sensitivity, being regarded as a stimulation-seeker. However, stimulation-seeking is now thought to be characteristic of the high psychoticism (P) scorer, P having some impulsivity content. Eysenck & Eysenck (1975) report that high P scorers are more likely to be drug addicted and alcoholic. Zuckerman, Neary & Brustman (1970) postulate a sensation-seeking motive, which is claimed to increase with age until adolescence and to be related to the impulsive form of extraversion. They report significantly higher scores on their sensation-seeking scale (SSS) from both male and female smokers than from non-smokers, with females significantly higher on 'Experience-seeking' and 'Disinhibition' factors, and males higher on the 'Thrill and adventure-seeking' factors. They also report that male and female smokers score higher on the 'Boredom susceptibility' factor, which fits well with the arousal modulation theory of smoking. Brown, Ruder, Ruder & Young (1974) report a significant correlation between the Change Seeker Index, a related measure, and cigarette smoking. Zuckerman *et al.* (1972) also report some significant correlations between SSS scores, primarily for the 'Disinhibition' factor, and alcohol use. This is of particular interest in view of the reported relationship between smoking and alcohol use. It is also noteworthy that scores for P and SSS intercorrelate positively, and that scores for both scales correlate positively with smoking, drinking and drug-taking (Zuckerman, 1979; Eysenck, 1980; Golding *et al.*, 1983).

These data suggest that the 'arousal seeker', i.e., the person for whom the environment does not normally offer a high enough level of stimulation, tends to produce 'highs' in a variety of ways: by maximising existing sources of stimulation, and by smoking, drinking and drug use, for example. It is equally plausible that such agents can also be instrumental in reducing levels of aversive arousal. Nicotine clearly has both a stimulant and a depressant effect on animal brains depending on dosage (Paton & Perry, 1953; Armitage, Hall & Sellers, 1969). Data from human EEG studies generally support the view that nicotine and smoking have stimulant effects (e.g. Philips, 1971) but there is some recent evidence for dose-related biphasic stimulant and depressant effects of nicotine on the contingent negative variation (CNV) (an EEG measure of cortical arousal) (see Appendix) (Ashton *et al.*, 1978), and also for personality-related biphasic stimulant and depressant effects (O'Connor, 1980). Also of relevance here is the observation that smokers can in fact use cigarettes to relax themselves under conditions of experimental stress, and, conversely, stimulate themselves under conditions of boredom or mild sensory deprivation (Mangan & Golding, 1978; Golding & Mangan, 1982a).

Nicotine addiction theorists, however, regard these postulated beneficial effects (of relaxation or stimulation) as a subjective rationalisation for the feeling of relief produced by the arrival of nicotine at depleted CNS sites. Thus, in learning theory terms, nicotine can be regarded as producing reward either more or less directly (arousal modulation) or by avoiding punishment (addiction). Since omission of punishment is regarded by some theorists (e.g., Gray, 1971) as equivalent to reward, the only way to resolve the relative contribution of beneficial arousal effects, compared with avoidance of aversive withdrawal effects, on smoking maintenance is to compare the effects of smoking on naive smokers, ex-smokers and current smokers. Critical studies on this issue, however, are lacking.

In addition to maintenance of the optimal arousal level, and perhaps as a consequence of this, nicotine itself and cigarette smoking facilitate performance in a number of tasks: vigilance (Frankenhaeuser *et al.*, 1971), and acquisition and retention in both animals (Garg, 1969) and humans (Andersson, 1975). The precise mechanisms involved are unknown (see Chapter 4: Effects of nicotine and tobacco smoking on performance). It may be that the effect can be accounted for simply in terms of increased arousal leading to narrowing of the attentional focus (Wachtel, 1967), with consequent improvement in performance. Additionally, cigarette smoking may be improving performance by bringing the smoker to the optimal part of the 'inverted-U curve' (see Appendix) relating cortical efficiency to arousal. Whatever the case, it seems obvious that an arousal modulation theory of smoking maintenance needs to be broadened to accommodate such effects on behaviour, with a consequent adaptive outcome.

Overall, the data indicate that smokers, relative to non-smokers, show more labile arousal levels, a suggestion reinforced by the recent observation that smokers are less able than non-smokers to control their EEG alpha in a bio-feedback experiment (De Good & Valle, 1978). Smoking could be an activity contributing to the maintenance of a 'steady state' which at times requires an increase, and at other times a decrease, in external stimulation. Reduction in levels of aggression and anxiety on the one hand, and release from boredom on the other, may be critical mood controls in the life space of the smoker.

Social learning theories

Social learning theories of smoking, which have emerged from the application of behaviour modification techniques (Pomerleau, 1980; Surgeon General, 1979, Ch. 16, p. 5) suggest that the habit is initially acquired under conditions of social reinforcement such as peer pressure. While the initial response to tobacco smoke may be aversive, habituation or tolerance of such aversion occurs, after sufficient practice, and this allows the behaviour to produce sufficient positive reinforcement in its own right to enable it to be sustained in the absence of social reinforcement, i.e., to be functionally autonomous. With continued smoking, discrimination learning occurs concerning situations in which smoking is socially punished and those in which it is ignored or favourably received. These circumstances begin to control smoking. Some stimuli or situations which are associated with smoking, e.g., cigarette packs, may also begin to serve as conditioned stimuli (CSs) which elicit covert responses (e.g., physiological discomfort, perceived as craving) and these, in turn, increase the likelihood of smoking. Eventually, smoking becomes ritualised and incorporated into many everyday activities and situations. Thus, for successful behaviour modification treatment of smoking, it is necessary to extinguish a wide range of conditioned stimuli, secondary reinforcers and discriminative stimuli which have become incorporated into the habit as a consequence of stimulus generalisation. Stimuli which trigger the desire to smoke must be eliminated in a wide variety of situations, e.g., when the smoker is alone, or at work, or drinking with friends, or has just finished a meal.

Social learning theories view smoking as a largely learnt behaviour. Although little emphasis is placed on the pharmacological determinants of smoking, the presumed reinforcing nature of nicotine can be accommodated within the social learning theory of smoking in various ways. Firstly, smoking is difficult to modify because of its ability to provide immediate reinforcement. Both the extreme rapidity (less than 10 s from each inhalation for nicotine to reach the brain) and the large number of reinforcements (73000 nicotine shots per year at 1 pack per day and 10 puffs per cigarette) produce a rapidity and frequency of reinforcement unmatched by any other drug, including injected heroin (see Russell, 1976).

Secondly, if the reinforcing nature of nicotine is considered from an addictive point of view, that is, smoking is seen in part as an avoidance/escape response to aversive withdrawal states, then the interesting suggestion is made that stimulus generalisation occurs from the aversive nicotine withdrawal states to other dysphoric states (e.g., anger, tension and boredom). Thus, the common observation that people smoke excessively when tense, bored or angry may be explicable in these terms, i.e., that the smoker responds to internal physiological cues of dysphoria as if they were caused by nicotine withdrawal. If response as well as stimulus generalisation has occurred, then smoking may indeed produce relief, and be regarded as a temporary coping response. We note here Schachter's (1973) rather similar 'attribution' model of the perceived calming effects of nicotine on stress (see Chapter 3: Reinforcing Mechanisms of Nicotine for Smoking).

Thirdly, social learning theories suggest that since the health disadvantages of smoking do not occur until many years later, the ultimate aversive consequences of smoking are delayed. Therefore, they have less influence over ongoing smoking behaviour than do the immediate consequences, which are pleasurable. In this respect, smoking has a much smaller immediate negative reinforcing component than alcohol (which, e.g., produces motor disruption and 'hang-overs'), and many other drugs of dependence.

Smoking typologies

In attempting to evaluate the evidence relating personality and psychosocial variables to smoking, a number of authors have noted the typically small differences found in most studies, approximately one-half a standard deviation on E and N, for example (McCrae, Costa & Bosse, 1978). This may be because the population of smokers is heterogeneous with regard to motives, i.e., the reasons why they smoke, and lumping all smokers together masks real differences between groups (Eysenck, 1982). This has prompted a number of researchers to sub-divide smokers into groups who smoke for different reasons, and to use more specific personality and behavioural criteria in examining such groups. This explains the emergence in the literature of smoking sub-groups, the so-called 'typologies', which sample the whole range of smoking motives proposed by the different theories we have described (see Table 15 for a review).

The best known of these typologies are those described by Tomkins (1968), Horn (1969), McKennell (1970), Russell, Peto & Patel (1974), Myrsten, Andersson, Frankenhaeuser & Elgerot (1975), Knott (1979a) and Crumpacker et al. (1979). There are, of course, common threads running through these different models. Horn (1969) initially noted six smoking factors, or 'motives', leading to types, and McKennell (1970) noted eight. McKennell combined these eight to generate six higher-order factors: inner need/relaxation, inner need/stimulation, habit, social pressure, handling and social pleasure. Perhaps the most reductionist model is that of Russell et al. (1974), who, on the basis of their Smoking Motives Questionnaire, describe the smoking motives psychosocial, indulgent, sensorimotor, stimulation, addictive and automatic, and derive a two-factor solution of pharmacological and non-pharmacological types from them. Crumpacker et al. (1979), using an extended version of this questionnaire, report the same factor structure across age, sex and class, but opt for a three-factor solution of pharmacological (the last three motives named above), non-pharmacological (psychosocial and sensorimotor) and indulgent types. We should note, however, that while identification of 'major' types of this sort may have undoubted value, at times critical information may be lost in the process of reduction. For example, McKennell comments that one of his factors, food substitution smoking, which loads his second-order inner need/relaxation factor, may play a particularly important role when a person is attempting to give up smoking, since nicotine is known to have a hunger suppressive effect.

Arguably, smoking typologies will attract little more than academic interest until systematic relationships can be demonstrated between such typologies and personality dimensions on the one hand, and these typologies and psychophysiological attributes on the other. Simply identifying pharmacological and non-pharmacological smokers on the basis of a fairly broadly-based 'reasons for smoking' questionnaire hardly advances our understanding of smoking dynamics, or suggests techniques which might help smokers to give up. For example, Russell *et al.* (1974) were able to distinguish a group of 'addicted' heavy smokers attending a smoking treatment clinic from a normal sample of smokers by virtue of the former group's higher scores on a 'pharmacological addiction' second-order factor, which is hardly a surprising outcome.

As regards the relationship between smoking typologies and personality/ psychophysiology, attempts have been made to link smoking motives with biological predispositions thought to underlie personality dimensions. The most influential theory of this genre is Eysenck's (1973) hypothesis suggesting that individuals who are under-aroused biologically will seek stimulation, and that those who are biologically over-aroused will avoid or seek to damp down stimulation. From this point of view, smoking can be regarded as a 'psychological tool' for regulating arousal towards a hypothetical optimum. Thus, according to Eysenck, it is the under-aroused extravert who smokes for stimulant effects, and the over-aroused introvert who smokes for tranquillising effects. There is some support for this proposition. Ashton, Millman, Telford & Thompson (1974) and Eysenck & O'Connor (1979) report that the more extraverted smoker obtains stimulant effects, and the more introverted smoker sedative effects from smoking when measured by electro-cortical responses (CNV), a finding which fits well with the concept that the extravert is under-aroused.

Knott (1979a) however, takes a somewhat different line. He identifies the low-arousal smoker who smokes when bored, and the high-arousal smoker who smokes when anxious or stressed, an observation which is directly supported by the Myrsten *et al.* (1975) study. This latter study demonstrated that smoking is beneficial in performance tasks for low-

Table 15. *Studies of 'smoking typologies': individual differences in smoking motivation and situation dependency*

Author(s)	Country	n	Type of analysis	Items	Results/factors, smoking motives or types revealed
Best & Hakstian (1978)	Canada	331	Factor (oblique) Cluster discriminant	63	11 factors (males): nervous tension, self-image, frustration, relaxation, automatic, social, discomfort inactive, time structuring, restlessness, sensory stimulation, concentration. Female factors are similar except for inclusion of 'food avoidance' and 'habit'. Cluster analysis reveals 4–5 types of smokers: heavy addicted smokers; moderate smokers with sedative versus stimulation-seeking motives; light smokers situation dependent; food avoidance (for females only)
Coan (1973)	USA	595	Factor analysis (oblique rotation)	43	6 (second-order) factors: compulsion, tension, incidental, affect management, attention regulation, unpleasant habit
		361 (175 smokers)	Factor analysis (oblique) 2-way ANOVA: sex × smoking	148	Smoking battery produced 19 first-order factors which were related to smoker/non-smoker differences. In addition, the 6 second-order smoking factors (above) are related to general personality and lifestyle variables in a consistent fashion
Crumpacker et al. (1979)	Sweden	909	Multivariate	44	3 factors: pharmacological, non-pharmacological, indulgent (see Russell et al., 1974)
J. S. Williams, P. W. Crumpacker & M. J. Krier, unpublished, cited	USA	–	Multivariate	–	3 factors: pharmacological, non-pharmacological, indulgent (see Russell et al., 1974)

Ikard, Green & Horn (1969)	USA	2094	Factor analysis (oblique rotation)	23	of cigarettes a day, high-arousal (HA) versus low-arousal (LA) situations. (Women fit the HA smoking motivation results best) 6 factors: habitual, addictive, negative affect reduction, pleasurable relaxation, stimulation, sensorimotor manipulation. Females show greater loadings on negative affect reduction
Knott (1979a)	Canada	100	T-test on HA versus LA smokers		Eysenck personality inventory and Vando reducing augmenting scale have a small but significant relationship with Myrsten et al.'s (1975) HA and LA scales which is against theoretical predictions
McKennell (1970)	England	1339	Factor (Varimax) analysis	42	'Smoking occasion' questionnaire, 7-factor solution: nervous irritation, relaxation, 'alone', activity accompaniment, food substitution, social, social confidence
McKennell (1973)	England	2000	Cluster, regression, factor (Varimax), sub-sampling replications	70	Replication of Ikard et al. (1969) & McKennell (1970) solutions mainly successful. Integration of these solutions to produce 6 factors: inner need/relaxation, inner need/stimulation, habit, handling, social, pleasure
Mausner & Platt (1971)	USA	30	Quantitative	[a]	Simple analyses reveal habit, affect (e.g., tension reduction, stimulation, etc.) and social support (e.g., with others, alone, activity, etc.) as the main components
	USA	45	Quantitative	[a]	
	USA	115	Quantitative	[a]	
	USA	31	Factor analysis	67	Analysis of smoking diary and questionnaire; 7 factors: tension reduction and pleasure, social and role, felt good, role, social, habit, stimulant

Table 15. (cont.)

Author(s)	Country	n	Type of analysis	Items	Results/factors, smoking motives or types revealed
Mausner & Platt (1971)	USA	248 (187 smokers)	Factor analysis	[b]	9 factors: tension reduction, pleasure, social self-image, habit, self-image, social stimulation, psychological addiction, stimulation, sensorimotor. Smoker versus non-smoker differences
Myrsten et al. (1975)	Sweden	16	T-test on HA versus LA smokers	20	High-arousal (HA) versus low-arousal (LA) questionnaire developed from Frith (1971b) and McKennell (1970). 8 HA and 8 LA smokers selected from pool of 90 subjects and tested under low and high arousing situations. Reaction time, pulse rate and mood ratings indicate that HA and LA smokers obtain 'real' smoking effects consistent with questionnaire predictions
Russell et al. (1974)	England	278	Factor analysis (oblique rotation)	34	6-factor solution: stimulation, addictive, automatic, psychosocial, indulgent, sensorimotor. These intercorrelate to form 2 second-order factors labelled pharmacological (first three factors) and non-pharmacological (last three factors)
Tomkins (1966, 1968)	USA	–	Observational		Theoretical basis for many subsequent smoking typologies. Suggested factors: habitual, positive affect, negative affect, addictive

[a] Most items are 'open-ended' or extracted from interview.
[b] A large combined series of test batteries, see Mausner & Platt (1971), page 56.

arousal, but not for high-arousal smokers under monotonous conditions, and for high-arousal, but not low-arousal, smokers under more stressful conditions. Knott, though, rearranges the personality/physiology/smoking nexus by proposing that high-arousal 'sedative' smokers are anxious extraverts, and that low-arousal 'stimulant' smokers are stable introverts, an observation which attracts some empirical support from the findings of Bartol (1975) and Barnes & Fishlinsky (1976).

When taken at face value, Knott's data propose some difficulties for personality/arousal modulation theories of smoking, although they are consistent with Eysenck's earlier (1963) prediction that high N should lead to indulgence in smoking only when coupled with extraversion. The rationale here is that if nicotine acts purely as a stimulant drug, then it should have a calming or normalising effect on highE/highN individuals by analogy with the reported effects of other stimulant drugs on these personality groups.

Eysenck's more recent theory, of course, would lead to substantially different predictions, namely, that the under-aroused extravert smokes for stimulant effects, the highly reactive introvert for sedative effects (Eysenck & O'Connor, 1979). Consider also the evidence that high N subjects smoke for sedative reasons (Warburton & Wesnes, 1978; Golding *et al.*, 1983). Taken in conjunction, these would lead us to expect Knott's high-arousal, sedative smoker to be introverted, anxious, or both, and his low-arousal, stimulant smoker to be extraverted, stable, or both.

Reasons for this conflict of evidence are not clear, though two possibilities, in particular, suggest themselves. First, however, we should comment that the extraversion/introversion and neuroticism/stability group differences reported by Knott, while statistically significant, are very small. Differences between means of 13.6 for E and 11.3 for N for the high-arousal group, and of 11.9 for E and 9.2 for N for the low-arousal group, in each case less than one-half a standard deviation, are hardly a secure basis for dichotomising groups.

One explanation for these conflicting findings may be that introversion/extraversion differences are irrelevant, the anxiety element in Knott's typology being the critical marker. Evidence from the studies reviewed so far in this section, however, does not indicate that anxiety is a stronger smoking motive than extraversion.

A second explanation may be that inspection of the different data bases from which these interpretations derive suggest a reason why introverts, who, in psychophysiology studies, smoke for sedative effects, yet on the basis of questionnaire data concerning reasons for smoking, judge their smoking to be stimulant. This reason is based on inferences derived from the activity theory of personality (Mangan & Paisey, 1980) which suggests very broadly that the biologically fixed optimal arousal level and the nature of the situational demands determine behaviour interactively. Thus, in a typical experiment examining the psychophysiological effects of smoking, where the subject is exposed to levels of stress or boredom arbitrarily fixed by the experimenter, the use of mood control drugs such as nicotine aims to provide a 'best fit' between these external and internal demands. This means that the chronically under-aroused (i.e., extraverted) subject will stimulation-seek when encountering boredom whereas the chronically highly aroused (i.e., introverted) subject will seek to damp down arousal under stressful conditions. This accounts for the reported relationships between extraversion and stimulation smoking, and between introversion and sedative smoking in psychophysiological experiments.

In real life, however, individuals strive to create psychologically comfortable environments. Thus the highly reactive introvert would be expected to opt for non-stimulating environments, the relatively inert extravert for stimulating environments. In this event, it is at least a plausible suggestion that the reactive introvert seeks some mild stimulation to escape from self-imposed boredom whereas the inert extravert needs to calm himself down after excessive stimulation-seeking. What we may be referring to here is finger-tip control for correcting arousal 'overshoot'.

Summary

A problem encountered in attempting to evaluate different theories of smoking is that each theory emanates from different data bases, all of which have some validity. As we noted before, if we regard smokers as a homogeneous group, then clearly we have a real conflict of evidence. On the other hand, if smokers are regarded as a heterogeneous group, then there is no reason why different motives should not be particularly relevant to particular sub-groups, or even for the same person at different times. In our view, there is no justification for assuming motivational identity throughout the population of smokers and across all situations.

This comment, of course, does not apply to addiction theories. Here, no 'motive', as such, is implied, insofar as maintenance of the habit is concerned, any more than in the case of the opiate addict. The same comment applies partly to genetic theories, except in the case of constitutional theories, where it is entirely possible that attributes such as neuroticism and stimulation-seeking, which may have strong genetic determination, may lead to different smoking motives, e.g., sedative in the case of neurotic individuals and stimulant in the case of the stimulation-seeker.

The problem is compounded by the fact that different motives may be relevant to recruitment and to persistence. For example, recruitment may be accounted for by social learning theory, the young person perhaps beginning smoking because of peer pressure, but continuing for a different reason, e.g., because he or she becomes addicted or because nicotine is an effective mood control agent. Again, recruitment may be determined directly by genetic predisposition (unlikely) or because of certain biological propensities which motivate the individual to drink, smoke and to abuse a variety of drugs. On the other hand, as we shall observe in our adolescent study (see Chapter 4), recruitment may be a response to acute, but relatively short-term disturbances in family and personal relationships which are expressed in higher scores on N and on a psychopathic deviance scale.

We choose the path of categorising theories on the basis of what might be described as 'determinism'. Addiction and simple genetic theories suggest that the individual, in either or both phases of the smoking habit, is the victim of forces outside his control. He may be persuaded to begin smoking for social (voluntary) reasons but continuance is outside his effective control. We see few grounds to sustain such a view. Other theories, particularly orality and arousal modulation theories, would suggest otherwise, particularly if we adopt a multiple drug usage model.

If we judge from a strictly pharmacological/reward point of view, the most impressive theory is the opponent-process theory, which is, in fact, a rather sophisticated version of simple addiction theory. We feel, however, that the most persuasive theories are the genetic and the psycho-biological theories, particularly where they 'fuse' in the constitutional and arousal modulation theories we have described. From the data reviewed, it seems clear to us that smokers and non-smokers differ markedly along a number of disease, personality and psychosocial dimensions, some of which, judging from the twin studies, have strong genetic determination. It is these predispositions which motivate individuals to smoke cigarettes, to drink alcohol and to engage in a variety of drug usages. It may be, of course, that continued, heavy smoking may ultimately introduce an element of addiction, but this is not the primary motivation maintaining this behaviour.

PART II

THE SOCIAL PHARMACOLOGY OF SMOKING

3

The psychopharmacology and psychophysiology of smoking

THE PHARMACOLOGY OF NICOTINE

Nicotine was first isolated from the leaves of tobacco by Posselt & Reiman in 1828 (Goodman & Gilman, 1980). It is colourless, volatile and strongly alkaline in reaction, readily soluble in water, alcohol and ether, and forms water-soluble salts. On exposure to air it turns brown and acquires the odour typical of tobacco. Under atmospheric pressure, it boils at 246 °C, and is consequently volatilised in the cone of burning tobacco at 800 °C. The free base is present in the smoke suspended on minute droplets of tar (0.3–1.0 μm) which are small enough to reach the small airways and lung alveoli. The nicotine molecule contains a pyridine and a pyrrolidine ring (Goodman & Gilman, 1971; Russell, 1976) (Fig. 3).

Lobeline (from *Lobelia inflata*) is the closest plant-derived analogue of nicotine, and shares many of its pharmacological properties to the extent of cross-tolerance. However, it is less potent than nicotine, and this may account for the fact that, apart from limited usage by some South American tribes, *L. inflata* has not enjoyed the international popularity of *Nicotiana tabacum* (Emboden, 1972).

Nicotine exists in both ionised and neutral forms, depending on the ambient pH. At body pH (7.36–7.44) it is mainly ionised, with a positive charge on the quaternary nitrogen (see Fig. 3), and it is in this form, as the nicotinium ion, that nicotine is pharmacologically active.

The structural basis for the pharmacological activity of the nicotinium ion would appear to be its resemblance to acetylcholine in terms of the spacing of positive and negative charges (Kier, 1968; Cynoweth, Ternai, Simeral & Maciel, 1973) (see Fig. 4). Acetylcholine (ACh) is a flexible molecule, and can take up different conformations which enable it to bind to two types of receptor, nicotinic receptors and muscarinic receptors.

97

These two types of receptors are named after the relative selectivity of activation by the cholinomimetic alkaloids which bind to them. Muscarine, pilocarpine and arecoline are closely related mushroom and plant-derived cholinomimetic alkaloids containing a positively charged nitrogen atom.

Fig. 3. Structure of nicotine and lobeline. Formation of the nicotinium ion and dissociation curve. (After Travell, 1960.)

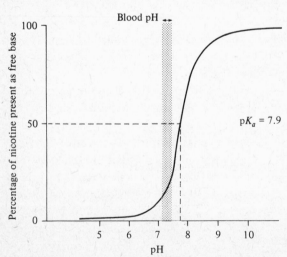

They are agonists for one of the types of cholinergic receptors whereas nicotine is selective for the other type (hence the names).

The failure of nicotine to bind to muscarinic receptors is due to the fact that the nicotine molecule has only one bond that can act as a major axis of rotation and thus achieves a much more limited range of conformations than the ACh molecule, which has four bonds that can act as major rotational axes. A variation of this model proposes that it is the ester-oxygen atom rather than the carbonyl-oxygen atom in ACh which provides the atom for hydrogen bonding in the case of ACh binding to a muscarinic receptor. On this basis, the different distances between the quaternary ammonium atom and the particular oxygen atom for hydrogen bonding define the nicotinic (0.59 nm for N^+ to carbonyl-O) as opposed to muscarinic (0.43 nm for N^+ to ester-O) modes of action of ACh (see Kier, 1968; Cynoweth *et al.*, 1973; Goodman & Gilman, 1980, p. 84, for a more detailed discussion).

Stimulation of the two types of cholinergic receptors can lead to totally different effects. Nicotine, in the range of doses absorbed from smoking, has relatively minor stimulant and depressant effects whereas the various muscarinic agonists can produce hallucinogenic effects in addition to straight stimulant effects. Muscarine comes from *Amanita muscaria*, the fly agaric mushroom, which has hallucinogenic properties. Arecoline, from

Fig. 4. Similarity of charge structure between the nicotinium ion and acetylcholine. (After Kier, 1968 and Cynoweth, Ternai, Simeral & Maciel, 1973.)

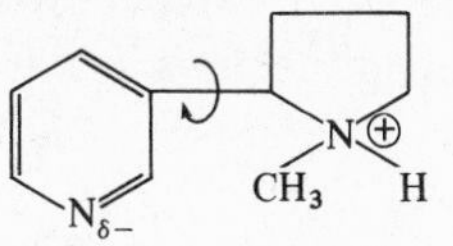

Nicotinium ion

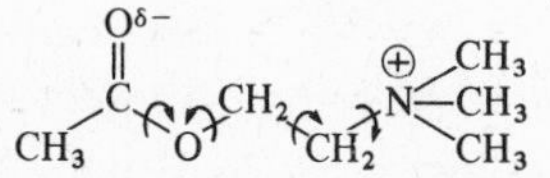

Acetylcholine

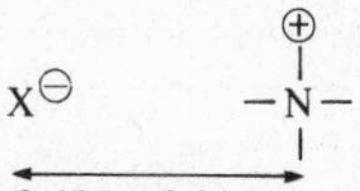

Critical charge spacing for nicotine agonists

0.485 ± 0.01 nm

(Rotational axes: methyl group rotations ignored)

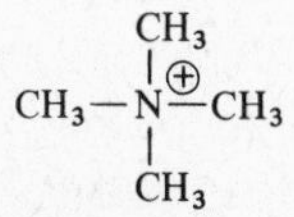

TMA, a synthetic nicotinic agonist
n.b. the negative charge may not be absolutely essential for activity since TMA does not possess it

the betel nut, is a mild stimulant, this property accounting for the habit of betel nut chewing in some countries (Emboden, 1972).

Nicotine acts mainly as a cholinergic agonist, mimicking the activity of acetylcholine on post-synaptic nicotinic receptors (Goodman & Gilman, 1971). This in turn can cause the secondary release of a variety of transmitters, depending on the type of neurone activated, including ACh itself (Armitage, Hall & Sellers, 1969), noradrenaline (NA) (Hall & Turner, 1972), serotonin (5-hydroxytryptamine, 5-HT) (Essman, 1973), possibly dopamine (Russell, 1976), and peptides (Lal et al., 1976). It is also possible that an additional action of nicotine is involved in the release of these various transmitters: nicotine may act pre-synaptically on receptors at the nerve terminal (Goodman & Gilman, 1980, p. 71). Studies of the nicotine-induced release mechanism of NA from hypothalamic synaptosomes (nerve-ending particles) (Yoshida, Kato & Imuro, 1980) indicate that this pre-synaptic effect may be the mode of nicotine action in Hall & Turner's (1972) original finding of nicotine-induced NA release. All the effects noted above can occur wherever these receptors and transmitters are found. Nicotine, therefore, has effects throughout the nervous system. Indeed, about the only receptors to escape a nicotine effect are the muscarinic (cholinergic) receptors, but even these may be affected indirectly via an action on preganglionic neurones.

The primary mode of action of nicotine on the brain is still uncertain, although it is probably similar to that observed on the more easily accessible and hence more intensively studied systems, the peripheral ganglia and the neuromuscular junction. When applied to peripheral ganglia or the neuromuscular junction, nicotine first facilitates, then blocks, impulse transmission (Paton & Perry, 1953). Acetylcholine shows similar dual action at these sites in the presence of an anti-cholinesterase. The classic differentiation of cholinergic receptors into two main types (nicotinic and muscarinic) may have to be modified with regard to the brain. There is some evidence, from iontophoretic application of ACh and various other cholinergic agonists and antagonists, that many cholinoceptive cells in the brain are responsive to both nicotinic and muscarinic agents (Cooper, Bloom & Roth, 1978; Segal, 1978). This may indicate the presence of 'mixed receptor types'. Further speculation about possible differences between central and peripheral types of cholinergic receptor results from the observation that classical nicotinic receptor blockers fail to prevent the dose-related stimulant (1 μg) and depressant (10 μg) effects of intraventricular injections of nicotine in the rat (Abood, Lowy & Booth, 1979). Indeed, some authors take the view that recent evidence from a variety of pharmacological, behavioural and binding studies suggests that many of the central actions of nicotine cannot be explained on the basis of 'traditional' specific nicotinic cholinergic mechanisms described here (Abood, Reynolds, Booth & Bidlack, 1981). Differentiation of nicotinic and muscarinic types of receptors is possible through the use of selective antagonists. Nicotinic receptors are blocked by antagonists such as tetraethylammonium (TEA), hexamethonium (C6), pentolinium and mecamylamine, whereas muscarinic receptors are blocked by atropine and scopolamine.

Nicotine action on the brain appears to mimic the nicotinic action of ACh on many brain synapses, i.e., an initial excitatory action followed by a possible later inhibitory one. This action has been observed by Phillis & York (1968), who injected nicotine (20 μg) into the brains of rats via arterial injection, and also used lung ventilation with cigarette smoke. After a brief stimulation of cortical neuronal firing, a more prolonged depression was noted. However, the nicotine effect is probably not exactly the same as that involved in the action of ACh on nicotinic receptors. This would typically end at the point of excitation, since cholinesterase would destroy and prevent any subsequent effects of prolonged ACh action on nicotinic receptors, i.e., inhibitory blockade through persistent depolarisation.

Much of the perplexity and paradox of nicotine effects results from the biphasic stimulant and depressant action at cholinoceptive sites. Confusion also arises from the fact that nicotine affects the balance of activity in a number of opposing systems within the brain as well as the balance between the peripheral sympathetic and parasympathetic systems. Thus, an increase in heart rate may arise either from a blockade of parasympathetic activity or from an increase in sympathetic activity. Compounded with this are variations in nicotine distribution, regional differences in dose-effectiveness, and the time-course of its action on opposing systems (Russell, 1976). In addition, it has been shown in animals that the starting state of the organism can modify the uptake, metabolism and neurochemical effects of nicotine (Essman, 1973), as well as the subsequent behavioural effects (Domino, 1973). This is not surprising, however, since the starting state of the organism is known to modify the effects of other drugs. For example, amphetamine will produce depression of high baseline rates and elevation of low rates of operant response in the rat (Kelleher & Morse, 1968). Such effects are often subsumed under the concept of 'Inverted-U' curves (see Appendix) relating performance to arousal.

Pharmacokinetics

Absorption

The pK_a of nicotine is 7.9, and over the pH range 7–9 the sigmoid dissociation curve accounts for over 80% of the ionisation of nicotine base to nicotinium ion (see Fig. 3). This has important consequences for both the absorption and the excretion of nicotine, since the nicotinium ion is far less permeable to membranes than the base, presumably because the presence of strong charges on the molecule makes it difficult for it to pass through the lipid phase of the membrane, ions being more stable in high (aqueous) than in low (lipid) dielectric constant environments. Thus alkaline conditions will favour the uncharged nicotine base and so lead to greater ease of absorption than acidic conditions, which favour the charged nicotinium ion.

Alkaline conditions are found in the smoke from air-cured pipe and cigar tobacco (pH = 8.5) and in the intestinal juices, whereas acidic conditions are found in the smoke from flue-cured cigarettes (pH = 5.5) and in the stomach (pH = 0.9–1.5 (Passmore & Robson, 1976)). Neutral conditions are found in the lung alveolar fluids (pH = 7.4). The pH of saliva and urine can vary over the ranges 5.6–7.6 and 5.2–6.5 respectively (pH data from Russell, 1976; Schachter *et al.*, 1977; and Russell & Feyerabend, 1978). These variations in pH have important consequences for the absorption and re-absorption of nicotine.

Thus, in the case of alkaline cigar and pipe smoke, an effective dose of nicotine, as indicated by such measures as rise in heart rate and femoral arterial pressure, or directly from plasma nicotine levels (Armitage, Hall & Morrison, 1968; Armitage & Turner, 1970; Armitage, 1978) may be absorbed by the small area of the buccal mucosa. However, this is contraindicated by Turner, Sillett & McNichol (1977), who report that non-inhaling pipe and cigar smokers show virtually no rise in plasma nicotine (and carboxyhaemoglobin, an index of amount of smoke inhaled) levels. This suggests that some degree of inhalation may be necessary for absorption of nicotine from cigar and pipe smoke. This may be one of the reasons why ex-cigarette smokers who switch to pipe or cigar smoking tend to inhale, the other reason, of course, being sheer habit.

By contrast, absorption of nicotine from acidic cigarette smoke by the buccal mucosa is zero. This is perhaps one of the factors favouring inhalation-style cigarette smoking, the much greater surface area of the lungs overcoming the difficulty of absorption from acidic cigarette smoke. Another important factor favouring inhalation of cigarette smoke as opposed to pipe or cigar smoke is simply that the latter (alkaline) smoke is far more irritating to the mucosal tissue than the milder (acidic) cigarette smoke.

Absorption through the lungs is very nearly as efficient as intravenous (i.v.) injection; more than 90% of the nicotine in inhaled tobacco smoke is absorbed by the lungs and this absorption is far faster and more efficient than buccal absorption (Armitage *et al.*, 1968; Armitage *et al.*, 1975) (see Fig. 5*a*). However, recent evidence indicates that absorption of nicotine from the nasal mucosa by the snuff taker produces levels of plasma nicotine approaching those achieved by inhalation-style cigarette smoking, and almost as rapidly (Russell, Jarvis, Devitt & Feyerabend, 1981; Russell, Jarvis, Feyerabend & Ferno, 1983).

Crucial variables for nicotine blood levels and consequent pharmacological effects are the rate and mode of nicotine absorption, in particular whether the dose is absorbed slowly and evenly, as in the case of buccal absorption from cigar or pipe smoke and chewing tobacco and of i.v. nicotine infusion, or rapidly in discrete doses, the so-called bolus form (see Appendix), as in the case of absorption from inhaled cigarette smoke and of rapid i.v. 'shots' of nicotine. It appears, from work on cats, that higher blood nicotine levels may be achieved after multiple bolus injections than after slow i.v. injections of the same amount of nicotine given over the same total time period (Turner, 1971). This, in turn, will cause much higher brain nicotine concentrations (see next section: Distribution of nicotine in the body).

Studies have also shown that the buccal absorption of nicotine is dependent on the pH of the buccal saliva, which can be experimentally varied by the use of buffered solutions (Beckett & Triggs, 1967). Since the pH of saliva shows diurnal variations (from 5.6 to 7.6 (Brawley, 1935)), and also changes before, during and just after a meal (Travell, 1960), it has been suggested by Russell (1976) that such pH fluctuations may affect buccal absorption of nicotine during smoking as well as salivary excretion and re-absorption of nicotine after smoking. It is interesting to note that American Indian tribes who were in the habit of chewing tobacco often added lime or pulverised shells, presumably with the objective of facilitating absorption by increasing the buccal pH. A similar strategy and mechanism occurs in the case of coca leaf chewing for cocaine (Brooks, 1953).

The probable reason why the ingestion of tobacco, as opposed to smoking, chewing and snuffing tobacco, has never become a popular habit, is that absorption of nicotine by this route is extremely slow and very inefficient. Thus, nicotine will not be absorbed easily from the stomach because of the extremely acidic environment. Travell (1960) found that nicotine injected into the ligated cat stomach at pH 8.6 in a dose of

20 mg kg^{-1} of body weight (at least twice the buffered fatal dose for cats) was fatal in 41 min, whereas 50 mg kg^{-1} of body weight injected into the stomach at pH 1.2 caused no effects. Absorption of effective doses of nicotine is delayed until the stomach contents pass into the intestines and are neutralised. Human data from Russell & Feyerabend (1978) indicate that ingested nicotine takes 3.5 h to appear in the plasma, although drinking some water (270 ml twice) improves absorption markedly, presumably by causing gastric emptying and dilution of the acidic gastric juices. However, huge doses (44 mg) of ingested nicotine were required to mimic the plasma nicotine levels achieved by smoking two 1.2 mg nicotine delivery cigarettes, implying that the aspiring tobacco eater would have to swallow mouthfuls of tobacco leaf regularly unless he took the precaution of consuming bicarbonate to neutralise his gastric acids. This could have serious consequences, since nicotine overdose can be fatal. A further explanation may be that even after ingested nicotine has been absorbed, a large proportion is subject to degradation by the liver, since,

Fig. 5. (a) Plasma nicotine concentrations in an inhaling smoker (filled circles) and a non-inhaling smoker (open circles) during and after smoking one cigarette which was discarded at time = 0 min. (From Feyerabend, Levitt & Russell, 1975.) (b) Arterial blood levels of [^{14}C]nicotine in habitual smokers, presumed to inhale deeply (subjects 1–4), in an occasional smoker presumed to inhale less deeply (subject 5) and in non-smokers (subjects 6 and 7) after smoking one cigarette labelled with [^{14}C]nicotine. (From Armitage et al., 1975.) (c) and (d) Arterial blood levels of [^{14}C]nicotine (filled circles) and [^{14}C]cotinine (open circles), and heart rate (squares), and blood pressure (BP) (asterisks), (c) during and after smoking a cigarette labelled with [^{14}C]nicotine and (d) during and after administration of 1 mg [^{14}C]nicotine given in 10 doses, each of 0.1 mg. (From Armitage et al., 1975.)

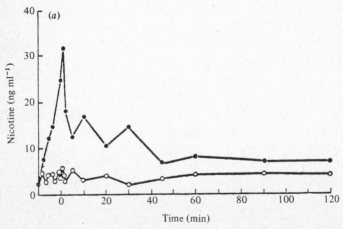

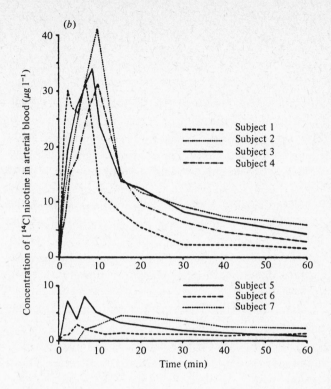

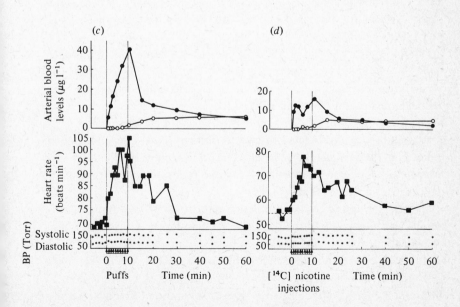

unlike nicotine absorbed by the mouth or lungs, all the nicotine absorbed from the gut will pass through the liver via the hepatic portal system before reaching the major target organ, i.e., the brain.

Blood levels

Advances in assay procedures such as gas chromatography, which distinguishes nicotine from its metabolites, have enabled the construction of fairly accurate time-based plasma nicotine profiles for smokers. Peak plasma nicotine coincides with finishing a cigarette for smokers who inhale (see Fig. 5a). The decay side of the curve has a half-life of less than 30 min, and probably separates into two stages. The initial rapid drop is caused by redistributions within the body, e.g., uptake by the brain and venous mixing. This so-called 'alpha' half-life lasts for 2–3 min (Russell & Feyerabend, 1978). The subsequent, slower 'beta' decline is caused by degradation of nicotine by the liver, kidney and lungs, and by nicotine excretion through the kidneys and, to a lesser extent, through the gut, salivary glands and sweat glands.

Considerable variations in plasma 'beta' half-lives have been reported, and these may represent true individual differences in rates of nicotine metabolism and excretion, and also reflect variations in smoking style, which will determine how rapidly the peak plasma nicotine levels are achieved and subsequently drop through the 'alpha' (redistribution) and 'beta' (metabolism and excretion) phases. Typical ranges of 'beta' half-lives are 24–84 min for (arterial) brachial blood nicotine (Armitage et al., 1975).

The major point of interest in the time-based plasma nicotine profiles is the extreme rapidity of the peak rise and initial drop (see Fig. 5a). This is a feature of absorption of nicotine by inhalation. A non-inhaling smoker puffing a cigar or pipe of air-cured tobacco (which will favour buccal absorption of nicotine) shows a much slower rise in plasma nicotine. This effect has been demonstrated in cats (Armitage et al., 1968) and, more recently, in humans using ^{14}C-labelled nicotine cigarettes and cigars with measurements of arterial nicotine (Armitage et al., 1975; Armitage, 1978; Armitage et al., 1978) (Figs. 5b, c, d).

The peak venous blood nicotine concentrations probably represent a serious under-estimate of the peak arterial blood nicotine concentrations which actually arrive at the brain, by a factor of 5 (Russell, 1976). Continuously repeated sampling of blood in the carotid artery would probably reveal a rising 'saw-toothed' curve, the 'teeth' corresponding to the nicotine blood boli produced after each inhalation of tobacco smoke.

This pattern of arrival of nicotine at the brain results in higher nicotine levels in the brain than would be possible if the blood levels in the carotid artery followed nicotine dispersion in the general circulation as is the case after slow intravenous infusion or buccal absorption. This in turn has implications for control, by the inhaling smoker, of nicotine intake, the 'puff-by-puff finger-tip control' described by Armitage (1978). It is suggested that this method allows the smoker to titrate himself with nicotine very accurately, whether to obtain a stimulant or depressant dose, or to maintain some 'set' nicotine level for a period of time. Furthermore, the great number of nicotine boli reinforcements available from inhalation-style versus non-inhalation-style smoking probably accounts for the greater popularity of inhalation-style cigarette smoking as opposed to cigar and pipe smoking, or chewing or snuffing. This is the so-called 'dependence on high-nicotine boli' described by Russell & Feyerabend (1978).

Distribution of nicotine in the body

Our knowledge of the distribution of nicotine in man, following smoking, is as yet largely inferential, since the techniques employed in animal research, i.e., nicotine assay of organs at various times post-smoking or post-injection, together with whole body autoradiographs with ^{14}C-labelled nicotine, are either inapplicable or potentially hazardous. (However, with sensitive radiation counters and the use of ^{11}C-labelled nicotine, which has a short half-life, investigators might reasonably attempt similar whole-body autoradiographs in man.)

The distribution of nicotine in the body depends very much on the route and rate of administration. Thus, any mode of nicotine administration which involves transmission through the portal venous system, i.e., ingested nicotine or intraperitoneal (i.p.) injections, will result in nicotine being concentrated largely in the liver and there degraded. On the other hand, absorption through the lungs, buccal mucosa or by i.v. injections, will favour initial concentration of nicotine in the brain and other organs because immediate nicotine metabolism in the liver is unavailable.

Absorption of nicotine from inhaled tobacco smoke into the blood flowing through the lungs is extremely rapid and efficient, as we have previously noted. From the lungs, nicotine follows the course of the circulation through the left side of the heart, whence it is pumped directly to the brain and other parts of the body. It is estimated that following inhalation of tobacco smoke, nicotine will reach the brain in about 8 s, and extremities such as the fingers and toes in about 20 s (Isaac & Rand, 1969; Russell, 1976). The high concentrations of nicotine in arterial blood that are achieved by smoke inhalation and subsequent nicotine equilibration between blood and brain produce high nicotine levels in the brain. There may also be a contributory effect from the brain and ganglia actively taking up nicotine.

Animal experiments indicate that the distribution of nicotine among body tissues is not uniform, and that the pattern of nicotine distribution changes rapidly. Thus, whole-body autoradiographs of mice injected intravenously with ^{14}C-labelled nicotine from cigarettes clearly show the rapid uptake of nicotine by the brain, liver, kidneys, salivary glands and cells in the fundus of the stomach (Schmiterlow et al., 1967). Five minutes post-injection, most of the nicotine is present in these organs and tissues. Thirty minutes post-injection, most of the nicotine assimilated by the brain has left and has been taken up by the liver, kidneys, salivary glands and stomach. The nicotine in the brain is concentrated in the grey rather than the white matter: particularly high levels occur in the cellular layers of the hippocampus (which has implications regarding the effect of smoking on the orienting response and memory, see later this chapter and Chapter 4: Consolidation). These findings have since been confirmed by studies in cats (Turner, 1969, 1971).

The study of Stalhandske (1970) using radioactively-labelled nicotine injections in mice supports and extends the above work. Through injection of ^{14}C-labelled nicotine by different routes, intravenously and intra-peritoneally, it was possible to demonstrate that the major part of the nicotine was concentrated in the first few minutes in the brain following i.v. injection, whereas following i.p. injection most of the nicotine went straight to the liver. With i.p. injections the blood level of nicotine was much lower (Fig. 6). This was presumably due to nicotine degradation by the liver.

Fig. 6. Nicotine concentrations in the brain (squares), liver (crosses) and blood (circles) of mice at various times after (a) an intravenous or (b) an intraperitoneal injection of [^{14}C]nicotine. Each value represents the average of at least three animals. (From Stalhandske, 1970.)

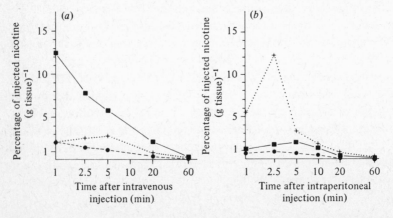

This interpretation is supported by the fact that phenobarbitone pretreatment, which is known to increase the rate of metabolism of many drugs, lowers brain nicotine levels obtained after i.p. injection but not the levels produced by i.v. nicotine. Phenobarbitone pretreatment enhances the liver metabolism of nicotine, and so differentially reduces the brain nicotine when the i.p. route of administration is employed (see also next section: Metabolism and Excretion of Nicotine). In addition, close consideration of the data from this experiment suggests that there may be an active uptake of nicotine by the brain against a concentration gradient. Active uptake of nicotine is known to occur in the superior cervical ganglion (of cats and rats) and to be further enhanced ('activation uptake') on nicotine-induced depolarisation of the cells of the ganglion (Brown, Hoffmann & Roth, 1969; Brown, Halliwell & Scholfield, 1971).

In principle, these results are extendable to the effects of smoking in humans. The time-course of such events, however, is a different matter, since the metabolic rate and circulation are much faster in smaller mammals. In addition, interspecies differences may be complex. Thus Japanese workers have shown species differences between dogs and monkeys for both nicotine degradation and nicotine uptake by the brain, liver enzyme activity being higher (Dohi, Kojima & Tsujimojo, 1973) and brain uptake of nicotine lower in monkeys because of the high affinity of nicotine for monkey skeletal muscle (Tsujimoto *et al.*, 1975). From animal studies we might note that the blood nicotine, which is estimated by decapitation and is thus the arterial rather than the venous level, has a half-life of about 5 min post i.v. injection in the mouse as compared with overall venous half-lives of 20–30 min (Russell, 1976) or overall brachial arterial half-lives of about 10–15 min in man (Armitage, 1978) (see also Fig. 5). On this basis blood nicotine clearance is 2–3 times faster in the mouse than in man. The nicotine half-life in the mouse brain is about 5 min (Stalhandske, 1970).

If we attempt some crude time-scaling between man and mouse (an arguable procedure) we arrive at a figure of about 10–15 min, or less, for the nicotine half-life in the human brain, after the finish of inhalation-style smoking. This half-life would be increased, of course, in the case of slow buccal absorption of nicotine following pipe or cigar smoking. This calculated value is similar to ^{11}C-labelled nicotine half-lives of approximately 10–15 min observed in monkey brain (Maziere *et al.*, 1979). This figure, if accurate, has serious implications for any theory suggesting that, in man, the purpose of cigarette smoking is simply to maintain nicotine at some steady-state concentration at brain receptors. Such a theory would be more applicable in the case of slow buccal absorption of nicotine from cigar and pipe smoking or from chewing tobacco. This point has been noted by such researchers as Russell (1976) and Armitage (1978), who suggest that different styles of smoking may reflect different underlying reasons for smoking.

Metabolism and excretion of nicotine

Nicotine is an extremely poisonous substance. The nicotine content of one cigar, about 60 mg, would be fatal to a human if injected intravenously. While the brain of the smoker actively takes up nicotine, the body attempts the task of expelling nicotine in two ways. These are: (a) metabolism to inactive forms and (b) excretion of the active molecule.

Metabolism. Nicotine is converted into two main metabolites, cotinine and nicotine-1'-N-oxide. These are formed by alternative pathways of oxidative metabolism involving either N-oxidation or *alpha*-carbon oxidation of the pyrrolidine ring (Fig. 7).

Conversion of nicotine to cotinine occurs in the liver, kidneys and lung, but not in the brain (Turner, Armitage, Briant & Dollery, 1975), and is the major pathway of nicotine inactivation. Under normal conditions of fluctuating urinary pH the amount of nicotine-1'-N-oxide excreted in the urine of smokers is about half that of cotinine (Beckett, Gorrod & Jenner, 1971a). The reduction of nicotine-1'-N-oxide to nicotine in the lower gastrointestinal tract is unlikely to be very important, since the re-metabolised nicotine will be largely degraded again by the liver during its first pass into general circulation.

Fig. 7. Alternative metabolic pathways of nicotine inactivation. (After Russell, 1976.)

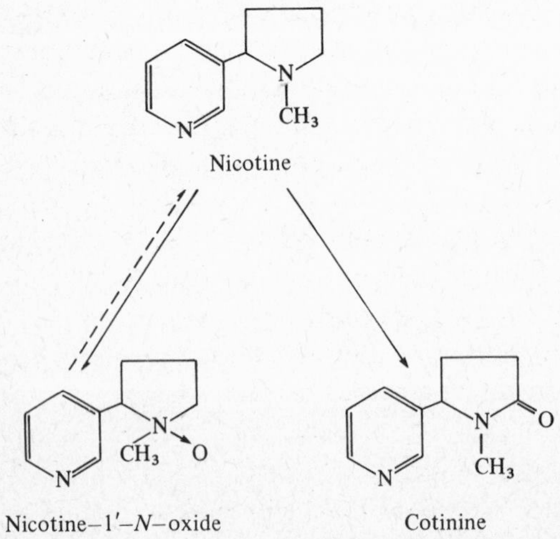

Nicotine

Nicotine–1'–N–oxide   Cotinine

There is now evidence that nicotine metabolism is increased by repeated exposure. Comparison of smokers and non-smokers reveals that the proportion of nicotine metabolites to unchanged nicotine excreted in the urine is much higher in smokers than in non-smokers (Beckett, Gorrod & Jenner, 1971*b*). This is not surprising, since metabolic tolerance due to induction of enzymes is well known for other drugs such as amphetamine, alcohol and cannabis. It is not known, however, how strong an effect this would have on the plasma or brain nicotine half-life of a heavy smoker, as opposed to a light smoker.

Excretion. The largest proportion by far of nicotine and its metabolites is eliminated from the body via urine, although they are also present in sweat, saliva and the milk of lactating women (Perlman & Dannenberg, 1942). This latter finding may be of significance for the breast-fed infant. In the cat 90% of the radioactivity of a given dose of labelled nicotine is excreted in the urine within three days, and 77% in the first twenty-four hours (Turner, 1969, 1971).

As in the case of absorption, the excretion of unchanged nicotine is pH dependent. When the pH is low (5.5 or less) the nicotine is almost totally ionised and cannot be re-absorbed through the kidney tubules. Under these conditions, 30–40% of an i.v. dose, and, by inference, of nicotine absorbed from smoking, is excreted in the urine as unchanged nicotine (Beckett *et al.*, 1971*a*; Goodman & Gilman, 1971). On the other hand, if the pH of urine exceeds 8.0, most of the nicotine is re-absorbed from the urine, not only through the renal tubules, but also through the bladder (Travell, 1960). Under normal conditions of fluctuating urinary pH, smokers excrete similar amounts of nicotine and cotinine in their urine, and about half as much nicotine-1'-N-oxide (Gorrod & Jenner, 1975). However, Feyerabend & Russell (1978), in commenting on their pH manipulation studies, state that, compared with the doses of nicotine administered, the amounts of nicotine (rather than metabolites) excreted in the urine were trivial, (< 12.5%), even under acidic conditions. They suggest that this is why major changes in urinary excretion rates of nicotine, which are markedly influenced by pH and urine flow rate, have relatively small (albeit statistically significant) effects on plasma nicotine levels.

Earlier, pH was implicated as a mediating variable in smoking style and for the input of nicotine to the system. Interestingly enough, as far as nicotine output from the system is concerned, pH crops up again as a possible mediator to account for observed increases of smoking rate during stress. Schachter (1978) has proposed that the observed decreases in urinary pH during stress, which lead to increased nicotine excretion, account for the increases in smoking rate of stressed smokers.

Regulation of nicotine intake

We have already noted the greater speed and efficiency of nicotine absorption and distribution to the CNS produced by inhalation-style smoking as compared to any other mode of tobacco usage. The speed with which nicotine reaches the brain potentially enables the smoker to make rapid adjustments of his smoking behaviour in order to achieve desired levels of nicotine, a so-called 'puff-by-puff finger-tip control' (Armitage, 1978). The manner in which the cigarette is smoked, i.e., the smoking style, is critically important for this. The quantity of nicotine extracted from the cigarette is determined by puffing frequency, puff duration and puff pressure, and subsequent nicotine absorption is determined by the depth and duration of smoke inhalation. The most direct and reliable method of recording smoking style involves the subject smoking through a special cigarette-holder. The internal space of this holder is connected via thin flexible tubing to a sensitive pressure recorder, enabling the measurement of puffing frequency and the recording of the puff pressure profile. The addition of a lightweight plethysmograph, such as a mercury strain gauge, around the smoker's chest, or an impedance pneumograph, allows measurement of chest wall movements, which can be calibrated against absolute volume of inhalation, using a spirometer (Guillerm & Radziszewski, 1978; Rawbone, Murphy, Tate & Kane, 1978; Golding, 1980). Provided the subject is sufficiently habituated, this experimental system does not induce any significant change in smoking pattern as assessed by comparison with smoking patterns obtained from the subject using remote infra-red sensing of the burning tobacco cone outside the experimental system (Guillerm & Radziszewski, 1978). Where increases in smoking vigour are noted in the laboratory, as compared to surreptitious observation outside, this is probably due to laboratory-induced stress, whether intentionally produced or not (Comer & Creighton, 1978). A specimen record of puffing frequency, puff pressure and subsequent smoke inhalation is shown in Fig. 8a. Analyses of smoking style patterns are shown in Fig. 8b.

Typically, there is a trend for the intensity of smoking to tail off over the course of smoking a single cigarette (see Fig. 8b). This suggests that smokers seek a rapid build-up of nicotine at the beginning of smoking and then attempt to maintain these brain nicotine levels. An additional reason for this tailing off is that the tobacco rod acts like a fractionation column, nicotine and tar becoming more concentrated in the tobacco towards the butt, over the course of smoking the cigarette (Surgeon General, 1979).

It is possible to observe increases in the vigour of smoking low-nicotine delivery cigarettes presumably because the smoker is attempting to obtain the habitual dose of nicotine (see Chapter 2: Simple Addiction Models). Similar changes can be observed under conditions of stress with normal nicotine delivery cigarettes (see Fig. 8b), perhaps because the smoker is attempting to obtain larger, and thus tranquillising, doses of nicotine (see later this chapter: Specific effects on neural/hormonal mechanisms, The Brain).

Fig. 8. (a) Specimen record of puffing patterns and inhalation. (b) Overall smoking style patterns as a function of time while smoking a single cigarette for subjects (n = 22) under White Noise Stress conditions (filled circles) and sensory isolation conditions (open circles). (Adapted from Golding, 1980.)

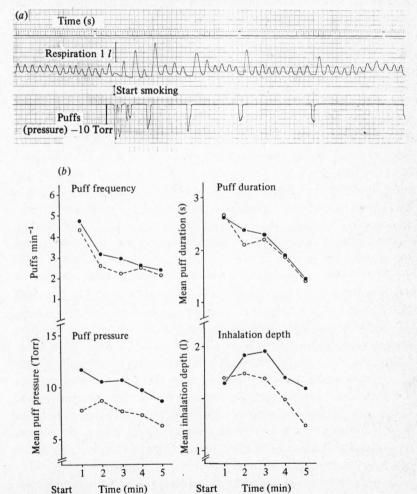

Observation of smoking style, in conjunction with other methods such as residual butt nicotine and exhaled carbon monoxide (CO) analysis, provides complementary data to those obtained more definitively by blood nicotine assays, and with considerably less distress to the subject. Moreover these techniques have important practical applications. By tape-recording individual smoking patterns and using these to control a puff duplicator or 'smoking robot', it is possible to find out how much tar, nicotine and CO the smokers' lungs are exposed to. In particular it appears that (apart from the absolute pressure of the puff) the shape of the puff pressure profile is an important determinant of tar and CO, but not nicotine, delivery. Slowly rising puff pressure profiles which peak at the end of the puff lead to the most tar and CO. Consequently it is of clinical relevance that there are large and consistent individual variations in smoking style (Golding, 1980), and, in particular, that female smokers tend to take smaller puffs than male smokers, with sharply rising pressure profiles, and tend to have lower tar to nicotine ratios (Creighton & Lewis, 1978; note the sex differences cited in Chapter 1: Smoking and morbidity/mortality).

Summary

The dissociation curve of nicotine base to the ionic form takes place over pH ranges encountered in the media from which nicotine is absorbed or re-absorbed: tobacco smoke itself, saliva, gastric juices and urine. Since the free base is much more easily absorbed than the nicotinium ion, this has important consequences for both the chosen route of nicotine absorption, i.e., inhalation-style versus buccal absorption, and, through re-absorption of nicotine from urine, for the half-lives of blood nicotine levels, and thus perhaps for smoking rates. Nicotine absorbed via the buccal mucosa (from pipe and cigar smoke) or lungs (from cigarette smoke) is less susceptible to inactivation in the liver than is ingested nicotine. However, the relative popularity of inhalation-style smoking, as opposed to buccal absorption by puffing, chewing or snuffing, cannot be totally explained in terms of the pH of tobacco smoke, since cigar and pipe smokers are frequently observed to inhale in some measure. A more convincing explanation is that inhalation-style smoking enables nicotine, in the form of a concentrated blood bolus, to reach the presumed major target area, the brain, very rapidly (less than 10 s), so that initially higher and more controllable brain nicotine levels can be achieved than via buccal absorption. This may imply that different styles of tobacco smoking are based on different nicotine 'needs'.

The extremely short brain nicotine half-lives (approximately 10–15 min post-smoking) estimated for man have important implications for any model attempting to explain cigarette smoking simply in terms of achieving nicotine homeostasis at brain receptors.

THE PSYCHOPHYSIOLOGY OF SMOKING

Given that nicotine has wide-ranging direct and indirect actions throughout the nervous system, and that it is absorbed efficiently and rapidly after cigarette smoking, it is not surprising that it has effects on nearly every physiological system studied.

A review of the major findings follows, with an attempt to interpret the results in terms of their possible reinforcing nature for the maintenance of cigarette smoking.

Specific effects on neural/hormonal mechanisms
The cardiovascular system

The effects on the cardiovascular system (CVS) of doses of nicotine equivalent to those obtained by cigarette smoking are predominantly stimulant, whether administered by injection (Lucchesi *et al.*, 1967), aerosol (Herxheimer, Griffiths, Hamilton & Wakefield, 1967) or, indeed, by cigarette smoking (Payne, 1914). The heart rate elevation usually observed after cigarette smoking appears to be due exclusively to the pharmacological action of the nicotine in the smoke, since the observed increases in pulse rate (and blood pressure) after nicotine has been absorbed do not occur when the vehicle of administration is aerosol propellant or inhalation of nicotine-free cigarette smoke (Herxheimer *et al.*, 1967). Nor do sham smoking or deep breathing (Elliott & Thysell, 1968) produce this effect.

The mechanism of action of nicotine on the CVS is a good example of the complexity of the pharmacological effects. Thus, nicotine can increase the heart rate by excitation of sympathetic, or paralysis of parasympathetic, cardiac ganglia. Of course, the opposite is also true, because of the biphasic properties of nicotine, although a nicotine-induced reduction of heart rate is in fact seldom observed. In addition, the effects of nicotine on the chemoreceptors of the carotid and aortic bodies and on medullary centres influence the heart, as do the cardiovascular compensatory reflexes resulting from changes in blood pressure caused by nicotine. It also appears that nicotine can directly stimulate the postganglionic nerve endings in the heart with local release of catecholamines in cardiac tissue. Finally, nicotine tends to produce a discharge of adrenaline from the adrenal medulla, and this hormone elevates the heart rate and raises the blood pressure (Goodman & Gilman, 1971). However, this adrenal gland release of adrenaline is not likely to be of major importance for cigarette smoking induced cardiovascular changes since the rise in circulating catecholamines occurs *after* the observed cardiovascular effects (Cryer, Haymond, Santiago & Shah, 1976).

In summary, nicotine itself and cigarette smoking, but not sham smoking, usually have an acute dose-related sympathomimetic effect on the CVS, increasing the pulse rate (the major effects lasting 10–15 min post-smoking) and blood pressure (which returns to normal in about 20 min), and decreasing peripheral blood flow as measured by decreased finger-tip temperature, toe temperature and foot blood flow (these latter effects lasting longer than the change in heart rate). These sympathomimetic effects can, however, be prevented by adrenergic blockade through the use of an *alpha*-blocker (phentolamine) and a *beta*-blocker (propranolol) (Cryer *et al.*, 1976). Recent evidence indicates that cigarette smoking increases cerebral blood flow in the brain of man, although the exact mechanism of action is not yet understood (Wennmalm, 1982).

Although nicotine-induced heart rate elevation following cigarette smoking is one of the most reliable correlates of cigarette smoking, a rapid receptor tolerance, tachyphylaxis, quickly ensues. This is often observed by the smoker, the first cigarette of the day having subjectively the strongest effects. Tachiphylaxis has been demonstrated in studies with rapidly injected nicotine designed to mimic the nicotine concentrations encountered by cigarette smokers (Russell & Feyerabend, 1978). It has also been observed as progressive decrements in heart rate acceleration produced by smoking successive cigarettes after elapse of an enforced short period of abstinence or after sleep (Frankenhaeuser *et al.*, 1968; Elliott & Thysell, 1968; Armitage, 1970). In these studies, the typical elevations in heart rate of 10–20 beats min^{-1} observed after the first cigarette are reduced to about 5 beats min^{-1} after only a few cigarettes. Such large reductions in heart rate are unlikely to be caused by a progressive decrease in the amount of nicotine extracted from each cigarette since successive rises in nicotine plasma levels due to cigarette smoking remain fairly constant (Russell & Feyerabend, 1978) provided that smokers are not forced to smoke cigarettes at unnaturally high frequencies. Further, neither the observed puffing rates nor the amount of each cigarette smoked (as assessed from butt nicotine content) decrease through the day (Armitage, 1970). It is also interesting to note that one of the few radiotelemetry studies of ad-lib smoking under 'unrestricted' conditions, by contrast with laboratory conditions, found little or no evidence that cigarettes increase the heart rate (Erwin, 1971). It would seem reasonable to suppose, therefore, that apart from the first few cigarettes of the day the smoker will tend to experience smoking-induced heart rate elevation not substantially different from the variations in heart rate resulting from normal day-to-day activities.

Over and above this, however, during the course of the day's smoking, the smoker will experience a gradual rise in tonic heart rate of the order of 10 beats min^{-1} (Armitage, 1970) compared with a small drop towards evening in non-smokers. This is probably due to the observed gradual accumulation of nicotine in the blood throughout the day (Russell & Feyerabend, 1978).

Release of catecholamines. As stated above, nicotine itself and cigarette smoking generally have a sympathomimetic effect on the CVS. The associated release of catecholamines from the adrenal medulla is sufficient but not necessary for these effects on the CVS, as Cryer *et al.* (1976) point out, since the time-course of adrenal stimulation is slower than that of heart rate elevation. The question thus arises of whether nicotine-induced release of catecholamines is important for the smoking habit.

The data of Cryer *et al.* (1976) are of particular interest, since, although there is general agreement that smoking produces release of adrenaline as measured in the blood (e.g. Hill & Wynder, 1974) or urine (e.g., Agué, 1974), this is one of the very few human studies which has found smoking-associated increments in circulatory as opposed to synaptic noradrenaline (NA) (the sympathetic neurotransmitter) in the blood (Hill & Wynder, 1974) and urine (Frankenhaeuser, Myrsten & Post, 1970; Frankenhaeuser *et al.*, 1971).

The latter studies demonstrate that the rate of excretion of adrenaline in urine increased by an average of 38% during a 90-min period following the smoking of two 1.3 mg nicotine cigarettes; with cigarettes of higher nicotine yield (2.3 mg nicotine/cigarette), urinary adrenaline was increased by 83%. There were corresponding dose-related decreases in NA excretion of 12% and 17% respectively.

The usual finding that smoking reduces circulatory NA levels may be related to the reduction of aggression by nicotine, a point which we have previously referred to (see Chapter 2: Behavioural traits and characteristics). This is because the NA to adrenaline ratio has been suggested as an index of the 'fight–flight' dimension of arousal (Ax, 1953; Funkenstein, 1955; Gray, 1971). It is possible that starting state is also important. Individuals with high NA levels could show smoking-related reductions of NA, and vice-versa for individuals with low NA levels. One study (Myrsten & Andersson, 1978) suggests that the starting state of the smoker is important in determining the final outcome of cigarette smoking. This investigation found that when a reaction-time task was performed under stressful conditions, which itself produced an increase in adrenaline, smoking produced no further increases in adrenaline.

We could regard this as a 'ceiling effect', or as a consequence of the smoker taking larger doses of nicotine during stress to obtain depressant effects. Nicotine has a biphasic action on the adrenal medulla. Small doses evoke the discharge of catecholamines and large doses prevent their release, in response to splanchnic nerve stimulation (Goodman & Gilman, 1971). The mechanism is no doubt complex since there is evidence that opioid peptides stored in the axon terminals of the splanchnic nerves located in the adrenal medulla may function as neuromodulators of ACh receptors located on chromaffin cells. The opiate peptides block the nicotine-induced catecholamine release (Kumakura, Karoum, Guidotti & Costa, 1980).

Excessive adreno-medullary activity is probably avoided by the smoker, since it would produce a decrement in behaviour efficiency as a consequence of the inverted-U relationship between arousal and behavioural efficiency (see Chapter 4: Performance of established behaviour).

The Surgeon General (1979, Ch. 14, p. 90) suggests that mobilisation of free fatty acids (FFA) and blood sugars occurs as a secondary response to circulatory catecholamines released by nicotine from smoking. However, the evidence on this point is not unanimous, particularly with regard to blood glucose (or insulin) (Cryer et al., 1976).

Release of other hormones and circulatory factors. Cigarette smoking does not significantly effect plasma glucagon, insulin, alanine, glucose or *beta*-hydroxybutyrate (Cryer et al., 1976). However, increments in plasma growth hormone, cortisol and antidiuretic hormone (ADH) have been reported (Cryer et al., 1976; Goodman & Gilman, 1971). The mechanism of action in each case probably involves a cholinergic final common pathway in the hypothalamus, for the following reason. The release of plasma growth hormone and cortisol are not susceptible to combined alpha- and beta- blockade by the alpha- and beta-blockers phentolamine and propranolol respectively (Cryer et al., 1976). The antidiuretic effect of nicotine, which is similar to that of ACh, is the result of stimulation of the hypothalamicohypophyseal system, with the consequent release of ADH (Goodman & Gilman, 1971). The nicotine-induced release of corticosteroids has been traced through a complicated sequence of events, and this detection provides a good example of the growing power of biological techniques (Jones, Hillhouse & Cole, 1978).

Skeletal muscle

There is evidence that smoking has a relaxing effect on skeletal muscle, and that this is largely due to nicotine. A report that smoking caused a dramatic transient reduction in skeletal muscle tone in spastic patients (Webster, 1964) together with the observation that smoking a tobacco cigarette reduced the amount of electromyogram (EMG) artefact during EEG recording of a very tense and anxious patient prompted Domino and his colleagues to explore this effect (Domino & von Baum-garten, 1969; Domino, 1973). Smoking a single cigarette produced a marked depression of the muscular contraction elicited by the patellar reflex. This effect was dose-related, and was also produced by inhalation of nicotine from an aerosol, but not by lettuce cigarettes or by nicotine-free

Fig. 9. Effects of inhaling a nicotine aerosol and a nicotine-free aerosol on the mean patellar reflex and electromyogram. (*a*) The mean patellar reflex; (*b*) electromyogram of the quadriceps femoris muscle. Both figures represent the value of 100% as the control for five to eight subjects. Note that inhaling the nicotine aerosol gave a greater depression than inhaling the nicotine-free aerosol. (From Domino, 1973.)

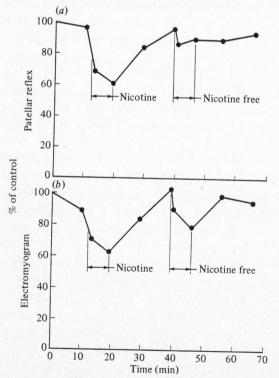

aerosol. The time-course of the reflex depression roughly follows that of the blood nicotine levels found after smoking (see Fig. 9).

Similar effects have been obtained in dogs by Isaac & Rand (1969) using i.v. nicotine and the introduction of tobacco smoke into the lungs. The mechanism of this depression of the patellar reflex is complex, involving both central and peripheral components. Ginzel, Watanabe, Eldred & Grover (1968) concluded, on the basis of their own and other studies, that small doses of nicotine (4–50 µg – close to 'real' smoking doses) injected intraventricularly into cat brains usually depressed the patellar and linguo-mandibular reflexes. Some degree of central involvement is certain, since high spinal transection abolishes the depressant effects of nicotine on reflexes. In addition, these depressant effects can be blocked by mecamylamine (a centrally acting nicotine blocker) but not by hexamethonium (a peripheral nicotine blocker).

The central mechanism is additional to the hypothesised mechanism of nicotine-induced depression of the patellar reflex (Domino, 1973). This mechanism proposes that depression of the patellar reflex is mediated by a direct stimulant action of nicotine on cholinergic receptors of the Renshaw cells in the spinal cord, such cells being inhibitory interneurones in the reflex arc. However, central, rather than peripheral, mechanisms of nicotine action are likely to be of great importance in accounting for the finding that nicotine and cigarette smoking reduce masseter muscle contractions of smokers exposed to noise stress (Hutchinson & Emley, 1973).

There is also a large amount of evidence indicating that nicotine itself and cigarette smoking increase muscle tremor (for review see Larson, Haag & Silvette, 1961). Animal experiments implicate both the central and peripheral actions of nicotine in the production of this increase.

In contrast to the evidence that nicotine and cigarette smoking reduce EMG activity in response to stimuli, the reports of Fagerstrom & Gotestam (1977) regarding trapezius muscle, and Golding (1980) regarding forearm extensor muscle, suggest that cigarette smoking, compared to sham smoking, increases tonic muscle activity. In addition, the latter study found no significant evidence that cigarette smoking, as opposed to sham smoking, increased the habituation rate of EMG responses (forearm extensor) to aversive stimuli (high intensity white-noise bursts).

There are various explanations for these contradictory results. Firstly, biphasic stimulant versus depressant effects of nicotine on EMG may be occurring. Secondly, as regards the Fagerstrom & Gotestam (1977) study, Domino (1979) has suggested that since the trapezius muscle (which is involved in holding up the head) may be involved in the orienting reflex, it is entirely possible that stimulant effects may occur in one set of muscles and depressant effects in others. In fact, a difficulty in using EMG as a response measure is the well-known principle of individual response specificity, i.e., the fact that individuals respond idiosyncratically in different muscle groups, and indeed in a variety of other response systems (Eysenck, 1977).

Respiration

Small doses of nicotine augment respiration reflexively by excitation of the chemoreceptors of the carotid and aortic bodies; larger doses act directly on the medulla oblongata. Excessive doses of nicotine may be lethal since they produce excitation followed by depression. Death results from failure of respiration due to both central paralysis and peripheral blockade of the muscles of respiration (Goodman & Gilman, 1980). In practice, i.e., for the average smoker, the effects are relatively small. Injections of small doses of nicotine into the human ascending aorta have been observed to have no effect on the rate of respiration, but to significantly increase the depth of respiration (Burgess & Rapaport, 1968). Some evidence indicates that the rate of respiration is slightly depressed by cigarette smoking (Dock, 1963) or by injection of the nicotine analogue lobeline (Bevan & Murray, 1963). However, the extent to which cigarette smoking causes respiratory depression is uncertain. Apart from a significant reduction in the respiration rate which is due to the immediate physical processes of cigarette smoking or sham smoking, i.e., to the interruption of the normal respiratory cycle by repeated inhalations of smoke (cigarette) or air (sham smoking), Golding (1980) found no significant effects for either the respiration rate or respiration irregularity.

The gastrointestinal tract

In contrast to the actions of nicotine on the CVS, which are mainly due to sympathetic stimulation, the effects of nicotine on the gastrointestinal tract are largely due to parasympathetic stimulation. The combined activation of parasympathetic ganglia and cholinergic nerve endings results in increased tone and motor activity of the bowel. Nausea, vomiting and occasionally diarrhoea are observed following systemic absorption of nicotine. Nausea and vomiting are caused by a complex of central (stimulation of the emetic chemoreceptor trigger zones of the medulla oblongata) and peripheral (stimulation of vagal and spinal afferent nerves which form part of the sensory input of the reflex pathways involved in the act of vomiting) actions (Goodman & Gilman, 1980).

Sensory receptors

Nicotine, like ACh, is known to stimulate a number of sensory receptors. These include mechano-receptors that respond to stretch or pressure of the skin, mesentery, tongue, lung and stomach, chemoreceptors of the carotid body, thermal receptors of the skin and tongue, and nociceptors (Goodman & Gilman, 1980).

The exocrine glands

Nicotine causes an initial stimulation of salivary and bronchial secretions which is followed by inhibition. Salivation caused by smoking is reflexively produced by the irritant smoke rather than by systemic effects of nicotine (Goodman & Gilman, 1980).

The electrodermal system

Electrodermal activity (sweat gland activity) is a commonly used measure of autonomic excitation. Tonic and phasic components of electrodermal activity are thought to reflect the excitation–inhibition balance of the limbic system (a major target area for nicotine), and in particular the hippocampus and amygdala (Rickles, 1972). While electrodermal activity is usually regarded as an index of central autonomic activity, systematic peripheral effects cannot be completely excluded in the case of cigarette smoking or nicotine. The immediate sympathetic innervation of the sweat gland is muscarinic and so should be unaffected by nicotine. Thus local iontophoresis of atropine blocks the skin conductance response (SCR) and reduces the skin conductance level (SCL) (see Appendix) (Venables & Martin, 1967). However, spinal actions of nicotine cannot be excluded, since studies on cats transected between spinal cord and brain indicate that close arterial injection of nicotine towards the right stellate ganglion causes cardioacceleration and/or sweat secretion from the right front foot pads (Aiken & Reit, 1968). While little work is reported regarding nicotine per se, cigarette smoking causes elevation of tonic activity (SCL) (Agué, 1974; Mangan & Golding, 1978; Golding & Mangan, 1982a), which appears to be dose-related (Golding, 1980) (see Fig. 10c). As can be seen by the effects of sham smoking in Fig. 10a, the purely sensorimotor aspects of cigarette smoking contribute to the smoking-induced elevation in the SCL. However, this is a relatively transient effect: a more sustained SCL elevation is achieved after 'real' smoking, presumably because of the nicotine absorbed by the smoker.

When the tonic SCL level is elevated under conditions of high arousal, for example during stress, the effects of cigarette smoking on the SCL appear to be minimal (see Fig. 10*b*). Thus the pre-smoking 'starting state' level of arousal of the individual modifies the outcome of cigarette smoking on the SCL, and this may account for one negative report concerning the effects of nicotine on the SCL. Subjects may have been relatively aroused in the experiment involving i.v. injections of nicotine, reported by Kumar *et al.* (1978), where no significant effects of nicotine on the SCL were recorded.

By contrast to its mainly stimulant effects on tonic electrodermal activity, i.e., on the SCL, cigarette smoking appears to have largely depressant effects on the phasic components of electrodermal activity such as skin conductance response (SCR) and spontaneous fluctuations (SFs) (Mangan & Golding, 1978; Golding & Mangan, 1982*a*, *b*). Similar findings have been reported by Izard, Grob & Rémond (1979), who note that the immediate activation of the electrodermal system during smoking is followed by a longer-lasting decrease in phasic electrodermal activity.

Body weight

The common observation that some smokers gain weight after giving up smoking probably derives from two sources. Firstly, appetite increases upon giving up smoking, partly as a consequence of the ability of smoking to prevent feedback of 'hunger-stimuli' such as hunger contractions of the stomach (Schendorf & Ivy, 1939) and, perhaps more importantly, because central nicotine action 'switches off' the feeding centres of the hypothalamus (Munster & Battig, 1975). There may also be an effect on fluid intake (Falkeborn, Larsson & Nordberg, 1981), which is perhaps unsurprising given that the CNS centres controlling drinking behaviour are also located in the hypothalamus.

Secondly, giving up smoking may be causing weight gain because smokers seem to expend calories less efficiently than non-smokers. Thus, weight gains after giving up smoking tend to occur even if calorie intake is reduced (Lincoln, 1969). This may be because smoking or nicotine increases the metabolic rate, perhaps by short-term increases in serum free fatty acids and triglycerides (Russell, 1976). Giving up smoking will consequently lower the metabolic rate and so cause weight gain irrespective of whether the ex-smoker attempts to curb his or her increased appetite.

The brain

The fact that doses of nicotine equivalent to those resulting from smoking increase CNS arousal is well attested from both animal (Armitage *et al.*, 1969; Cheshire, Kellett & Willey, 1973) and human studies (Murphree, Pfeiffer & Price, 1967; Philips, 1971; Brown, 1973; Knott &

Venables, 1977), arousal being measured by EEG desynchronisation, attenuation, or a frequency shift of alpha activity. A similar inference might also be derived from studies reporting decreased arousal as one consequence of smoking deprivation (Knapp *et al.*, 1963; Ulett & Itil, 1969; Hall *et al.*, 1973; Knott & Venables, 1977). This cortical arousal is probably secondary to the effect of nicotine on the reticular activating system and the hippocampus (Domino, 1973), where particularly high levels of nicotine occur after absorption. Bilateral lesions of the mid-brain reticular formation in cats will completely abolish the cortical desynchronisation produced by nicotine even in doses as high as 100 μg kg^{-1} of body weight (20 μg kg^{-1} of body weight normally being sufficient (Domino, 1973)). In addition, iontophoretic injection of nicotine into the brainstem activates some

Fig. 10. (*a*) Skin conductance levels (SCLs) for real smoking of a 1.3 mg nicotine delivery cigarette (filled circles), sham smoking (squares), and situation control (open circles) for 24 subjects during 16 min of sensory isolation. Start and finish of smoking are marked on the figure. Note that the real cigarette produces a larger and more long-lasting stimulant effect on the SCL than does sham smoking. (From Mangan & Golding, 1978.) (*b*) Effects of real smoking (1.3 mg nicotine cigarette) (filled circles) (n = 12) and sham smoking (open circles) (n = 6) on the skin conductance level (SCL) during stress and during sensory isolation conditions. Start and finish of smoking are marked on the figure. Note that whereas smoking produces stimulant effects during sensory isolation, it has no effect on the SCL during stress. (From Golding, 1980.) (*c*) The effects of smoking two successive high-nicotine (1.8 mg) (filled circles) or two successive low-nicotine (0.36 mg) (open circles) cigarettes on the skin conductance level (SCL) for ten subjects in each group. Start and finish of smoking are marked on the figure; the total time elapsed between finishing the first cigarette and starting the second cigarette is 22 min. Note the greater stimulant effect of the high-nicotine cigarette on the SCL for both the first and second cigarettes smoked. (From Golding, 1980.)

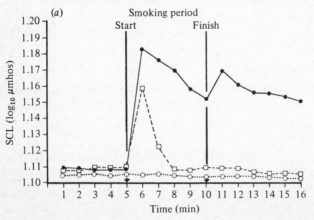

neurones, thus providing direct evidence of nicotine action. Unlike many other stimulant drugs, the arousal due to nicotine or tobacco smoking closely resembles normal arousal produced by natural stimulating conditions (Domino, 1973; Russell, 1976). In a very well-controlled study, Cheshire *et al.* (1973) found that nicotine administered intravenously in doses of 1 or 5 μg kg^{-1} of body weight min^{-1} produced a dose-related EEG desynchronisation in monkeys which was indistinguishable from 'normal arousal' produced by visual or auditory stimulation. By contrast, other stimulants such as D-amphetamine (0.1 mg kg^{-1} of body weight, and 0.5 mg kg^{-1} of body weight given orally) and caffeine (50 mg kg^{-1} of body

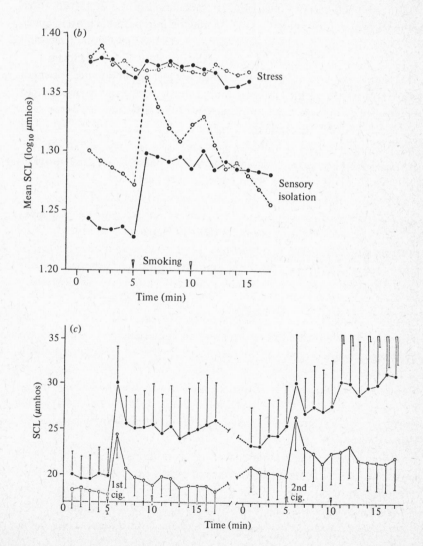

weight given orally), while producing the same order of magnitude of overall EEG desynchronisation over a longer time-course, resulted in significant differences in particular EEG bands from normal arousal, and from arousal produced by nicotine.

Nicotine also causes a release of ACh from the cortex. This, too, is secondary to effects in other areas since ACh is not released when nicotine is applied directly to the cortex. The EEG arousal is short lived whereas the cortical ACh release is more prolonged, lasting for an hour or more. This suggests that these two effects of nicotine are mediated by different mechanisms (Armitage et al., 1969).

Although activation of the EEG is emphasised in the literature, there are reports of depressant effects. These may be interpretable both in terms of (1) the known biphasic dose-response curves for the action of nicotine at the synapse and in terms of (2) the starting state of the organism.

(1) Armitage et al. (1969) found that the most common effect of small frequent doses (2 μg kg^{-1} of body weight every 30 s) of i.v. nicotine in anaesthetised cats was desynchronisation of the EEG and an increase of cortical ACh. By contrast, larger doses given less frequently (4 μg kg^{-1} of body weight every 60 s) could increase or decrease EEG activity with a corresponding increase or decrease in ACh release. This dose range is equivalent to that obtained from cigarette smoking.

Although human smoking studies have generally regarded EEG activation as the rule, the exceptions, in terms of smoking producing EEG synchronisation, may be more frequent than is generally admitted. Thus, Murphree et al. (1967) noted that some subjects showed increases in EEG alpha activity following cigarette smoking although stimulant effects predominated in the sample. Similar 'mixed' stimulant and depressant effects have been reported by Knott (1978), Rémond, Martinerie & Baillon (1979), Golding & Mangan (1982a), and Izard et al. (1979), the latter study indicating that mixed effects were more characteristic of the alpha EEG band whereas the beta bands tended to show the more stimulant effects of smoking.

(2) The starting state is known to modify the effects of many drugs, including nicotine, on the CNS (Domino, 1973; Ashton et al., 1981). This has been suggested by Murphree et al. (1967) to explain some paradoxical depressant effects of nicotine.

It is plausible to suggest that under some conditions (such as a high basal state of arousal) the depressant actions of nicotine may predominate. This is supported by the observation that the starting state, whether in terms of personality differences (Ashton et al., 1974; Eysenck & O'Connor, 1979) or situation (Ashton & Watson, 1970), may direct both the rate of nicotine intake and, probably as a consequence, physiological outcome.

Further support for this hypothesis comes from a series of studies (Mangan & Golding, 1978; Golding, 1980; Golding & Mangan, 1982a) in which subjects were observed when smoking cigarettes during high arousal (white noise stress), middle arousal (boredom situations) and low arousal (sensory isolation). In general, smokers tended to obtain depressant effects from cigarette smoking during stress conditions, mixed stimulant and depressant effects during boring conditions, and stimulant effects during sensory isolation conditions, arousal being measured in terms of EEG and electrodermal activity (Figs. 10 and 11). In addition, there

Fig. 11. Effects of smoking a 1.3 mg nicotine delivery cigarette (real cigarette) (filled circles), sham smoking (activity control) (squares) and situation control (open circles) on EEG alpha activity during (*a*) relaxing and (*b*) stressful conditions for 24 subjects in each condition. EEG alpha activity is expressed as the percentage deviation from baseline EEG alpha activity levels measured at the beginning of each condition. Note that smoking decreased alpha activity during relaxation (stimulant effect) but increased alpha activity during stress (depressant effect). (From Mangan & Golding, 1978.)

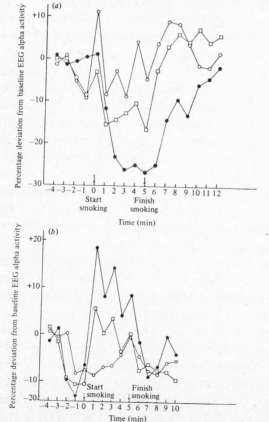

appeared to be a systematic relationship between the vigour with which a cigarette was smoked and the level of situation-induced arousal. Smokers under stress smoked their cigarettes significantly more vigorously (as assessed by puff number, duration and pressure, depth of inhalation, and residual butt weight) than during sensory isolation. This observation is consistent with the hypothesis that high rates of nicotine intake tend to favour depressant rather than stimulant effects.

However, the view that large doses of nicotine favour depressant effects is not unaminous. Izard *et al.* (1979) observed that those smokers who wish to stimulate themselves or arouse their cerebral cortex automatically take a considerably higher dose of nicotine. It may be that the contradiction is more apparent than real, in that studies of the stimulant versus depressant outcome of nicotine dosage between individuals (see Izard *et al.*, 1979) are different from those studies utilising within-subject variations caused by situational stress. In particular, it may be noted that Izard *et al.* (1979) found that non-smokers and light smokers tended to obtain depressant effects whereas heavy smokers (who obtained higher blood nicotine levels) tended to show more stimulant effects. Tolerance to the effects of nicotine in the heavy smoker may be a crucial confounding factor.

The complexity of analysis of the final outcome of cigarette smoking in terms of the biphasic dose–response effects of nicotine interacting with the starting state of the brain is further increased by consideration of smoking behaviour itself. The behavioural as opposed to nicotine contribution of smoking to EEG effects can be considered at three levels:

(i) Effects from the initiation of the behaviour (whether driven by internal attempts at nicotine homeostasis or arousal modulation, or direct external cues such as the social suggestion of other smokers).

(ii) The direct effects of activity; motor and sensory feedback from lighting up, taste, inhalation and the smell of smoking.

(iii) Conditioning of the feedback stimuli from smoking behaviour to the direct pharmacological effects of nicotine.

Any or all of these possible contributors to the EEG effects of smoking are important, and are often lumped together as 'secondary reinforcing' effects of smoking. Thus mecamylamine, a centrally acting nicotine antagonist, will completely block EEG desynchronisation in the cerebral cortex and olfactory bulb of both alert and *encéphale isolé* cats which has been caused by nicotine injection, but will not totally blockade those effects when nicotine is administered via smoke into the lungs (Hall, 1970). It would appear from this result that the stimulus of the smoke itself is sufficient to cause some degree of EEG arousal. Olfactory bulb stimulation by tobacco smoke is likely to be important since this is the only 'direct' sensory route into the brain. 'The olfactory system breaks all the laws that seem to govern the organisation of other sensory mechanisms. It is, as we have noted, the only system known in which the primary sensory neurons lie at the body surface. There is no transducing element, as there is in say, Corti's organ; the olfactory epithelial cell itself is buffeted by the external environment' (Nauta & Feirtag, 1979). Similarly, in humans, there is evidence that smoking behaviour, as opposed to nicotine, provides some of the observed effects of smoking on EEG activity. Thus, controls such as inhalation of nicotine-free smoke or sham smoking with a glass tube filled with cotton wool can produce similar effects to those found when humans smoke cigarettes containing nicotine, namely, an upward shift of dominant alpha frequency by 1 or 2 Hz (Hauser, Schwarz, Roth & Bickford, 1958), and reduction of EEG alpha activity (Murphree *et al.*, 1967).

The picture is complicated by individual differences in the degree to which these 'secondary reinforcing' effects occur. Hauser *et al.* (1958) noted that while over 80% of all subjects showed this frequency shift after cigarette smoking, 30% of the subjects showed the shift during the initial inhalation (i.e., before nicotine could arrive at the CNS). These subject differences may reflect some conditioning of smoking behaviour to pharmacological effects, and may help to explain why pharmacological control of central nicotine levels, whether by the use of nicotine blocking agents or by the pre-loading of subjects with nicotine, does not affect smoking rates to the extent we might expect.

Phasic electroencephalogram: evoked potentials, photic driving, contingent negative variation

By contrast with the generally stimulant effects of nicotine and cigarette smoking on tonic EEG activity, both depressant and stimulant effects have been reported on phasic EEG activity. For average evoked potential amplitudes, stimulant (Hall *et al.*, 1973; Friedman, Goldberg, Horvarth & Meares, 1974*a*) and depressant effects (Vasquez & Toman, 1967; Knott & Venables, 1978) of smoking, compared to smoking deprivation, have been reported. Depressant effects of smoking can be inferred from the Vogel, Broverman & Klaiber (1977) study on photic driving. They found that after 3 h of deprivation, smokers exhibited a greater frequency of EEG 'driving' responses to photic stimulation than non-smokers, and that smoking one cigarette resulted in a reduction of EEG driving responses to a level comparable to that of non-smokers. These findings in humans are congruent with animal studies; smoking dosages of nicotine (12.5 μg kg^{-1} of body weight) reduce evoked potential amplitudes in the cat auditory cortex while simultaneously increasing general CNS excitation (Pradhan & Guha, 1976).

Knott & Venables (1978) suggest that smoking may be able to stimulate CNS inhibitory mechanisms (without simultaneous reductions in CNS excitatory processes) and that this results in the 'screening out' of irrelevant and irritating sensory input from consciousness. This suggestion agrees with the finding that tobacco smoking increases the rate of habituation to intense auditory stimuli, measured by EEG alpha-blocking response (Friedman, Horvath & Meares, 1974b). In addition, animal work suggests a possible site of action of nicotine on these inhibitory processes. Relying on previously reported studies (Bhattacharya & Goldstein, 1970; Nelsen, Pelley & Goldstein, 1973) which implicated the hippocampal limbic system as the major target area for nicotine, Nelsen, Pelley & Goldstein (1975) examined the hypothesis that if the reticular formation and limbic arousal systems are mutually inhibitory (Routtenberg, 1968), then nicotine-induced limbic (hippocampal) system arousal should counteract the behavioural disruption resulting from electrical stimulation of the reticular formation. Administration of nicotine (100 μg kg^{-1} of body weight) did, indeed, attenuate the behavioural disruption caused by

Fig. 12. Mean dose-response curve in six subjects showing the effect of intravenous (i.v.) nicotine (each dose given as five 'shots') expressed as the change in mean magnitude of CNV relative to mean saline control. Note the biphasic shape of the curve: smaller doses produce an increase in CNV magnitude (stimulant effect) and larger doses produce a decrease in CNV magnitude (depressant effect) relative to saline control. Correlated T-test for significance of difference between mean CNV with nicotine and mean CNV with saline for each dose: *p < 0.05; **p < 0.01. (From Ashton *et al.*, 1978.)

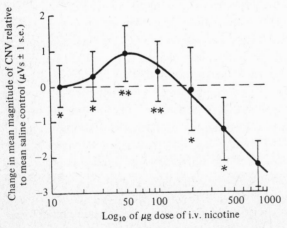

stimulation of the reticular formation in rats executing a visual performance task. From these results the authors suggested that a possible reinforcement for smoking is a reduction in reticular activation when this is manifested as over-arousal in excessively stimulating environments.

However, the two studies mentioned at the beginning of this section clearly indicate stimulant rather than depressant effects of cigarette smoking on the evoked potential. One possible explanation for these results may be that, given the variations in subject population and smoking style, these smokers absorbed doses of nicotine which were in fact stimulant. Support for this contention comes from the studies of Ashton *et al.* (1974, 1978, 1980) concerning the effects of cigarette smoking and dosages of nicotine on the contingent negative variation (CNV) in man. The results of this work clearly demonstrate that smoking can produce stimulant or depressant effects on the CNV, the direction of which is dependent on the rate of smoking or the dose of nicotine (Fig. 12).

Reinforcing mechanisms of nicotine for smoking
The importance of nicotine as a reinforcer

The evidence that nicotine is the primary reinforcer for tobacco consumption comes from three main sources.

(1) There is the circumstantial evidence that smoking is almost exclusively practised when there is the consequent absorption of some psychoactive drug, e.g., an opiate, cannabis or nicotine itself. In addition, there is the observation that the absorption of nicotine is the common denominator of cigarette, cigar and pipe smoking, and the snuffing or chewing of tobacco, rather than some other agent derived from tobacco, e.g., tar or CO. Also consistent with this view is evidence that the most popular mode of tobacco consumption, inhalation-style cigarette smoking, leads to the quickest and most efficient absorption of nicotine.

(2) There is the evidence, reviewed earlier (Chapter 2: Simple addiction models), that experimental manipulation of the availability of nicotine to the postulated target receptors in the CNS by means of 'pre-loading' the smoker with oral or i.v. nicotine, by using selective nicotinic receptor blockers, or by reducing/increasing cigarette nicotine delivery, produces variations in the predicted direction (plus or minus) in cigarette consumption or in the vigour with which the cigarette is smoked.

(3) There is evidence that nicotine is self-administered by animals, although it is far less powerful as a reinforcer than is amphetamine or cocaine (see Chapter 4: Animal models).

These three strands of evidence, of which the circumstantial evidence is arguably the strongest, suggest that nicotine is the primary reinforcer for the smoking habit. However, the relative importance of nicotine as a reinforcer no doubt varies between individuals. Thus, some smokers, particularly non-inhaling pipe smokers, appear to absorb relatively small quantities of nicotine. The main reinforcer for these smokers may be the taste and smell of tobacco smoke (including the effects of nicotine on sensory receptors), with the additional pleasurable aspects of sucking on the pipe. Such 'oral' type behaviours apparently can be extremely pleasurable in the absence of any reinforcement by psychoactive drug or nutritive substance, as evidenced by the popularity of chewing gum.

It is also probable that the importance of nicotine as a reinforcer may vary over time and circumstances. Thus, some of the failures to demonstrate significant control of smoking behaviour by means of varying nicotine availability to central receptors may be explicable if an 'Arousal Modulation' rather than a simple 'Nicotine Addiction' model of smoking is advocated. The former model postulates that nicotine assumes greatest importance as a mood control agent when the smoker is over-excited or anxious or drowsy and fatigued. Under more 'neutral' conditions, cigarette smoking continues by virtue of the secondary reinforcing properties acquired from nicotine action under more extreme states of arousal.

Specific reinforcing mechanisms

Many effects of nicotine could in fact be reinforcing. These include the alerting and muscle relaxant effects, the facilitation of memory or attention and the decrease of appetite and irritability. Before these are analysed in any great detail it is as well to acknowledge, however, that nicotine overdose can be extremely aversive and even fatal. Such unpleasant effects as nausea, vomiting and diarrhoea may occur when the novice tries his or her first cigarette. This may deter some people from taking up the habit. Indeed, the aversive consequences of nicotine overdose have been employed with mixed success in 'rapid smoking' regimes as one smoking-cessation intervention technique (see Chapter 5). However, nicotine as taken by the average smoker, i.e., in small doses, would appear to be highly reinforcing. The possible reinforcing mechanisms of nicotine are analysed in terms of the peripheral and central physiological effects and effects on mood and performance (the latter being dealt with in greater detail in Chapter 4).

The cardiovascular system. It is possible that increased heart rate and associated effects of nicotine on the CVS represent one of the reinforcers of the smoking habit. The most obvious mechanism for reinforcement is that smokers have chronically low heart rates which they wish to elevate to cope with their day-to-day activities. However, evidence does not bear this out. Larson & Silvette (1971), from a review of the available data, conclude that smokers, on average, have similar pulse rates to non-smokers. Unfortunately, no longitudinal data on heart rate of smokers before commencement of the habit are available, as far as we are aware, so that the non-significance of any differences could possibly be ascribed to chronic effects of nicotine on the smoker's heart rate.

Schachter (1973) makes the interesting suggestion that, paradoxically, the 'calming' effects ascribed to cigarette smoking may be due to the general sympathetic arousal caused by cigarette smoking, of which heart rate is one measure. This essentially 'attribution' theory of the calming properties of smoking suggests that in a fearful situation the smoker will light up in order to ascribe the feedback of sympathetic responses he is experiencing, as a result of his fears or anxieties, to the sympathomimetic effects of the cigarette. Thus, the smoker relabels the visceral sensations he is experiencing as pleasurable.

Apart from Schachter's cognitive hypothesis, an explanation of the calming effects of smoking can be inferred from the Law of Initial Value: 'high autonomic excitation preceding stimulation is correlated with low autonomic reactivity upon stimulation' (Lacey, 1956). According to this view, smoking will exert a calming influence by increasing autonomic excitation, thus reducing autonomic reactivity to further aversive stimulation. Similar explanations might be couched in terms of Lacey's (1967) hypothesis that 'sensory-rejection is associated with heart rate acceleration', together with the subsequent work by Hare (1975), which supports the notion that heart rate elevations in anticipation of shock may form part of a defensive response (Sokolov, 1963), this being indicative of a coping response to a stressor.

However, there are two major difficulties with any model of smoking behaviour in which heart rate elevation is a primary reinforcer for the habit. Firstly, a rapid cardiovascular tolerance occurs over the course of a few cigarettes, and so will attenuate any major cardiovascular effects after the first few cigarettes of the day, although it is true that 'tonic' heart rate will rise through the course of a day's smoking. This can be seen in Schachter's own experiment in which the second cigarette produces relatively little further heart rate elevation (Fig. 13).

Secondly, adrenergic blockade with *beta*-adrenergic blockers, such as oxprenolol, largely prevent the sympathomimetic effects of smoking, but do not prevent the subjective pleasurable effects (Carruthers, 1976). In fact, it is established that these blockers themselves have anxiolytic properties (Turner, Granville-Grossman & Smart, 1965; Taggart & Carruthers,

1972), probably because they damp down sympathetic over-activity associated with stress.

Such considerations reinforce the view that the pleasures associated with smoking are mainly due to direct stimulation of the central nervous system which is relatively unaffected by *beta*-blockade, rather than the easily suppressible peripheral consequences of increased sympathetic activity.

Release of catecholamines. As stated above, the peripheral sympathomimetic effects of nicotine can be blocked by a variety of agents. However, the work of Carruthers (1976), discussed above, suggests that oxprenolol, a *beta*-receptor blocker with mainly peripheral effects, does not appear to diminish the subjective pleasurable effects of smoking, which are presumably centrally mediated. Thus peripheral catecholamine changes associated with cigarette smoking may reflect more important CNS effects, rather than being major reinforcers for the smoking habit in their own right, although the evidence is far from conclusive.

Release of other hormones. Release of ADH has not been suggested as a reinforcer for smoking. Similarly, the motivation for coffee and alcohol consumption, which are often associated with smoking behaviour, has not been interpreted in terms of the known diuretic effects of these stimulants

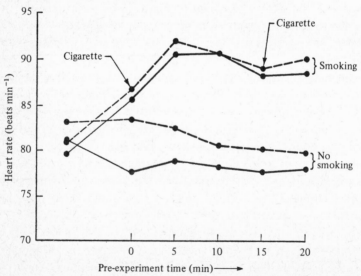

Fig. 13. The effects of electric shock and smoking on heart rate. Dashed lines, electric shock treatment; solid lines, no electric shock. (From Schachter, 1973.)

(by inhibition of reabsorption from the kidney tubules and inhibition of ADH release from the posterior pituitary, respectively) (Laurence, 1973). However, ADH is also released in the brain itself and may be involved in facilitating memory (*Lancet*, 1979b). This may explain some of the known effects of smoking on memory (see Chapter 4: Consolidation).

The reinforcing aspects of growth hormones would appear to be rather long term and can probably be disregarded as a factor of major importance in the maintenance of smoking behaviour.

By contrast, the nicotine-induced release of corticosteroids has been suggested as a putative reinforcer of smoking. Stimulation of adreno-cortical activity by enhanced corticotrophin release (Kershbaum *et al.*, 1968) has been suggested to act as a reinforcer for smoking by increasing the output of corticosteroids in individuals with slow or inadequate corticosteroid production in face of stress (Grant, 1968). If this is true, we would predict that smokers, compared to non-smokers, should show less corticosteroid release to stress, and that smoking should augment the inadequate stress-induced corticosteroid release in the smoker.

Conversely, if the corticosteroid levels of heavy smokers are substantially elevated, we might argue that some of the minor withdrawal effects experienced by heavy smokers when giving up the habit may be due to rebound loss of corticosteroid production. High blood levels of steroid prevent release of corticotrophin (negative feedback achieved either by acting directly on the pituitary or indirectly on corticotrophin-releasing factor (CRF) release from the hypothalamus), which in turn results in corticosteroid hypofunction (Laurence, 1973). Some of the minor with-drawal effects of 'giving up' in a heavy smoker may thus be analogous to the catastrophe which can follow sudden withdrawal of clinical steroid therapy.

Unfortunately, there appear to be no experiments which directly examine these hypotheses, although the study of Tucci & Sode (1972) on a group of 94 non-smokers and non-deprived light and heavy smokers revealed no significant differences in plasma cortisol and urinary cortico-steroid levels between any of these groups. This type of study, although useful, illustrates the importance of including deprived smokers as controls, since we could postulate that the basal level of corticosteroid production by the deprived smoker would be lower than that of the non-smoker. However, the authors note that there were no significant differences in circadian variation of corticosteroid levels between smokers and non-smokers. Since the smoker will not be smoking for some part of the night, this acts as a partial non-smoking smoker control, and reinforces the view that corticosteroid release is not an important reinforcing factor in smoking. The same study did demonstrate a slight non-significant elevation of urinary adrenaline and depression of noradrenaline in heavy smokers as compared to non-smokers, as might be expected (see above: Specific effects on neural/hormonal mechanisms, release of catecholamines; see also Chapter 2: Simple addiction models, and later this chapter as regards the possible release of central 'opiate' peptides concurrently with cortico-trophin release).

Skeletal muscle. Although the relaxing effect of cigarette smoking on skeletal muscle has been suggested as reinforcing for the habit, especially in stressful situations (Russell, 1976), the evidence and its interpretation are uncertain. Firstly, although the depressant effects of cigarette smoking on muscle reflex are well proven, and, unlike cardiovascular system changes, do not seem to be subject to rapid tolerance (Domino, 1973), it is not known for certain whether tonic muscle activity is reduced as well. Indeed, the few reports examining the effects of cigarette smoking on tonic EMG activity suggest that this is not the case (Fagerstrom & Gotestam, 1977; Golding, 1980).

Secondly, the extent to which the observed increase of EMG activity (especially phasic) during stress and anxiety merely reflects central events is arguable. There is also the question of whether the feedback from increased muscle tension can contribute to, or modulate, the perception of stress. Analogously, this question also arises when considering the reasons for the effectiveness of the benzodiazepine minor tranquillisers. These are relatively selective for the limbic system, which is concerned with emotional control (probably by modulating GABA, an inhibitory neurotransmitter (see *Trends in NeuroSciences*, 1978)). The benzodiazepines also have central muscle-relaxant effects (Laurence, 1973) which may be secondary to, or independent of, the former mechanism, and so contribute to the final anxiolytic effects.

A similar central versus peripheral debate arises in the case of progressive desensitisation therapies for phobias and EMG biofeedback for anxiety states. Some theorists take the view that reduction of muscle tension is incompatible with states of anxiety, and so reduces anxiety. By contrast, there is experimental evidence that feedback from voluntary muscle can throw 'noise' into the system and scotomise perception of stressful situations (Murphy, 1970). This idea can be traced back to Wilhelm Reich's (1949) concept of 'character armour' and to the Eastern martial arts, where muscle relaxation is emphasised, in part, to prevent the individual 'scotomising' his environment, which would reduce his capacity to observe any impending attack.

The smoking-induced increase in muscle tremor discussed earlier is likely to be a disadvantage to the smoker carrying out any activities requiring precise muscle control, e.g., threading a needle, fine drawing, pistol shooting.

In summary, therefore, it is difficult to state with any confidence whether a reduction in tonic muscle tension in the stressed cigarette smoker will be reinforcing. Moreover, the well-known phenomenon of response specificity (idiosyncratic responding in muscular, visceral or cardiovascular systems) (Barrell & Price, 1977; Eysenck, 1977) indicates that only a certain proportion of smokers will respond maximally in the muscular system. Many individuals will have a greater response in the cardiovascular system or viscera.

The electrodermal system. Perception of smoking effects on electrodermal activity (a small increase in sweating) by the smoker is unlikely to have major reinforcing value. Electrodermal effects are best regarded as reflecting central stimulant actions of nicotine on tonic autonomic responding and depressant actions on phasic autonomic responding respectively. Decreased phasic autonomic responding may reflect the 'filtering out' of distracting or aversive stimuli. Indeed, Knott (1979*b*) presents some electrodermal, evoked potential and performance evidence to support his contention that smokers, compared to non-smokers, may be rather poor at stimulus filtering and so use cigarettes as a 'stimulus barrier'.

Body weight. The appetite-suppressant effects of nicotine provided by cigarette smoking may be regarded as rewarding in the classic 'drive reduction' sense for the hungry smoker. Moreover, the possible weight gain of the smoker who gives up, caused by increased appetite and lowered metabolic rate, may be a serious deterrent to giving up smoking, especially for women.

The brain. Although the physical activity of smoking itself may effect changes in the CNS, these can be considered secondary in importance compared to the effects of the postulated primary reinforcer, nicotine. The EEG changes and the behavioural arousal which follow nicotine injections are prevented by mecamylamine. This shows that they are mediated by cholinergic mechanisms (Domino, 1967; Hall, 1970). However, as mentioned earlier, this direct cholinergic action of nicotine can lead to the release of many central neurotransmitters. Considering the rapid clearance of nicotine from the brain, which is of the order of a few minutes, compared with the much longer time intervals usually experienced between smoking successive cigarettes, it is plausible to argue that the secondary changes induced by these neurotransmitters are the main determinants of smoking behaviour.

Nicotine-induced noradrenaline release (Bhagat, 1970; Hall & Turner, 1972) is of particular interest, since activity in the hypothalamic reward system seems to involve catecholamine release (Stein & Wise, 1967). However, nicotine also has a direct influence on hypothalamic electrical self-stimulating behaviour in a biphasic dose-dependent manner (Domino, 1973). We might thus view the reinforcing nature of nicotine as being due to secondary release of central catecholamines signalling reward in a manner analogous to the reinforcing role of amphetamine.

However, while at a crude level of analysis this view of the major reinforcing effect of nicotine is attractive, it ignores the still little-understood relationship between arousal and reward-punishment systems. Since the immediate effects of reward are well known to be arousing (Gray, 1971), although ultimately de-arousing in the classic 'drive reduction' sense of appetitive behaviour, we can account for the stimulant effects of nicotine on tonic EEG measures. Similarly, increased arousal seems to focus attention (Wachtel, 1967), thus inhibiting responses to irrelevant stimuli, which could account for the increase in habituation rates found by Friedman *et al.* (1974). A similar 'stimulus filter' model has been proposed by Knott & Venables (1978) on the basis of their own and other experiments on evoked potentials and photic driving.

Alternatively, the reverse viewpoint is equally plausible, i.e., that nicotine, by virtue of its biphasic stimulant and depressant effects can shift arousal to a hypothetical 'arousal optimum' (Berlyne, 1971), and so signal reward. The resolution of these two viewpoints may involve the exact nature of the stimuli impinging upon the smoker. Thus the nicotine-induced shift from reticular to limbic system control of cortical activity found by Nelsen *et al.* (1973) may reflect the activation of an arousal system which focuses mainly on those stimuli in the environment which have rewarding value. This explanation of limbic versus reticular system involvement in nicotine reinforcement is based upon the two-arousal-system theory of Routtenberg (1968). Such a model would simultaneously account for the hypothesised directly rewarding effects of nicotine by stimulation of 'reward systems' and for the filtering out of irrelevant or unpleasant stimuli which, in turn, would signal reward.

At a pharmacological level the relationship between the attentional aspects of arousal and reward-punishment systems becomes even closer, even though imperfectly understood. The link between noradrenaline and reward is probably much more complex than suggested by the original experiments of Stein & Wise (1967) relating noradrenaline release to electrical self-stimulation behaviour in the 'reward pathways' of the hypothalamus. There is evidence that specific lesioning of noradrenergic pathways with 6-hydroxydopamine does not interfere with the ability of rats to learn simple behaviours for food reward, nor with avoidance of direct and indirect punishment, but does interfere with extinction and those tasks involving complex environmental stimuli. Mason (1979) suggests that the noradrenergic pathways are not directly involved with reward and punishment per se, but are concerned with the direction of attention, i.e., 'stimulus sampling' by reward and punishment systems. Further pharmacological analysis of this issue in terms of smoking behaviour awaits a fuller understanding of the precise mechanisms involved. These no doubt include dopamine, 5-HT and peptides.

Finally, some evidence points to the involvement of 'opiate-like' peptides in the rewarding effects of nicotine. We have already noted suggestions that nicotine may cause the release of 'internal opiates', this being based on the observation that *beta*-endorphin and adrenocorticotrophin are secreted concomitantly in the pituitary gland (see Chapter 2: Simple addiction models). There is some evidence, admittedly patchy, supporting this. Thus naloxone (a specific opiate antagonist) appears to prevent a postulated nicotine-mediated endorphin release associated with variations in respiratory rate due to smoking (Tobin, Jenouri & Sackner, 1982). While this piece of evidence may not be immediately convincing as regards the rewarding nature of smoking, it is suggestive of some opiate peptide involvement in nicotine action. More persuasive is the demonstration that naloxone, as opposed to a double-blind placebo, reduced cigarette consumption by 30% in a group of habitual smokers who were ad-lib. smoking, and also reduced their subjective desire to smoke (Karras & Kane, 1980). The authors suggest that nicotine-induced *beta*-endorphin release is the positive reinforcer for smoking; blockade with naloxone prevents the rewarding effects of the opiate-like peptide and thus removes the motivation to smoke. However it is equally plausible to suggest that, under these conditions, smokers should increase their smoking in an attempt to overcome the opioid blockade, an effect consistent with the results obtained using central nicotine blockade (see Chapter 2: Simple addiction models; Stolerman *et al.*, 1973b; and Chapter 4: Animal models). One resolution of this theoretical dilemma is to postulate that such increases in smoking are relatively transient, occurring before the smoker gives up in the absence of direct pharmacological reinforcement. Certainly it is a common observation that rats lever-pressing for food reward on a partial-reinforcement schedule will show transient increases in lever-pressing before the behaviour finally extinguishes. The involvement of an opiate-like peptide release as a reinforcer for smoking, if true, suggests obvious addiction analogies and also possible smoking cessation strategies (see Chapter 5: Drug therapy).

SUMMARY

Nicotine has biphasic dose-related effects at nicotinic cholinergic receptors, being stimulant in small doses and depressant at larger doses. However, it is difficult to predict whether a given dose of nicotine, that is stimulant or depressant at the receptor level, will be similarly stimulant or depressant at higher levels of neural organisation. This is because nicotine action leads to the release of a wide variety of central and peripheral neurotransmitters and hormones (ACh, NA, Ad, 5-HT, ACTH) which themselves may have excitatory or inhibitory actions. Thus, depressant effects may be caused by stimulation of inhibitory systems and vice-versa.

Nicotine is most rapidly and efficiently absorbed by inhalation-style smoking of cigarettes in quantities sufficient to produce easily observable effects. These include increased heart rate; the release of circulatory hormones such as Ad, ADH and corticosteroids together with mobilisation of free fatty acids and perhaps glucose; depression of simple muscle reflexes together with stimulant and depressant effects on muscle tone and activity; increased bowel activity under some circumstances; stimulation of peripheral sensory receptors, particularly in the mouth; increased sweating activity under most conditions; and, finally, both stimulant and depressant effects on a variety of measures of central activity such as EEG, evoked potentials, photic driving and the CNV. While some of these actions of nicotine may be strictly peripheral (e.g., stimulation of sensory receptors) central actions of nicotine appear to be of primary importance.

The sensorimotor aspects of smoking (smell, taste and physical manipulation) may have important central effects, especially with regards to olfactory stimulation. These effects, together with possible classically conditioned responses, formed through association between the sensorimotor stimuli and subsequent arrival of nicotine at the target receptors, are often referred to as the 'secondary reinforcing' properties of smoking.

For the cigarette smoker, probably the most important reinforcing feature of nicotine obtained from a cigarette is its dual nature as both a tranquilliser and a stimulant. Moreover, there is some evidence that smokers may alter their smoking behaviour in a manner consistent with obtaining stimulant or depressant actions appropriate to their prior state of arousal.

4

Smoking recruitment and maintenance

We have already described putative smoking motives, and explored, in some detail, the reinforcing effects of nicotine. In this chapter, we plan to assess the empirical support offered for these different propositions. As a preliminary, however, we shall make a brief excursion into animal smoking models to see whether these offer any clues about factors underlying human smoking.

Animal models

Self-administration of nicotine and tobacco smoke are, of course, not confined to humans. In his monograph *The Descent of Man* (1871), Charles Darwin recorded that many monkeys 'smoked tobacco with pleasure', as well as having 'a strong taste for tea, coffee and spirituous liquors'. Similar anecdotal accounts are given by a number of authors (see Gritz & Siegel, 1979, for review). However, it is often noted that animals in the wild are much less likely to ingest tobacco intentionally than when captive or domesticated. It has been suggested that this may be because stress or 'despair' predisposes the animal in captivity to tobacco usage (Marais, 1936), or, more simply, that captive and domesticated animals self-administer tobacco and its products only because they are provided by humans, who, in fact, provide all nutritional needs (Gritz & Siegel, 1979).

For whatever reason, difficulties have arisen in constructing animal 'models' of smoking, although somewhat more success has been achieved in demonstrating self-administration by animals of nicotine via injection. Various studies have shown that both monkeys (Deneau & Inoki, 1967) and rats (Clark, 1969; Hanson, Ivester & Morton, 1979) will self-inject nicotine for its own sake. The amounts (weight-corrected) of nicotine self-injected approximate those obtainable in human smoking. Further parallels with human smoking are that monkeys tend to cease self-injection at night, when the lights are out, and also appear to have 'preferred' levels of nicotine. Thus, self-injection of doses of nicotine below 10 μg kg^{-1} of body weight fails to reinforce lever pressing for injection, while doses greater than 500 μg kg^{-1} of body weight actively prevent self-injections in most cases (Deneau & Inoki, 1967).

As in the case of human smoking (Stolerman *et al.*, 1973*b*), mecamylamine (a central nicotinic blocker) but not pentolinium (a peripheral nicotinic blocker) produces a temporary increase in the rate of nicotine self-administration in rats (Hanson *et al.*, 1979), presumably as the rats try to overcome the blockade of the central effects of nicotine. Omission of nicotine causes extinction of the operant behaviour (bar-pressing) for self-injection, but this extinction is slow. In most cases, 'priming' with free nicotine reinforcements promotes self-administration (Deneau & Inoki, 1967; Hanson *et al.*, 1979), an effect similar to that reported for electrical self-stimulation of the brain in animals (Rolls, 1975). The exact function of 'priming', in terms of increasing arousal and thus 'activating' or 'reminding' the animal, is, however, uncertain. A close analogy can be made with the concept of incentive motivation (Hebb, 1949) or 'drive induction', best observed under zero-drive conditions, to explain why a small 'free' reward will often increase the motivation (or 'drive') of an animal to perform some operant task in order to obtain more of this same reward. This can be observed in humans as well as in animals, and is commonly referred to as the 'salted-peanut effect'. Consumption of one or a few peanuts increases the appetite of that individual for more peanuts. Conventional drive theory, on the other hand, predicts the opposite, i.e., the more peanuts eaten, the lower the hunger drive observed. Eventually, of course, this is in fact true.

Although nicotine is self-administered by animals, it is far less powerful as a reinforcer than amphetamine, cocaine, opiates and barbiturates (Yanagita, 1977; Hanson *et al.*, 1979; Goodman & Gilman, 1980). The reasons for this are unclear. However, it is possible that nicotine does not produce as great a release or elevation of central catecholamines thought to be involved in reward as amphetamine and cocaine; nor does nicotine cause equivalent relief from withdrawal symptoms, since the nicotine withdrawal syndrome is in no way as great as that observed for opiates and barbiturates. Moreover, it is clear that animals can discriminate between the effects of nicotine and those of other psychoactive drugs such as lysergic acid diethylamide (LSD) (a hallucinogen), morphine and arecoline (a muscarinic agonist (Rosencrans, 1979)). Rats trained on a two-lever operant discrimination task for food reward, in which the discriminant stimulus (nicotine versus saline, and morphine, or vice versa) is associated with food reward on one of the two levers, show up to 85% discrimination accuracy. Interestingly, the discrimination between nicotine and D-amphetamine is not so accurate, which suggests that part of the central effect of nicotine is similar to that of D-amphetamine. This could well be the central catecholamine release known to be caused by both drugs (see Chapter 3: Pharmacology of nicotine). Consistent with this view was the observation that, apart from central nicotinic blockade itself, a catecholamine synthesis blocker (*alpha*-methyl-tyrosine) was alone in disrupting the discriminant response to nicotine amongst a wide range of other selective antagonists (peripheral alpha- and beta-adrenergic, peripheral nicotinic, 5-HT synthesis and muscarinic).

Given the relative difficulty in demonstrating self-administration of nicotine by animals, as opposed to other psychoactive drugs, it is not surprising that great difficulty has been encountered in producing voluntary smoking behaviour in animals. Those medical experiments in which animals have been forced to inhale tobacco from cigarettes fitted to face masks, from trachea tubes (e.g., the smoking beagles) or by placing the whole animal in a smoke-filled chamber (see Gritz & Siegel, 1979, for review), do not represent animal models of voluntary smoking.

'Voluntary' smoking behaviour has been demonstrated with monkeys who are initially trained to suck air from tubes using rewards such as sweetened water. A number of studies have shown that monkeys, in a free choice situation, will preferentially suck tubes delivering air passing over heated tobacco rather than air passing over an empty heated chamber (Van Laer & Jarvik, 1963), or, under appropriate conditions, will 'smoke' cigarettes mounted on plexiglass plates or vapours distilled from tobacco. This behaviour can be maintained with no other reward, and on a free-choice basis (Jarvik, 1967, 1973). Similar results have been demonstrated for cannabis smoke (Pickens & Thompson, 1972).

Since there is great intersubject variability in this 'smoking' behaviour, some experimenters have utilised reinforcements such as sweetened liquids to shape and maintain the monkey's puffing activity in order to obtain more stable puffing rates (Ando & Yanagita, 1981). However, this so-called 'schedule-controlled' smoking, while producing a more invariable and robust 'smoking' activity, removes the voluntary element in smoking. It is doubtful, therefore, whether data of these sort can provide an empirical base for an animal model of smoking.

A more important general criticism of monkey smoking models refers to the extent to which this type of smoking behaviour actually resembles human smoking. In one important characteristic it does not, as monkeys tend to take many hundreds of small puffs; 'sucking' rather than 'smoking' behaviour might be a more appropriate term. It may be that monkeys have insufficient voluntary control of their respiratory apparatus to enable satisfactory inhalation of smoke compared with humans, who have developed better voluntary control of respiration since this is necessary for speech. We note here the lack of success in teaching primates to speak, as opposed to the more successful attempts to teach them 'sign language'. Nevertheless, smoking monkeys have achieved significant levels of plasma nicotine, whether it be by puffing, swallowing or inhaling. In some cases these plasma nicotine levels are comparable to nicotine levels achieved by human smokers (Ando & Yanagita, 1981).

The situation as regards the control of monkey smoking behaviour by means of nicotine pre-loading or use of nicotine blocking agents is more confused. Thus Jarvik (1973), commenting on the observation that injections of mecamylamine (a central nicotinic receptor antagonist) reduce monkeys' preference for cigarette smoke, suggested that mecamylamine blocks the action of nicotine, precluding its rewarding effect and thus resulting in a loss of preference for the smoke. The opposite result in human cigarette smokers, i.e., that mecamylamine produces an increase in smoking rate, has been explained as the attempt to overcome central nicotine blockade (Stolerman *et al.*, 1973*b*). On the face of it, these explanations are contradictory.

Such contradictions may have prompted Russell (1979) to question whether nicotine is rewarding, or whether it is in fact aversive. He suggests that much of the evidence concerning the role of nicotine in the smoking habit is explicable from the reverse point of view. If nicotine is regarded as aversive, particularly at higher dosage levels, then it is quite obvious why smokers should reduce their smoking after nicotine pre-loading or after increased cigarette nicotine delivery, and, conversely, why they should increase their smoking when challenged with central nicotine blockers or reduced nicotine delivery cigarettes. However, the most likely explanation is that certain levels of nicotine are rewarding and that levels above and below are aversive and frustrating respectively.

There is a simple explanation which might account for the uncertainty concerning the role of nicotine blockers. Assuming that nicotine, albeit in small doses only, is rewarding, then the effect of blocking this reward on the operant behaviour of smoking, either by use of selective antagonists such as mecamylamine, or by omission of nicotine (e.g., hot air only), is predictable from general learning theory. Omission of reinforcement will initially produce an increase in responding, especially if the behaviour has been reinforced on a partial reinforcement schedule (the so-called invigorating effects of 'frustrative non-reward' (Gray, 1971)). However, should this increase in response rate produce no reward, then eventually response extinction will occur. The latter happens when nicotine is omitted altogether (e.g., herbal cigarettes) or is presented in such low doses (e.g., some ultra-low tar brand cigarettes) as to make smoking simply not worth the effort. Similarly, it is highly probable that the human smokers subjected to nicotinic blockade in Stolerman, *et al*.'s study (1973*b*) would eventually have stopped smoking if the blockade had been complete and had lasted for a longer period of time; no doubt they would have behaved similarly to Jarvik's monkeys.

It is obvious that a good deal of progress has been made in the past decade in developing animal models of smoking behaviour, although a number of difficulties still need to be resolved. While the comment 'This work has so far not revealed anything about smoking in humans which could not be done equally with human subjects', made by Russell (1976) regarding animal smoking as compared with nicotine self-injection undoubtedly has some substance, there is no reason for doubting the importance of such a development in the future, as indeed is proving to be the case in other problem areas such as schizophrenia research. Experiments which, on ethical grounds, are difficult to conduct with human subjects would then be possible. For example, subjects could be exposed to high and continuous levels of stress, as was Brady's 'executive monkey', and the use of drugs such as nicotine under these circumstances could then be examined. It would also be of interest to determine, in a monkey smoking group, the role of imitation of adult smoking in the recruitment of young animals to the habit.

Recruitment to smoking
There is little doubt that recruitment occurs mainly during very early to middle adolescence (Surgeon General, 1979, Appendix A, p. 14; Bewley *et al*., 1974), that boys tend to smoke more than girls (although this sex difference is reducing) and that the percentage smoking increases with age: by the age of 17 years, nearly 30% of boys and 25% of girls in the UK smoke. The figures vary between regions, ethnic groups and countries; in Japan, for example, there is a much greater sex discrepancy in cigarette smoking (males smoking more than females) than in other developed countries (Todd, 1978). To take another example, Bewley, Johnson, Bland & Murray (1980) present survey data demonstrating that smoking prevalence has significantly decreased from 25.1% in 1974 to 19.7% in 1977 for girls aged 14–15 years whereas smoking prevalence for boys remained relatively constant and only decreased from 24.8% to 24.1%

over the same period. Bewley *et al.* (1980) comment that this sex trend in adolescent smoking prevalence is at variance with many other studies both in the UK and in other countries, and suggest that regional variations may be important.

Most individuals have either tried smoking or had the opportunity of accepting a cigarette during their adolescence or teens. The factors which determine in what way a smoker emerges from the initial encounter with tobacco, are not clear, however. At first sight, factors of primary importance appear to be social rather than genetic, whether these are exercised by the peer group or the family, or by culture through schools and the mass media. This is indicated by the recent increase in smoking by women which occurred concurrently with emancipation in terms of status, jobs and social acceptance of what in the past was regarded as 'masculine' behaviour. Of relevance here is the recent World Health Organisation (WHO) report of smoking in 23 countries (the majority being developed countries), in over half of which a dramatic, relative increase in smoking prevalence rates for girls compared with boys is recorded (Masironi & Roy, 1982). Nobody would suggest that the gene pool has changed radically over the past twenty to forty years.

Nevertheless, as we have previously inferred in our discussion of theories of smoking and smoking motives, there may in fact be a second-order genetic effect if we espouse an arousal modulation theory of smoking, which we think is supported by a good deal of evidence. Assume that the anxious, or stimulation-seeking young person is the one more likely to continue smoking. In this case, a genetic argument could be advanced to account in part for the reasons why some adolescents, after their first encounter with a cigarette continue, while others give up, since anxiety and stimulation-seeking have been shown to have strong genetic components. Possibly a more convincing argument, in view of the mildly noxious effects of first encounter with a cigarette, is that certain exogenous factors such as peer group influence initially maintain smoking, but that these motives are superseded by other more 'psychobiological' motives. There is no reason to doubt, of course, that different motives, at least in the early stages, run a parallel course.

A number of studies (see reviews in Surgeon General, 1979, Ch. 17; Bewley, Bland & Harris, 1974; Cherry & Kiernan, 1978) have demonstrated the importance of influences such as smoking by parents, siblings and peers, and of personality and behavioural traits such as rebelliousness, extraversion and anxiety. The relative importance of some of these factors is revealed in a recent large-scale Australian study of 10- to 12-year-olds (O'Connell *et al.*, 1981). Important predictors of smoking were smoking by friends (peer group) and siblings, and approval of tobacco advertising. Far less important predictors of smoking were (male) sex, having more pocket money and parental smoking.

The relative importance of peer group smoking has also been emphasised in a number of other studies (e.g., Bynner, 1969; Levitt & Edwards, 1970). Unfortunately, personality variables were not investigated in the O'Connell *et al.* (1981) study and so their importance relative to peer group, sibling smoking and attitude towards tobacco advertising cannot be assessed. Evidence from a longitudinal study of personality and smoking habits indicated that individuals destined to become smokers were significantly different from future non-smokers on personality traits such as E and N (Cherry & Kiernan, 1978). This suggests that the relationship between personality and smoking might be causal. Also of interest is the observation that loss of a parent is related to smoking (Holland, Halil, Bennett & Elliott, 1969). Social class trends are apparent in adult smoking, and appear to reach back to about the age of 14 years, smoking being more prevalent in the lower socioeconomic status (SES) groups (Holland *et al.*, 1969; Mausner & Platt, 1971). Relatively clear-cut evidence, noticed as early as 1910 (Meylan, 1910; Johnson, 1918), suggests that low academic achievement is predictive of smoking (Bewley & Bland, 1977). However, there may be some confounding effects of SES, which is certainly not a reflection of differences in intelligence (Clarke *et al.*, 1972). This suggests that non-cognitive factors may contribute to both under-achievement and smoking. The influences of school environment, including whether or not teachers smoke, educational anti-smoking programmes, and the mass media are as yet unclear. However, it seems to be the case that merely increasing adolescents' knowledge of the harmful consequences of smoking does not markedly deter them from taking up the habit. Indeed, great difficulty has been found by smoking prevention campaigns in effectively penetrating the complex interactions within the family and peer group (see also Chapter 5: School education/prevention).

A schematic representation of the most important factors underlying smoking recruitment is given in Fig. 14.

A study to assess which variables are predictive of smoking

Relatively few studies have attempted multivariate analysis of a broad battery of questions in order to assess which variables, or combination of variables, are the most predictive of smoking. The study reported here was directed to this end.

General plan of research

The study was planned in two phases. In phase I (1974–5), an inventory of 450–500 items measuring a wide range of biographical, socio-cultural, personality and behavioural variables was administered to representative samples of 12- to 13-, 14- to 15-, and 16- to 17-year-old boys and girls (n = 752) attending Oxfordshire comprehensive schools (details of items may be found in Mangan & Golding, 1983*a*). The data were analysed by stepwise multiple regression and multiple discriminant analysis, which identified sets of items, within each age–sex group, differentiating smokers from non-smokers, and, within the smoking groups, predicting number of cigarettes currently smoked (the still-smoking group) or smoked before giving up (the given-up group).

In phase II of the study (1975–6), short-form item sets, derived from the multiple discriminant and regression analyses of Phase I, were administered to similar age–sex groups drawn from matched schools (n = 1550, approximately equal numbers of boys and girls).

In this second phase, as before, multiple discriminant and regression analyses were run for combined boys' and girls' groups, and for separate groups of still-smoking, given-up and never-smoked subjects.

Results

The percentage of smokers (using the definition of at least 1 cigarette per week) were: 12- to 13-year-olds, 18% of boys and 13% of girls; 14- to 15-year-olds, 41% of boys and 33% of girls; 16- to 17-year-olds, 18% of boys and 24% of girls. The relatively low proportions of smokers in the 16- to 17-year-old group probably reflect the fact that many pupils had left school before this age. Given the known interrelations between scholastic achievement, SES and smoking, it is reasonable to suggest that

Fig. 14. Factors influencing recruitment to smoking.

GENETICS

SEX

PERSONALITY

FAMILY

PEER GROUP

CULTURAL

Smoking as an early marker of LIFESTYLE leading to

OTHER DRUG USE: ALCOHOL TEA/COFFEE TRANQUILLISERS ETC.

IRREGULARITY OF MEALS

DIVORCE

CHANGE OF EMPLOYMENT ETC.

the smoker tends to leave school early. Otherwise the percentages were similar to those in the UK reported by other authors (Bewley *et al.*, 1974).

It was apparent that the currently smoking and ex-smoker categories did not have fixed boundaries. The given-up group included a substantial proportion of undecided smokers. Many had only recently given up. Fifty-five per cent of the 12- to 13-year-olds, and 52% of the 14- and 15-year-olds reported quitting within the previous six months. Undoubtedly some of these later resumed smoking. The item

'If you have given up, do you intend to take up smoking again?

(a) yes   (b) undecided   (c) no

was given an a/b endorsement by 35% of the 12- to 13-year-olds, and 31% of the 14- and 15-year-olds. Of interest here is the observation by Bewley & Bland (1977) of only 63% consistency in reported smoking status by 10 to $12\frac{1}{2}$-year-olds on a six-month follow-up. There is no doubt that some of the upswing in prevalence rates between the ages of 13 and 15 is attributable to resumption of smoking by some ex-smokers. The issue is further confused by the possibility that some of the current non-smokers in the study will be recruited, and that some smokers, who are merely 'experimenting' with tobacco, will give up later as a result of parental, mass media and similar types of intervention.

On the other hand, while it might be true that for some proportion of still-smoking groups group membership could be reflecting relatively transitory, and possibly highly idiosyncratic factors operating at the time of testing, the alternative of combining the given-up and never-smoked groups, which is the practice normally adopted, may mask some aetiologically significant factors. Just as it is true that a certain proportion of both groups are 'waverers', the hard core of each group might be expected to retain membership under 'normal' circumstances.

As far as causal factors for recruitment are concerned, there appears to be no simple, direct and unequivocal data source. Granted, we can ask subjects to indicate the reason why they started smoking, and provide a number of options, and this is the procedure usually adopoted. One such item was included in the present schedule. The results are presented in Table 16. More than 50% of subjects in most groups, and over 60% in many groups, reported that they started smoking 'because I was offered a cigarette'; Bewley *et al.* (1974) similarly report a figure of over 50% for their sample of 10- to $11\frac{1}{2}$-year-old boys. These data, however, have little aetiological significance. They reflect occasion, rather than cause. If we accept the proposition that the majority of children, at some stage, are offered a cigarette, the critical questions that we need to ask are why some refuse and then why some smoke irregularly and infrequently while others again become regular smokers. That is, we need to establish those

Table 16. *Percentage figures of reasons for recruitment to smoking at each age–sex level among Oxfordshire schoolchildren*

	16–17 years Boys+ girls	14–15 years Boys+ girls	12–13 years Boys+ girls	16–17 years Boys	14–15 years Boys	12–13 years Boys	16–17 years Girls	14–15 years Girls	12–13 years Girls
Those still smoking (SS)									
To be grown up	10	5	4	17	2	4	0	9	5
To be like others	14	21	25	25	27	35	0	15	12
Others in family smoked	0	14	8	0	17	2	0	10	15
Was offered a cigarette	76	59	63	58	54	59	100	66	68
Those given up (GU)									
To be grown up	11	5	8	17	8	11	8	3	3
To be like others	33	33	18	50	27	17	25	37	19
Others in family smoked	6	7	15	0	4	14	8	9	16
Was offered a cigarette	50	55	59	33	61	58	59	51	62

underlying factors which determine which of these options will be exercised, and why. Items such as 'to be like others', 'others in the family smoked' and 'to be grown up' may be more important aetiologically, although less frequently given as reasons for starting to smoke than 'was offered a cigarette'.

To give a convenient overall picture of the results, summary statements of the regression and discriminant analyses for still-smoking and given-up versus never-smoked subjects in all age–sex groups are presented in Tables 17 and 18.

In general terms the multiple regression and multiple discriminant analyses closely resemble each other. The notable exception is for the still-smoking 16- to 17-year-old girls: discriminant analysis suggests that as a group they appear more relaxed and composed and regression analysis suggests that the heavy smoker is more tense. A similar conflict of evidence about neuroticism has been noted by Warburton & Wesnes (1978) in the adult population; it is suggested that it is the sub-group of heavily smoking females who are more neurotic (see Chapter 2: Personality and smoking).

Since anxiety appears to be a critical predictor in a number of analyses reported in Table 18, it seems appropriate, at this point, to report the results of a secondary analysis of data collected after the inventories had been completed. Subjects in the 12- to 13- and 14- to 15-year-old groups were asked to note down on a separate sheet 'what things you worry about most'. Responses were sorted by three independent judges, who were able to identify four clear categories: poor home relationships, psychosexual anxiety, anxiety about present scholastic and future vocational achievement, and concern about peer-group acceptance. In addition there was a dump category for idiosyncratic responses. These data are presented in Table 19.

Discussion

Twelve- to thirteen-year-old groups. Analysis of combined data (boys and girls taken together) indicates that current heavy smokers are anxious, frustrated, rebellious, have high P scores, drink excessively compared with their peers and report that their close friends are scholastically well motivated, which might suggest that they themselves are anxious about achievement.

From the separate analyses, it is clear that heavily smoking boys disapprove of co-education, have weak tactual imagery, report that a sister smokes heavily, appear to be anxious and judge that their fathers lack understanding. The observation that the still-smoking boys tend to have sisters who smoke heavily is at variance with the report by Bewley & Bland (1977) of no association between a child's smoking and that of siblings of the opposite sex. There is no obvious explanation for this conflict of

Table 17. *Variables predicting present or former cigarette consumption rates in still-smoking or given-up groups at each age–sex level among Oxfordshire schoolchildren (multiple regression analyses)*

Group	Still smoking	Given up
16–17 years. Boys+girls	High alcohol consumption; extraverted; permissive	High alcohol consumption; has used cannabis; permissive
16–17 years. Boys	Enthusiastic/happy-go-lucky; steady/responsible; positive home relationships	Enthusiastic/happy-go-lucky; risk-taker
16–17 years. Girls	Poor mood control; values new experiences; tense	Large age gap to next sister; values new experiences; relaxed/composed
14–15 years. Boys+girls	Oral dependent/stimulation-seeker; older brother heavy smoker; aggressive/dominant; high P	Oral dependent/stimulation-seeker; aggressive/dominant; high P; older brother heavy smoker
14–15 years. Boys	High alcohol consumption; socially compliant; parents divorced; outgoing/participating; permissive; anxious	High alcohol consumption; outgoing/participating; authoritarian; unconcerned about health; anxious
14–15 years. Girls	Older sister smokes heavily; extraverted/socially compliant; earns from part-time job	Older sister smokes heavily; socially compliant; values freedom from worry; receives generous pocket money; anxious
12–13 years. Boys+girls	Anxious; tense/frustrated; rebellious; undemonstrative; high P; high alcohol consumption; close friends academically oriented; vivid imagery	Aggressive/dominant; places little value on having fun; friends not academically oriented; wants to leave home; unconcerned about health
12–13 years. Boys	Disapproves of co-education; weak imagery, particularly tactual; older sister smokes heavily; anxious; group dependent/socially bold	Disapproves of co-education; poor imagery, particularly olfactory; strong tactual imagery; father rated as not understanding; parent absent through death or divorce; group dependent/socially bold
12–13 years. Girls	Threat-sensitive/anxious; wants to leave home; internally restrained; number of younger brothers at home; seeks advice from teachers	Poor imagery; parent absent from home through death or divorce; authoritarian; group-oriented

Table 18. *Variables distinguishing smokers from never smoked and given up smokers from never smoked[a] at each age–sex level among Oxfordshire schoolchildren*

Group	Still smoking versus never smoked	Given-up versus never smoked
16–17 years. Boys + girls	High alcohol consumption; has used cannabis; good auditory imagery	Moderately high alcohol consumption
16–17 years. Boys	Emotionally more stable; extraverted	Fairly emotionally stable; fairly extraverted
16–17 years. Girls	More relaxed/composed; seeks new experiences; vivid auditory imagery	Fairly relaxed/composed
14–15 years. Boys + girls	High alcohol consumption; laughs at authority; socially extraverted; parents divorced; heavy tea/coffee consumption	High alcohol consumption; brother smokes; less dominant; loving father; moderately high tea/coffee consumption
14–15 years. Boys	High alcohol consumption; less concerned with health; more younger sisters living at home; less self-pity; bright dresser in clothes	High alcohol consumption; less concerned with health; fewer friends than others
14–15 years. Girls	Sister smokes heavily; values freedom from worry; follows the peer group; very empathic; unconcerned with poor schoolwork; peer group is not work orientated	Sister smokes moderately; values freedom from worry; follows the peer group; fairly empathic
12–13 years. Boys + girls	Unconcerned with health; aggressive and starts fights; frustrated and worried; extraverted and energetic; peer group dislikes school; low expectation of academic success	Unconcerned with health; aggressive and starts fights; worried and has stomach aches; extraverted and energetic
12–13 years. Boys	Sister smokes heavily; does not believe in co-education; father not understanding; life is full of worry; strong peer group identification	Does not believe in co-education; low empathy; father not understanding; strong peer group identification
12–13 years. Girls	Wishes to leave home; more younger brothers at home; zestful in peer group interaction; parents divorced	Wishes to leave home; more younger brothers at home; zestful in peer group interaction

[a] Variables have significance $p < 0.05$ or better as revealed by stepwise multiple discriminant analysis. The polarity of each item loads towards the still-smoking or given-up group as appropriate, e.g., 16- to 17-year-old smokers drink much more alcohol than never smokers whereas the given-up smokers only drink moderately more alcohol than never smokers.

evidence. The current heavily-smoking girls show high levels of anxiety, and a strong desire to leave home. For this group, we also note a strong High School Personality Questionnaire (HSPQ) Factor J endorsement. This trait description is 'individualistic, circumspect, internally restrained, obstructive'. The Cattells observe that high Factor J scores are 'clues to watch for in anticipating delinquency' (Cattell & Cattell, 1973).

It is difficult to interpret the critical item content for these groups unequivocally. It is obvious enough that currently smoking girls of this age are unhappy at home, but the reasons are unclear. Note, however, that other significant items in the list refer to the number of younger brothers living at home, and to the fact that these girls tend to seek advice from teachers rather than parents. From this, we might infer that sibling rivalry and/or conflict, particularly with younger brothers, is the main source of unhappiness at home. This view is reinforced by the content of the anxiety responses reported by this group (Table 19), which refers to conflict with parents, in many cases owing to parental expectations, often from working mothers, that these girls will take care of younger brothers and sisters, i.e., the 'little mother' syndrome. Presumably younger brothers present more disciplinary problems.

As far as the boys are concerned, critical items, such as disapproval of co-education and weak tactual imagery, could denote a high level of psychosexual anxiety. This is supported by information on sources of anxiety in this group reported in Table 19.

For the given-up groups, the combined analyses suggest that those who smoke heavily tend to be assertive, dominant and stubborn, that they are disinterested in school, and that they wish to leave home, although not to the same extent as still-smoking girls. There is little real evidence of psychopathology in this group, rather considerable disaffection with their present lot and disinterest in school.

For given-up boys, the most predictive items are disapproval of co-education, weak imagery, especially tactual, strong dependence on the peer group and the fact that their fathers lack understanding, items all applicable to the still-smoking group of boys. However, there is a substantial loading of the item revealing absence of a parent from the family for a variety of reasons (Table 20). The aetiology of smoking with this group, therefore, could also be linked with problems in the family.

For the given-up girls, the critical items are poor imagery and absence of a parent through death, divorce or separation. There are small loadings on authoritarianism and group orientation. As in the case of the given-up boys, there is no evidence in this group that heavy smoking is associated with high levels of anxiety, or with a desire to leave home. The precise

Table 19. *Anxiety sources reported by 12-to 13-year-old and 14- to 15-year-old smokers and non-smokers among Oxfordshire schoolchildren (numbers are % of responses in each age, sex and smoking status group, where SS indicates still smoking and GU indicates Given up) (multiple discriminant analyses)*

	Poor home relationships		Psychosexual		Scholastic/ vocational achievement		Acceptance by group		Miscellaneous	
Smokers	SS	GU	SS	GU	SS	GU	SS	GU	SS	GU
12–13 years. Boys	18	26	52	24	12	14	12	25	6	11
12–13 years. Girls	42	25	22	23	10	12	16	16	10	24
14–15 years. Boys	19	15	41	36	22	27	7	12	11	10
14–15 years. Girls	14	13	24	21	27	30	21	26	14	10
Non-smokers										
12–13 years. Boys	10		23		36		14		17	
12–13 years. Girls	21		23		27		9		20	
14–15 years. Boys	18		32		34		7		9	
14–15 years. Girls	16		15		30		16		23	

significance of the parental absence item, therefore, is unclear. From the data shown in Table 19, there are no indications of any particularly significant source of anxiety. Perhaps in this group, as with the given-up boys, the item simply denotes lack of control and discipline, leading to exaggerated peer/reference group identification, thus making more likely the acquisition of peer-related behaviours, of which smoking is an example.

Fourteen- to fifteen-year-old groups. The most predictive items for the combined and boys' still-smoking and given-up groups are two 'oral dependency' and/or stimulation-seeking items: the number of cups of tea or coffee drunk per day for the total group, and the amount of beer drunk per week for the separate boys' groups. However, the extent to which these items reflect 'oral dependency' is arguable. Frequency of drinking, which might be expected to reflect oral dependency needs, is not a critical item. On the other hand, frequency could be largely a function of opportunity to drink, which, in the group, may be limited.

In view of the P-item weights, a more convincing explanation might be that heavy smokers are stimulation-seekers. Both smoking and drinking can be viewed as arousal/control behaviours, their function being to maintain a homeostatic arousal level. As we have previously noted, this is suggested by the fact that smoking rates for both currently-smoking and given-up boys are also predicted by items measuring anxiety.

There are, of course, other important dimensions suggested in the combined and separate boys' lists. In the combined groups, both still-smoking and given-up subjects report that an older brother smokes heavily and test out as being dominant and aggressive. In the still-smoking boys' group, heavy smokers are anxious, strongly group dependent, and express 'liberal' attitudes to sex. There is a high incidence of parental divorce as

Table 20. *Parental absence revealed by still-smoking, given-up and non-smoking groups of 12- to 13-year-old boys and girls among Oxfordshire schoolchildren* (*figures given are percentages*)

Reason for parental absence	Still smoking		Given up		Non-smoking	
	Boys	Girls	Boys	Girls	Boys	Girls
Death	7.1	4	3.1	6.7	5.7	2.0
Divorce	9.5	32	0.0	6.7	5.7	4.9
Separation	11.9	16	9.2	5.0	2.9	2.0
Father works away	23.8	8	24.6	11.6	11.4	8.8
All reasons combined	52.3	60	36.9	30	25.7	17.7

in 12- to 13-year-olds, suggesting lack of parental supervision and control. Forty-one per cent of anxiety responses refer to psychosexual anxiety and 19% to poor home relationships (Table 19). The content of these responses reveals that for these boys, fear of getting their girlfriends pregnant and feelings of sexual inadequacy, the latter an important facet of the male psyche at this age, are main sources of anxiety.

Data for the given-up boys show no evidence of poor home relationships. These boys show disapproval rather than acceptance of birth control. Thirty-six per cent of anxiety responses are psychosexual in origin (Table 19). The content of these responses reveals anxiety about sexual adequacy, this uncertainty referring to future rather than present behaviour.

The separate 14- to 15-year-old girls' groups presents a quite different picture. For both still-smoking and given-up girls, the most predictive item concerns an older sister who smokes heavily. Strong peer/reference group identification, which implies the acquisition of peer-related behaviours such as smoking are indicated by weights for extraversion and group dependency. In both groups, financial considerations are important in order to support an expensive habit. A number of still-smoking girls have a part-time job, and of the given-up group have generous allowances from their parents. In neither of these groups is there much evidence of stimulation-seeking/arousal control or psychopathology.

Sixteen- to seventeen-year-old groups. Here, interpretation of results is relatively straightforward. The quantity of beer drunk per week, and items relating to permissiveness and extraversion identify the still-smoking combined group. These items take up almost all the variance accounted for in the regression analysis. From the results of the analyses, there are no grounds for assuming that heavy smoking refers to level of social dysfunction. More likely, it reflects stimulation-seeking/oral dependency, or can be regarded as a socially facilitative behaviour. This is supported by the strong weight for extraversion, and the fact that frequency of drinking, rather than amount of beer drunk, emerges as the best predictor for all 'smokers'.

High School Personality Questionnaire F Scale items, reflecting a happy-go-lucky, group-oriented, extraverted personality, almost exclusively predict consumption rates amongst still-smoking boys. For the girls, items referring to mood control and desire for new experiences, which are the best predictors, suggest that smoking may function as an arousal modulator.

Former heavy smokers in the combined group of given-up smokers report that they drink excessively and are permissive. They also report that they have used cannabis in the past, which might suggest that these individuals are 'experience' as well as stimulation seekers.

Predictive items for the given-up boys are largely items from HSPQ Factor F, which loads second-order extraversion and an item referring to risk-taking. The latter we might regard as one aspect of stimulation-seeking, as Zuckerman et al. (1972) and Eysenck & Eysenck (1975, 1976) suggest. On the other hand, the 16- to 17-year-old given-up girl represents herself as relaxed and non-anxious. She values having new experiences. The significance of a large age gap between herself and a younger sister is unclear, but it could suggest a degree of independence and lack of sibling conflict in the home.

In general, the data suggest that the 16- to 17-year-old schoolboy or schoolgirl smoker is an 'adjustive' smoker, that smoking is both a stimulation-seeking and a socially facilitative behaviour. The mood control function of smoking and drinking appears to be restricted to the group of still-smoking girls.

Summary

Overall, there is little doubt that heavy smoking in the youngest age group is symptomatic of some psychopathology which penetrates relatively deeply into the psychical structure. On the other hand, amongst given-up smokers, heavy smoking appears to be one of a symptomatic cluster centring round rebelliousness to parents and authority. With 14- and 15-year-old smokers, there is also some evidence of psychological disturbance, but we note the intrusion of items reflecting stimulation-seeking. Sixteen- to seventeen-year-old school-attending smokers, however, test out as relatively 'normal', the most outstanding feature of their profiles being high levels of alcohol consumption.

In line with previous suggestions, there are grounds for proposing that between the ages of 12 and 15, which cover the initiation and transitional phases of smoking, different motives for smoking emerge and assume particular significance. In the initiation phase, which probably embraces the majority of the 12- to 13-year-old smokers, motives are largely sociocultural and psychological. Where the smoking habit is more firmly entrenched, however, as in the case of the 14- to 17-year-old smoker, these motives are more likely to be psychological and psychobiological.

Finally, we might comment that, neglecting for a moment the 16- to 17-year-old group, which, as we have noted, is a special case, the content of the critical items in the various analyses reported has a good deal in common with that recorded by Cederlof et al. (1977) in their B Series analyses (see Table 11). They report, with mainly adult samples, that smoking is associated with 'psychosocial discord', measured in terms of excessive drinking and use of sleeping pills and tranquillisers, divorce, 'instability', a high level of coffee consumption, a poor employment record and so on. Clearly, some of these indices are inappropriate with the present age samples. However, some items were adapted from adult psychopathy inventories (Robins, 1966). For example, the quality of home relationships was substituted for marital relationships (divorce?) and academic achievement for work history, and it is many of these items, particularly excessive drinking and poor home relationships, which differentiate the still-smoking and given-up from the non-smoking groups amongst 13- and 15-year-olds. (With regard to drinking, we might add that solvent abuse may become an important alternative predictor of smoking in some regions of the UK.)

Smoking maintenance and the effects of nicotine and smoking on performance

Whereas the most immediate influence on smoking recruitment seems to be a psychosocial factor, it is probable that smoking is maintained by additional factors. The principal reinforcer for the maintenance of smoking is doubtless nicotine, the possible rewarding actions of which have been discused earlier, both in general terms and at the pharmacological/psychophysiological level. In this section we examine the effects of nicotine and smoking on performance and their implications for the maintenance of smoking. For convenience, performance variables are sub-set into the following categories:

(i) Learning: acquisition of behaviour
(ii) Consolidation of memory (in the absence of overt behaviour)
(iii) Performance of established behaviour.

Learning

Nicotine has a biphasic dose-dependent effect on animal learning, which is in keeping with its known biphasic effects at EEG and synaptic levels. Provided the 'correct' dosage is chosen (usually within weighted equivalent dosage levels obtained by smokers), and this may depend upon the particular starting state (individual differences, strains and species of animal), nicotine can be shown to facilitate the acquisition of shock avoidance (Evangelista, Gattoni & Izquierdo, 1970; Domino, 1973), operant behaviour such as bar-pressing to obtain water (Morrison, 1967, 1968), visual discrimination (Bovet-Nitti, 1969) and maze learning (Garg, 1969; Battig, 1970). While dosage comparisons between different experiments are difficult to evaluate, primarily because different investigators have employed different routes and rates of nicotine injection, one finding in particular seems relatively unambiguous and clear-cut. Small doses of nicotine (40 μg kg^{-1} of body weight injected subcutaneously) facilitate, and larger doses (80 μg kg^{-1} of body weight injected subcutaneously) inhibit acquisition of active avoidance (pole-jump response) in the rat (Domino, 1973).

Fig. 15. Effects of smoking a 1.3 mg nicotine cigarette (treatment) (filled circles) versus control (open circles) immediately prior to acquisition of paired associate learning (PAL) of (*a*) low-interference word pairs and (*b*) high-interference word pairs, 12 subjects in each group. PAL learning curves are plotted as the number of errors per trial. Trials 1–13 on the left of each figure represent PAL acquisition to error-free criterion. Trials 1–5 on the right of each figure represent re-test (recall) to error-free criterion, 30 min post acquisition. Note that smoking impairs acquisition of low-interference word pairs but facilitates acquisition of high-interference word pairs. Smoking enhances later recall for both low- and high-interference word pairs. (From Mangan & Golding, 1978.)

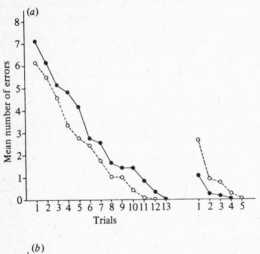

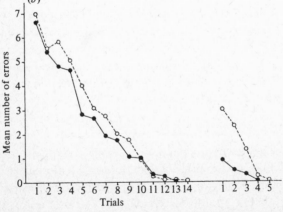

With human subjects, there is evidence that smoking has little effect, overall, on verbal learning, but improves subsequent recall (Andersson, 1975). Mangan & Golding (1978) and Mangan (1983) report no significant effects of smoking either a 0.7 mg or a 1.3 mg nicotine yield cigarette on acquisition of verbal paired associates. However, significant improvement in subsequent recall was recorded with both strengths of cigarette versus the control. Evidence has also been reported that, in a serial learning task, smoking significantly improves recall in the primacy, but not in the intermediate and recency categories (Mangan, 1983). These results, taken together, indicate that smoking has more clear-cut effects on consolidation than on acquisition.

It appears, however, that smoking, and, inferentially, nicotine, has a facilitatory effect on acquisition in more 'difficult' tasks, which is probably explicable in terms of the effect of nicotine to narrow the attentional focus (Johnston, 1965, 1966). Thus, while acquisition of simple verbal rote learning (Andersson, 1975; Mangan, 1983), and immediate memory for digits (Williams, 1980) may be slightly impaired or unaffected by cigarette smoking, the data reported by Andersson & Hockey (1977) and by Mangan & Golding (1978) and Mangan (1983) suggest that, with the inclusion of more 'irrelevant' material in the learning task (thus making the task more 'difficult'), the major effect of smoking is to focus the subject's attention on the immediate task, and to prevent him from attending to irrelevant background stimuli. In the above experiments, this effect was shown in a smoking-induced impairment of incidental learning (memory for the position of words on a screen) while having no effect on immediate serial recall of the words themselves (Andersson & Hockey, 1977), and by a non-significant impairment of acquisition of low interference paired associate and a non-significant improvement of high interference paired associate word lists (Mangan & Golding, 1978; Mangan, 1983) (see Fig. 15) (see also Appendix: Paired associate learning). This finding is supported by the observation of Kleinman, Vaughn & Christ (1973) that deprivation of tobacco for twenty-four hours facilitated learning of easy paired associates, but impaired performance with hard pairs. The possible physiological basis for this attentional focussing effect of cigarette smoking has been discussed previously (see Chapter 3: Reinforcing mechanisms of nicotine for smoking, The electrodermal system, The Brain, and also Specific effects, The brain).

Consolidation of memory

'Consolidation' refers to the postulated transfer of memory traces from the 'short-term memory stores' to the 'long-term memory stores'. The former operate over time-scales of seconds, the latter over time-scales of minutes to days. In practice, the consolidation process can be examined by re-testing for the required behaviour at various intervals following acquisition.

While learning and memory have been tested on smokers, mainly by smoking prior to acquisition, it is possible that the findings of improved recall in experiments detailed earlier (see Learning) are less due to an effect of smoking on the acquisition process, which involves mainly short-term memory and attention, and more due to an effect on the postulated consolidation process occurring between acquisition and subsequent re-testing. Provided the initial training is short in duration relative to the clearance of nicotine and subsequent transmitter release, cigarette smoking prior to acquisition may be acting directly upon this consolidation process.

A number of studies have attempted to examine systematically the effects of smoking/nicotine, post-learning, on memory consolidation. In the only human study reported, Mangan & Golding (1983b) report that cigarette smoking immediately post-acquisition of paired associate material improves recall after one-month re-test. In animal studies, post-trial injections of nicotine have been shown to facilitate retention of maze learning in rats (Garg & Holland, 1968; Evangelista et al., 1970). However, nicotine is not alone in possessing this property, since the same experimenters have found post-trial injections of amphetamine, strychnine, picrotoxin and hexamethonium to be also effective in facilitating retention. Evangelista et al. (1970) make the unusual suggestion that improved consolidation may be mediated by stabilisation of autonomic reflexes by peripheral ganglion blocking. Some such explanation seems necessary to explain the effects of hexamethonium, which functions solely as a peripheral ganglion-blocker. Presumably, the process of consolidation can be improved by removing interfering stimuli during the consolidation process, in this case peripheral autonomic feedback. However, in view of the current ignorance about the physiological basis of memory, there is no need to postulate a unitary mechanism encompassing all these drug effects. Thus, nicotine is known to release ADH (see Chapter 3: Specific effects on neural/hormonal mechanisms, release of other hormones and circulatory factors), which has been implicated in memory consolidation (*Lancet*, 1979b). In addition, both nicotine and amphetamine can cause release of NA (see same section of Chapter 3), which has been implicated in the grossest possible form of learning – cortical plasticity during development (Pettigrew, 1978).

Bearing on this latter mechanism, nicotine has been shown to induce theta activity in the hippocampus (EEG activity related to arousal, the orienting response and learning), and to increase hippocampal RNA levels (Daroqui & Orsingher, 1972). While the former effect is probably more related to acquisition than to consolidation, the latter increase of RNA, in an organ implicated in attentional and memory processes, is suggestive of a possible nicotine action on consolidation through prior NA release, since RNA and associated protein synthesis have been proposed as the final stage of consolidation (see Cooper *et al.*, 1978; Dunn, 1980; for recent reviews). These EEG and RNA changes in the hippocampus have been shown to depend on noradrenergic pathways, since both changes are prevented by *alpha*-methyl-tyrosine, which is a specific inhibitor of catecholamine synthesis and predictably reverses the amphetamine or nicotine-induced facilitation of learning (Orsingher & Fulginiti, 1971). However, the evidence is far from unanimous. Thus, in demonstrating that post-trial administration of nicotine could reverse amnesia induced by anisomycin (a protein synthesis inhibitor) in mice learning a passive shock avoidance task, Flood *et al.* (1978) found no evidence that the overall degree of protein synthesis inhibition produced by anisomycin was affected. Post-trial caffeine administration had similar beneficial effects on memory to those produced by nicotine whereas post-trial administration of depressant drugs such as chloral hydrate and sodium phenobarbitone tended to augment the amnesic effects of anisomycin, these stimulants and depressants producing their effects on memory with no appreciable influence on the overall protein synthesis inhibition. Flood *et al.* (1978) and Mangan & Golding (1983*b*) make the suggestion that variations in arousal during the post-trial time period, produced in this case by drugs, can critically affect memory consolidation.

Understanding of the mechanism by which cigarette smoking and, by implication, nicotine, affects the consolidation process awaits a greater knowledge of the physical basis of memory, which no doubt involves all the known transmitters, including peptides, and also Ca^{2+} and cyclic AMP, before the hypothetical final RNA and protein synthesis stages (see also reviews of the neurochemistry of learning in Alpern & Jackson, 1978; Drachman, 1978; and Dunn, 1980). This understanding will be at least as important as the understanding of the encoding of 'evolutionary memory' on the DNA molecule.

Performance of established behaviour

Animal studies: effects of acute injection of nicotine. Acute injections of nicotine have been shown to produce mixed effects of facilitation and depression on a number of operant response measures in the rat, including electrical self-stimulation of the lateral and posterior hypothalamus (Olds & Domino, 1969; Pradhan & Bowling, 1971; Newman, 1972; Domino, 1973), bar-pressing for water reward (Morrison, 1967, 1968; Armitage *et al.*,

1968), conditional pole-jump behaviour in the rat, and shock-avoidance behaviour in the monkey (Domino, 1965). The range of doses employed was typically 25–600 μg nicotine kg^{-1} of body weight injected subcutaneously and 100–800 μg nicotine kg^{-1} of body weight injected intraperitoneally. For comparison, 25–50 μg kg^{-1} of body weight injected subcutaneously is quite similar to doses produced by inhalation of cigarette smoke in man (Domino, 1973). These mixed stimulant and depressant effects on operant responses can be explained in terms of the known biphasic dose-response effects of nicotine at synaptic and EEG levels (see, e.g., Armitage *et al.*, 1968; Domino, 1973). In general, it would appear that while small doses produce a stimulant effect, larger doses will produce depressant actions. As discussed earlier, the starting state of the animal also appears to mediate the direction of nicotine effects. Domino (1973) suggests that nicotine will tend to reduce the self-stimulation rate in rats with high rates of response, and vice-versa. This effect is not specific to nicotine, but also occurs for amphetamine.

The direction of the nicotine effect is often time-dependent, medium doses producing initial depression followed by facilitation after a few minutes (Domino, 1973). This is crudely explicable in terms of the biphasic dose-response curve for nicotine, since within a few minutes following injection, the brain levels of nicotine rapidly fall, judging from data indicating a half-life of 5 min post i.v. injection in the mouse brain (Stahlhandske, 1970). However, 'active' mechanisms involving short-term adaptation to secondary transmitter release, e.g., NA and ACh, followed by rebound effects, cannot be excluded, since time-based rebound effects of CNS activity in the *opposite* direction to those at the behavioural level have been found in the EEG of the cat. Thus, Domino (1973) observed a transient EEG activation, occurring within one minute after i.v. injection of nicotine (20 μg kg^{-1} of body weight) into rabbits, cats and dogs, which was followed by spindle bursts (i.e., EEG de-activation) within four minutes. Presumably the reverse type of rebound can also occur, i.e., depressant followed by stimulant effects, after acute nicotine injection. They certainly do occur over the long time-scales involved in chronic nicotine administration (Morrison & Stephenson, 1972; Stolerman, Fink & Jarvik, 1973a). Although these latter effects are usually described in terms of long-term tolerance to nicotine depressant effects, it is not unreasonable to suggest that a short-term reversible tolerance to the depressant effects of nicotine may be contributing to the initially observed depressant effects and then to stimulant effects on operant response after acute nicotine injection.

The pharmacological bases of these depressant and stimulant effects appear to be primarily central ACh and NA release (although other transmitter systems may be involved). Thus, physostigmine (an inhibitor of cholinesterase which crosses the blood-brain barrier) but not neostigmine (a peripheral cholinesterase inhibitor) will potentiate the depression of operant response rates caused by high doses of nicotine (Morrison, 1968). Since, in a similar way, the stimulant effects of even small doses of nicotine on operant response rates are reduced or abolished, it is possible that the depressant actions of nicotine are mediated largely by ACh release, and that the stimulant effects may be mediated by different mechanisms, e.g., NA release. Some support for this view is suggested by the differential interactions with nicotine of a variety of nicotinic and muscarinic agonists and antagonists on electrical self-stimulation behaviour (SS). Newman (1972) suggests that nicotine may be stimulating a central 'GO' mechanism (as measured by increased SS rates) via release of NA, the mechanism probably being post-synaptic, i.e., via prior ACh release. On the other hand, any decreases in SS rates (e.g., as observed by Domino, 1973) following higher doses of nicotine are mediated by nicotine-induced release of ACh onto muscarinic, as opposed to nicotinic, receptors, a so-called 'NO-GO' system.

Animal studies: effects of chronic injection of nicotine. There is some evidence that chronic as opposed to acute injection of nicotine in rats will have additional effects. At the pharmacological level, there is some evidence that chronic exposure to nicotine over long time-periods may cause subtle alterations in the physiology of the brain. For example, reductions in the number of nicotine binding sites in the midbrain and also reductions in 5-HT levels in the hippocampus have been observed (Balfour & Benwell, 1981; Falkeborn *et al.*, 1981). These and other changes in brain functioning, together with increased activity of hepatic detoxification mechanisms (see Chapter 3: Metabolism and excretion of nicotine) may account for the development of tolerance to nicotine. Behavioural tolerance to the depressant effects of chronic nicotine administration appears after a few days (Morrison & Stephenson, 1972) (see Fig. 16). This tolerance has also been reported by Stolerman *et al.* (1973a). It would appear that chronic nicotine administration either in drinking water, or through implanted subcutaneous reservoirs, or by i.p. injections within equivalent weighted human dose ranges, produces a tolerance lasting for at least 90 days following regular treatment with nicotine (as measured by spontaneous locomotor activity in a Y maze). Although Stolerman *et al.* (1973a) suggest that this long-lasting tolerance may be related to relapse to tobacco usage in man, they also state that a nicotine abstinence syndrome was not detected.

A stronger 'animal model' for relapse to tobacco in smokers who have 'given up' is provided by Hall & Morrison (1973). Rats which have been helped by nicotine to learn a difficult and stressful shock avoidance task more rapidly, and to perform it more efficiently, seem to depend on the continuation of nicotine to maintain proficiency. When nicotine is withdrawn, their ability to perform the task deteriorates progressively until eventually their performance is no better than that of novices. This is not simply a learning dissociation phenomenon (state-dependent learning) whereby the animal is unable to remember what was learned under the influence of nicotine, because the disruption was relatively slight on the first day of withdrawal and deteriorated progressively. Nicotine may be acting as a tranquilliser in this situation, since if a conditioned 'safety-signal' is presented during withdrawal from nicotine, then the decrement in performance does not occur. This suggests that nicotine may be reducing the stressful aspects of the shock avoidance situation, and can thus be compared to other tranquillisers, although it is arguable whether an analogy should be drawn with 'major' tranquillisers, e.g., chlorpromazine and opiates, or with 'minor' tranquillisers, e.g., alcohol, barbiturates and valium (see Gray, 1971; Domino, 1973).

Fig. 16. Effects of chronic nicotine (triangles), amphetamine (filled circles) or saline (open circles) on mean activity-box scores for groups of eight rats tested for 30 min during ten trials over 14 days. Animals were tested each day immediately after the injection of nicotine (0.8 mg kg^{-1} of body weight) amphetamine (0.8 mg kg^{-1} of body weight) or saline (control). Note the decrease in activity-box scores for nicotine (depressant effect) and the increase for amphetamine (stimulant effect) versus saline control on Day 1. Subsequently the activity-box scores for nicotine increase, indicating the development of tolerance to the depressant effect of nicotine, and revealing an ultimate stimulant effect. (From Morrison & Stephenson, 1972.)

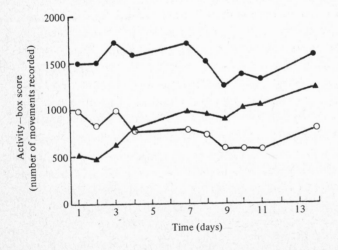

In addition, chronic nicotine administration ($100 \mu g \text{ kg}^{-1}$ of body weight, by injection three times daily) appears to have effects on what might be loosely termed 'attention' in rats performing a visual discrimination task for food reward (Nelsen & Goldstein, 1973). It would appear that, while impairing acquisition by increasing 'omission' errors, after criterion performance has been reached nicotine causes a significant decrease in errors of 'commission' (bar-pressing when the cue light signalling reward availability was not on), although having no significant effect on 'omission' errors (failure to make correct response when cue light signalling reward availability was on). This finding is explicable in terms of Routtenberg's (1968) two-system theory of cortical activation, in which the reticular formation and limbic system are mutually inhibitory, controlling 'Drive orientated arousal' and 'Incentive orientated arousal' respectively. Chronic nicotine administration has indeed been found to favour limbic system versus reticular system control of the cortex in the rat (Nelsen *et al.*, 1973) and the rabbit (Bhattacharya & Goldstein, 1970). This provides support for the view that chronic nicotine may be favouring 'Incentive orientated arousal', i.e., base-rate operant response via the limbic system, while inhibiting 'Drive orientated arousal', i.e., acquisition of new learning.

Finally, there is some evidence that attentional systems are disrupted following withdrawal from chronic nicotine treatment. This is indicated by concurrent changes of slow cortical potentials, which correlate with the attentional aspects of auditory discrimination performance in rats (Ebenezer, 1982).

Human studies. While some of the effects of cigarette smoking on established human performance might be inferred from animal studies, there are obviously limits to the extent of extrapolation possible. This is primarily because it is difficult to determine in any precise way the baseline performance for particular tasks. This difficulty usually reduces to the question of whether we are studying the effects of smoking deprivation, which would be analogous to the chronic nicotine studies referred to above, or to the effects of smoking per se, as represented in the acute nicotine administration studies. The two may not be the same. Unfortunately, there are insufficient data from which to draw firm conclusions as to whether smoking is genuinely improving the performance of the smoker, or merely preventing 'nicotine hunger' from disrupting a deprived smoker's level of performance efficiency.

One of the few performance studies to compare the performance of non-smokers with that of smokers smoking and deprived of smoking is that of Tarriere & Hartemann (1964). In a $2\frac{1}{2}$-h signal detection task simulating car driving, the initial performance of non-smokers, smoking smokers and deprived smokers was similar. However, whereas the smoking smokers' performance remained relatively constant, the performance of both the non-smokers and deprived-smokers deteriorated over time. We may also note here the performance enhancement effects, detailed later in this section, of oral nicotine in both non-smokers and deprived smokers (Wesnes & Warburton, 1978).

However, comparing smokers with non-smokers does not fully resolve the question raised earlier, since smokers differ from non-smokers in respects other than smoking itself, for example personality (see Chapter 2). Personality differences themselves can correlate with variations in performance and so are likely to act as confounding variables (Warburton & Wesnes, 1978).

With human data there are suggestions that cigarette smoking has a stimulant action on critical flicker frequency (see Appendix) (Warwick and Eysenck, 1963). It is presumably because of similar stimulant effects that smoking also appears to offset boredom and fatigue-induced decrement in tasks such as driving simulation (Heimstra, Bancroft & De Kock, 1967; Ashton & Watson, 1970), reaction time (Myrsten & Andersson, 1978), visual and auditory vigilance (Mangan & Golding, 1978; Wesnes & Warburton, 1978; Mangan, 1982*a*), and spiral after-effect (Golding & Mangan, 1982*b*).

The effects of smoking on human performance, however, are not uniformly enhancing, the type of effect probably depending on complex interactions between the starting state of the individual performer (perhaps reflecting a biological predisposition represented in high extraversion (E) or psychoticism (P) scores, for example), nicotine dosage, levels of situational stress and what actually constitutes task 'difficulty'. In a variety of simple, non-stressful tasks, moderate doses of nicotine may improve learning, as previously noted, and enhance performance simply by narrowing attention, in line with the general finding that increased arousal, whether produced by pharmacological or non-pharmacological means, will focus or narrow attention (Wachtel, 1967). Narrowed attention and reduced distractability probably explain the finding that nicotine tablets (0 mg, 1 mg or 2 mg of oral nicotine given to deprived smokers and non-smokers) decrease the interfering effects of colour and word (e.g., 'BLUE' written in red colour) in the Stroop Test (see Appendix) (Wesnes & Warburton, 1978). It may also explain the finding that smoking improves vigilance by suppressing 'false positives' (Mangan & Golding, 1978; Mangan, 1982*a*), through a shift to limbic system arousal (Nelsen *et al.*, 1973), (see Fig. 17).

Fig. 17. Effects of smoking (treatment) a 1.3 mg middle-nicotine (filled circles) or a 0.7 mg low-nicotine (squares) cigarette, and control (open circles), immediately prior to an auditory vigilance task lasting 30 min (12 subjects in each group). Correct detection rates are shown in (a) and false detection rates (errors of commission) are shown in (b). Note that overall vigilance performance was improved by smoking, but that the low-nicotine cigarette improved correct detections, whereas the middle-nicotine cigarette suppressed false detections. (From Mangan, 1982a.)

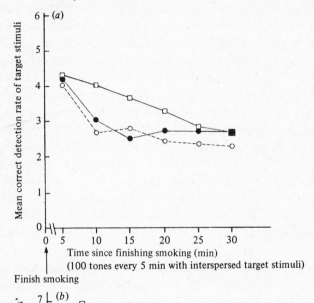

In practice, the class of interfering stimuli which smoking suppresses in human learning and performance may have to be broadened to include preoccupations with failure acting as distracting stimuli which will interfere with the main task in anxious subjects (Warburton & Wesnes, 1978). This type of smoking effect can be viewed as depressant, i.e., anxiolytic. Similarly, for those smokers whose response to difficult and stressful tasks is one of irritation or anger rather than anxiety, smoking may exert a calming influence and so enhance performance (Heimstra, 1973; see also Chapter 2: Behavioural traits and characteristics). It is entirely possible, given the evidence reviewed earlier (see Chapter 3: Specific effects on neural/hormonal mechanisms – phasic electroencephalogram: evoked potentials, photic driving, contingent negative variation), that a subject may be able to titrate himself with the correct dose of nicotine to inhibit interfering stimuli, both emotional and non-emotional, while leaving cortical excitation undiminished for the main task.

Arguing from the stimulant properties of nicotine, however, we would be hard put to account for the fact that smoking *deprivation*, while not affecting smokers' performance on simple sensori-cognitive-motor tasks, does in fact improve performance on more complex cognitive tasks such as Raven's Matrices (a series of non-verbal tests of reasoning ability) (Elgerot, 1976). Inferentially, smoking should decrement or have no effect on performance in such tasks.

A possible interpretation involves the Yerkes–Dodson Law (see Appendix). Since optimal arousal is lower for more complex tasks, a decrement in performance might be anticipated if the dose of nicotine is 'over-arousing'. However, smokers, through self-titration, should be able to vary the effects of nicotine, whether stimulant or depressant, and thus be able to lower arousal and enhance performance for complex tasks. Such control is sometimes possibly inefficient, and it may be that the optimal level of (low) arousal can be achieved only in high stress situations. Some evidence for this proposition is offered by Myrsten *et al.* (1975), who used questionnaire methods to divide smokers into two groups, 'high-arousal' smokers who felt the need to smoke when over-excited or stressed and 'low-arousal' smokers who needed to smoke in low-stimulation, boring situations. These two groups of smokers were then tested in boring and stressful situations. The results support the view that smokers can increase their performance on a complex sensorimotor task, but only when their starting states are taken into account. Smoking during low situational arousal (boredom) improved the performance only of 'low-arousal' smokers, whereas that of 'high-arousal' smokers was improved only during high situational arousal. Williams (1980) has also related the predominantly enhancing effects of cigarette smoking on letter cancellation speed (the speed with which the subject can cross out a particular target letter wherever it occurs when reading through a section of printed text, without making mistakes) to the inverted-U relationship (see Appendix) between performance and arousal.

Finally, smoking appears to have some protective action against the disruptive effects of alcohol intoxication on human performance. Thus smokers who were allowed to smoke when they drank alcohol had faster reaction times and performed better on mental arithmetic tasks than when they drank without smoking (Myrsten & Andersson, 1975). A similar opposing effect between alcohol and smoking has been demonstrated on critical flicker frequency (CFF) (see Appendix) although the protective action of smoking on alcohol-induced reductions in CFF performance are preferentially shown over long rather than short versions of the task (Leigh, 1982). The stimulant properties of nicotine in small doses presumably offset the depressant actions of alcohol. Interactions of this sort may contribute in part to the commonly observed pattern of association between alcohol consumption and smoking.

Summary

In animals, nicotine can facilitate or impair the learning and performance of a variety of tasks, including bar-pressing, maze-learning and active avoidance of electric shock. In general, small doses facilitate and larger doses impair performance. The pharmacological basis of such effects is probably the biphasic dose-related nature of nicotine, being generally stimulant at low doses and depressant at high doses. Nicotine also appears to increase the consolidation of memory traces after learning, an effect similar to that observed with many other stimulant drugs. The mechanism of this effect is conjectural.

In human learning and performance, the situation is much less clear. Smoking appears to impair (slightly) the learning of simple material, but to enhance (non-significantly) the learning of difficult material, and to improve consolidation. The latter effect is probably due to the specific effect of nicotine on structures which are known to be intimately involved in recall and consolidation.

As far as the effects of nicotine and cigarette smoking on human performance are concerned, some issues are unresolved. One obvious problem is that we need to differentiate task difficulty, due to monotony or interference, from difficulty as a function of intellectual demand, and to take account of the starting state of the individual performer. With simple, non-stressful tasks, nicotine has a generally enhancing effect, as a consequence of narrowed attention and the screening out of interference. With difficult tasks, however, the outcome may depend on the success of the smoker in shifting himself towards the optimum of the inverted-U curve relating arousal to performance efficiency.

PART III

PREVENTION AND CESSATION

5

Intervention and termination strategies

INTERVENTION STRATEGIES
Introduction

Intervention and termination strategies can be divided into those of a general nature, e.g., mass communication of anti-smoking propaganda, and those of a more specific nature such as programmes involving small groups or individual smokers. We shall examine the more specific programmes first.

The period 1965–80 was characterised by a great burgeoning of studies which compared and evaluated different smoking cessation strategies. This is clearly reflected in the 1979 Surgeon General's Report, which cites 453 references. Orleans, Shipley, Williams & Haac (1981) cite 335 studies. Despite an enormous research effort, however, it is unfortunately the case that we still know comparatively little about the relative efficacy of treatments, so that the replicability and general utility of almost all procedures can be no more than tentatively assessed. This is because many of the outcome studies in this field are flawed by methodological errors and deficiencies, a surprising state in view of the fact that smoking is such an obvious candidate for outcome research.

The most critical problem concerns the validity of the treatment results. The majority of studies rely on unverified self-report as the dependent measure. The inappropriateness of such a procedure hardly warrants comment. Not unexpectedly, there is clear evidence of false reporting by both children and adults in smoking cessation programmes (Pechacek, 1979). Clearly, data of this sort need to be supported by objective measures, of which the most impressive are biological assays of various types. These are, basically, levels of plasma nicotine, urinary nicotine and metabolites (see Chapter 3: Pharmacokinetics), plasma carboxyhaemoglobin (COHb), exhaled carbon monoxide (CO), which is directly proportional to plasma COHb concentration, and thiocyanates (SCN) in urine, blood and saliva. Each of these assays has advantages and disadvantages. Samples of exhaled CO, saliva (SCN) and urine (nicotine and metabolites) are easier to obtain than blood samples. There is considerable variation in the post-smoking half-lives of the compounds in question. These range from minutes to a few hours for nicotine and metabolites, to $2\frac{1}{2}$–4 h for CO (Goldsmith & Landaw, 1968), although CO levels show high diurnal variability, to approximately 14 days for SCN concentration (Vogt, Selvin, Widdowson & Hulley, 1977). On this basis, the SCN technique is obviously preferable. However, there are now rapid, accurate and inexpensive methods for measuring exhaled CO, and this is increasingly becoming the method of choice.

Singly, or in combination, these techniques seem necessary adjuncts to self-report data. This is well illustrated, for example, by a report from the Toronto Smoking Withdrawal Study Centre (1973) of 29% successful abstinence at one-year follow-up. However, COHb assessments revealed that 21% of the reported ex-smokers had levels above 5%, which strongly suggests smoking. We can only guess at what other assay procedures might have revealed.

Over and above the problem of the questionable validity of self-report data, many of the early and some of the later studies are rendered almost uninterpretable by very basic faults, e.g., lack of appropriate designs and experimental controls, especially attention-placebo, lack of attempts to generalise treatment effects from clinical to real-life settings, and lack of multidimensional analysis of data to tease out the complex interactions which might allow the simultaneous testing of different theoretical issues.

Another major fault is the lack of comprehensive follow-up of participants in cessation programmes. Many studies report dramatic post-treatment effects, but long-term follow-up data from the few available studies invariably show rapid relapse, particularly in the first 3–4 months post-treatment. It could be argued that a one-year, or at least a six-month, follow-up should be an absolute requirement. In addition, of course, it is important to consider the early treatment dropout rate, since this inflates remission percentages. It is also possible that survivors are the most highly motivated subjects, so that it is debatable as to whether it is the treatment, the high level of motivation, or both, that is producing cessation.

Finally, we should mention the possibility that lack of replicability may be in part a function of variability due to the smallness or unrepresentativeness of the samples being tested. Thus, how subjects are recruited and selected, and their personality characteristics, may be as important as treatment effects. In some programmes the success of the therapist in achieving rapport may be a critical factor.

Overall, the quality of the more recent studies has improved considerably; nevertheless, many are deficient in some important respect. With this caveat in mind, we give a brief review of the intervention literature. The proliferation of studies makes a full review impracticable, so we have restricted ourselves to those studies which meet minimal validity criteria. These can be conveniently categorised under the following headings: Behaviour modification, Drug therapy, Individual counselling and Group counselling (including Smoking clinics). We should, of course, note the distinction between intervention techniques which treat the smoking response (behaviour modification and drug therapy) and those which treat the smoker (counselling therapies).

Behaviour modification

This approach refers to a number of treatment methods derived from learning theory, all of which can be subsumed under the rubric 'Behaviour therapy' (Eysenck, 1960), or 'Behaviour modification' (Ullmann & Krasner, 1969). In a very broad sense, it encompasses a wide range of techniques designed to suppress or substitute for unwanted, maladaptive behaviours such as phobic fears or excessive use of alcohol. Historically, this approach is rooted firmly in behaviourism, which asserts that maladaptive, like adaptive behaviours, exemplify the laws applying to all learning and conditioning. Modification of maladaptive behaviours can therefore be effected by counter-conditioning or deconditioning procedures, which presuppose a knowledge of, and application of, these laws. This modern conception of neurotic disorder and its treatment thus owes a great deal to Watson, to Wolpe & Skinner, and to Eysenck (for further details consult Eysenck, 1968).

Although the take-off point for behaviour therapy as a discipline can be traced to Wolpe's seminal (1958) work, a considerable number of techniques which subsequently became incorporated into the armamentarium of the behaviour therapist had been reported considerably earlier. For example, Mary Cover Jones' (1924) account of the dismissal of a phobic fear of a rabbit in a number of young children by a process of 'direct conditioning', i.e., counter-conditioning, and by a rough-and-ready systematic desensitisation technique, and Dunlap's (1932) report of the suppression of a motor (typing) error by massed practice, a technique which was subsequently adapted by Yates (1958) in treating a facial tic, are good cases in point. However, it was only when a more 'formal', systematic approach to behaviour modification was attempted, primarily due to Eysenck and Wolpe, that the importance and relevance of these examples became apparent. An important impetus to this development was provided by Eysenck (1968), who, in his general theory of socialisation, proposed that introverts, because of certain biological predispositions, are prone to 'surplus' conditioning, and thus tend to be anxious and withdrawn. Behaviour modification is a way of dealing with this surplus conditioning.

It is self-evident that the framework within which the effectiveness of behaviour modification must be evaluated is that of outcome research. This is possible only when specific, measurable, i.e., target, behaviours are identifiable, so that it is possible to manage problems of control, measurement and comparison of the relative efficacies of different treatment methods. This approach has been successful in dealing with social anxiety (Paul, 1966) and with a number of phobic disorders (Rachman, 1967). If we regard smoking as a maladaptive behaviour, it offers an appropriate target behaviour that is likely to be sensitive to control techniques, considered within the limits of outcome research. The behaviour is observable, it occurs in discriminable units and has a high frequency in the population at large.

On the whole, most of the early controlled intervention research produced unimpressive results. This is well borne out in a number of reviews published in the late sixties (e.g., Krutzer, Lichtenstein & Mees, 1968; Bernstein, 1969; Schwartz, 1969). A good illustrative study is that of Schwartz & Dubitzky (1968a, b) which showed that at one-year follow-up, none of the seven experimental conditions which they employed, and which, at that time, were considered to be the most promising intervention strategies, was superior to the no-contact or minimal-contact control conditions. Recent studies have employed better designs, and the validation criteria mentioned above have been more nearly met. Even with these studies, however, there are a number of vexing problems, particularly that of extensive enough follow-up.

This is particularly applicable to dissertation research, for which smoking cessation has been a particularly attractive field (Surgeon General, 1979). This, in the USA context, means that follow-ups have to be limited to 1–3 months. A good deal of well-meaning effort, therefore, has produced inconclusive results.

In briefly describing behaviour modification techniques we should distinguish the operant (self-control) procedures, which are designed to detect the environmental stimuli which control the smoking response, and to extinguish such control, from the more invasive, directly suppressive techniques, such as electric shock aversion.

Self-control techniques

The most simple self-control technique is self-monitoring of individual smoking behaviour. The subject is provided with increased awareness of target behaviour, and of the controlling stimuli, and then is acquainted with specific self-management skills to control the target behaviour. Self-monitoring is sometimes combined with stimulus-control treatments. Here, subjects are taught to reduce the relevance/strength of cues which prompt smoking, either by eliminating smoking from an increasing number of situations, or by making time intervals the controlling cue.

Coverant control (covert + operant = coverant), an operant procedure originally described by Homme (1965), requires the smoker to generate an inventory of thoughts that are incompatible with the thought of smoking. These 'coverants' are low probability behaviours (e.g., thoughts about cardiovascular disease, cancer as a consequence of smoking, or more 'personal' consequences such as bad breath) which are systematically triggered by a high probability behaviour (such as coffee drinking or sitting down in an office chair) also selected by the smoker. This triggering is made contingent upon first holding in mind one item from the coverant inventory. The underlying theory relates to Premack's (1959) differential probability hypothesis, which is itself a variant of dominance theory, as expounded in the Soviet psychological literature and by Razran (1955), and which states that for any set of responses, the more probable one reinforces the less probable one.

Contractual management (contingency contracting), described initially by Tooley & Pratt (1967), involves negotiation of behavioural contracts or pledges, whereby the smoker agrees to meet certain non-smoking obligations in exchange for social rewards and approval. One variant is that in which subjects are required to deposit money, say US $20, which is refundable at the end of the treatment if the subject is successful at quitting. If not, the money may be donated to a nominated charity.

Systematic desensitisation is a technique originally based on the assumption that smoking is frequently cued by anxiety-provoking stimuli ('negative affect' smoking). Thus smoking will diminish if the antecedent and proximal stimuli leading to smoking are desensitised, that is, reciprocally inhibited, by being paired with deep relaxation. Normally subjects are trained in the Wolpe–Lazarus method of relaxation (for details see Eysenck, 1968). Hierarchies of smoking situations are obtained from questionnaires, and these situations are then imagined by the smoker under relaxing conditions. The assumption is that if the anxiety which 'causes' smoking is inhibited or reduced by whatever means, the smoker will experience less desire to smoke (Koenig & Masters, 1965).

A variant of systematic desensitisation is a form of counter-conditioning. This presupposes that, if a response other than smoking can be conditioned to stimuli which ordinarily lead to smoking, and the link between these stimuli and the response of smoking is weakened, then the smoker will have at his disposal an alternative strategy or response (Pyke, Agnew & Kopperud, 1966).

Operant self-control programmes based on techniques used with alcoholics and obese subjects have also been employed. Many variants of this are possible. One well-used technique (Ober, 1968) involves supplying subjects with a pocket-sized stimulator, subjects being instructed to shock themselves whenever they crave a cigarette.

Empirical studies of self-control techniques. Pechacek (1979) has comprehensively reviewed most of the stimulus-control cessation literature and concludes that smokers rarely reduce their consumption to fewer than 10 cigarettes a day, and that these gains are not maintained. At this point, presumably each cigarette becomes more reinforcing, and smoking becomes increasingly more difficult to give up. However, a number of carefully controlled studies employing a variety of skills have produced more encouraging results (Brengelmann, 1975, 1977; Pomerleau & Pomerleau, 1977; Pomerleau, Adkins & Pertschuk, 1978).

The contractual-management or contingency-contracting technique has also been more successful in later studies. Figures ranging from 84% (Elliott & Tighe, 1968) to 50% (Winett, 1973) abstinence at treatment termination have been reported. The Elliott & Tighe (1968) procedure, however, was a multi-component technique involving public pledges, stimulus-control techniques and group support. Some success has also been reported within a treatment-by-mail programme. Forty-seven per cent of those responding to a fifteen-month follow-up reported abstinence (Brengelmann & Sedlmayr, 1977). However, an obvious problem in such studies is the perennial one of the validity of self-report. There is also the problem of the non-responder. Overall, it seems that as a single technique, contingency contracting may initiate some behavioural change, and may be of value when used in combination with other procedures to prevent relapse.

Systematic desensitisation and coverant control have been shown in the more recent literature to be relatively ineffective (Pechacek, 1979).

Controlled smoking has also been studied. This involves helping smokers to migrate from high tar and nicotine cigarettes to pipes and cigars. Frederiksen (1976), Frederiksen, Peterson & Murphy (1976), Frederiksen & Frazier (1977) and Frederiksen, Miller & Peterson (1977) have shown that risks associated with smoking can be reduced by helping subjects change the topography of their behaviour. Smokers can be taught to change the amount of smoke inhaled, the number of puffs taken and the length of the cigarette smoked.

Overall, the self-management and stimulus-control techniques have been shown to be only temporarily superior to control conditions insofar as long-term cessation is concerned. There is the common pattern of immediate and often substantial temporary reduction followed by rapid relapse in long-term abstinence rates which do not differ significantly from those expected from unprompted quitting. Results, at best, could therefore only be described as moderately encouraging.

Aversion techniques

Some of the self-control techniques described above could be regarded as aversive. However, aversion therapy, as such, invariably involves much more radical and, in some cases, traumatic procedures.

One seldomly used technique involves the use of apomorphine, a centrally acting emetic. The nausea and vomiting caused by this drug is preceded by the smoking of a cigarette (Raymond, 1964).

A commonly used aversive stimulus in behaviour modification of maladaptive behaviours such as excessive drinking and sexual 'deviance' is electric shock. In smoking cessation the usual procedure is the delivery of a shock to the smoker, on an intermittent schedule, while he is inhaling smoke from a cigarette.

Covert sensitisation was first described by Cautela (1970). The smoker is trained to imagine the smoking act while receiving the suggestion that he is experiencing some highly unpleasant sensation such as vomiting.

Moving down the scale of aversiveness, we have another technique in which a ventilator is used to blow a mixture of hot air and smoke into the smoker's face, concurrent with his lighting a cigarette, such conditions being maintained until the cigarette is extinguished. Once the cigarette has been extinguished, a positive reinforcement, cool, mentholated air, is delivered, and the subject is encouraged to pick up and consume a mint (Wilde, 1964).

Negative practice, originally devised by Dunlap (1932), has been employed by Eysenck (1953) and subsequently used in a large number of studies concerned with smoking cessation (Leventhal & Cleary, 1980). In the presence of the experimenter, the subject rapidly smokes several cigarettes (at a puff rate of one every 6 or 12 s) while paying particular attention to sensory and psychophysiological reactions, and keeping in mind his desire to stop smoking. This technique is usually referred to as rapid smoking.

These latter three techniques could be regarded as variants of a 'satiation procedure', in which the subject is flooded or overwhelmed by the aversive stimulus, thus developing a residual, and, presumably, a long-lasting aversion.

The breath-holding method is infrequently used, but is reported to be reasonably effective. The subject is simply required to hold his breath for a short time concurrent with imagining the inhalation of a cigarette.

Empirical studies of aversion techniques. While chemical aversion techniques, using apomorphine or antabuse, have proved reasonably successful in treating alcoholism (Nathan & Briddell, 1977), there are no recent smoking cessation studies using chemical aversion reported in the current literature (Pechacek, 1979).

As we mentioned previously, the most commonly employed aversive stimulus is electric shock. Generally speaking, both the early and the later studies agree that this technique has failed to produce long-term abstinence (Pechacek, 1979). The comment of Russell, Armstrong & Patel (1976) that traditional electric shock conditioning procedures do not contribute significantly is apposite, and finds strong support in the contemporary literature. While some success has been reported, for example by Berecz (1976), who used imaginal urges rather than real smoking, this is an aberration from the general finding that, as a sole treatment, shock aversion therapy fails, mainly because the effects do not usually generalise outside the therapeutic context. Of interest here is Nathan & Briddell's (1977) complementary finding that electric aversion therapy does not produce enduring behaviour or attitudinal change towards excessive alcohol consumption.

As far as satiation techniques are concerned, despite some early encouraging results, recent data have been almost entirely negative. Rigorously controlled studies indicate that the technique is little superior to control procedures, and that long-term abstinence is poor (Pechacek, 1979).

The ventilated air technique has not proved popular in smoking cessation. A number of researchers have found the smoke-blowing apparatus inconvenient, the technique clumsy and the outcome uncertain (Lichtenstein *et al.*, 1973). They have therefore opted for the rapid-smoking-only condition, owing to its early effectiveness, convenience and simplicity. Results, however, have been mixed and variable. Danaher's (1977) review reports a wide variation in results, with some studies showing minimal or no long-term success, others showing moderate success and a few approximating the follow-up data of earlier studies. Pechacek (1979), from his review, reports essentially the same finding. Perhaps this procedure is potentially very effective. However, the intervention is complex, depending as it does on the subject's active revivification of the aversion, warm person–client relationships offering social reinforcement, positive expectations and flexible or individualised treatment scheduling to ensure total abstinence prior to the termination of treatment.

More encouraging results have been reported from combined treatments. For example, Schmahl, Lichtenstein & Harris (1972) report 100% termination abstinence and 57% abstinence at six-month follow-up where subjects were required to smoke rapidly and continuously (every 6 s) while facing into the blown smoke until further smoking could not be tolerated.

Overall, there is some unanimity that the recent sensitisation studies have produced disappointing results (Elliott & Denney, 1978; Glasgow, 1978). Production of only physiological aversion and conditioning effects are apparently insufficient to produce long-term abstinence.

Drug therapy

As we have previously noted, the ultimate reinforcement for smoking would appear to be the psychopharmacological effects of nicotine. While the exact nature of the reward involved is problematical, there seems little doubt that the known depressant and stimulant effects of nicotine provide the primary reinforcement. This being the case, it could be argued that drugs having the same pharmacological effect as nicotine should either substitute for smoking or minimise withdrawal symptoms.

The two main classes of drugs used have been nicotine itself or the lobeline compounds, i.e., drugs which simulate the effects of nicotine, and either tranquillisers, which are employed to suppress the symptoms of nervousness and irritability, or stimulants, such as amphetamines, which offset fatigue, these being states which often accompany smoking cessation.

This approach to smoking cessation has generally been unsuccessful. Lobeline has been the most approved substitute, but its effectiveness seems to be no greater than that of an appropriate placebo (Davison & Rosen, 1972). Most of the reported studies have produced no evidence to question the conclusion advanced in the 1964 Surgeon General's Report: 'Acceptable evidence that the extinction of the tobacco habit can be effected solely by the use of tobacco substitutes has not yet been presented.' As far as the second class of drugs is concerned, again the evidence is discouraging.

Drugs such as meprobamate and valium have been shown to have little effect on smoking cessation.

Another technique has been to employ nicotine chewing gum. Double-blind studies have shown that it is more effective than a placebo, but beyond the control of withdrawal symptoms, its effect seems to be a relatively small component in the overall success (Schneider, Popek, Jarvik & Gritz, 1977; Raw, Jarvis, Feyerabend & Russell, 1980). Of course, one aspect of treatment may be the actual chewing. To the extent that smoking is an oral fixation behaviour, sucking or chewing any substance could be to some degree a substitute behaviour (see Chapter 2: Psychobiological theories). It may also be true that greater success rates are achieved with nicotine chewing gum with the heavy 'addicted' smoker (Jarvis, Raw, Russell & Feyerabend, 1982). Another factor of relevance to the recently reported (Jarvis *et al.*, 1982) success of nicotine chewing gum is that in the UK it is available only on doctor's prescription and thus the treatment has the added force of personal medical advice.

A recent large-scale trial of 1550 patients attending hospital clinics with smoking-related diseases indicated that nicotine, versus placebo gum, versus advice booklets, produced no significant improvement on physician's advice, in terms of cessation rates at one year (Thoracic Society, 1983). COHb and plasma-SCN measures indicated that roughly a quarter of the patients who denied smoking were, in fact, still smoking. The relatively low final success rate (approximately 10%) in this study was much lower than the 38% success rate for nicotine gum reported by Jarvis *et al.* (1982). The authors (Thoracic Society, 1983) suggest that differences in the motivation to quit smoking, perhaps because of subject preselection by the therapist, are critical in determining final success rates. It may be, of course, that nicotine gum has a significant advantage as a treatment tool only in highly motivated heavy smokers. The use of other smoking substitutes, such as snuff or nasal nicotine solution, which produce higher nicotine plasma levels more rapidly than nicotine gum, may lead to greater success with therapies of this type (Russell *et al.*, 1983).

A rather less successful outcome has been reported for anti-smoking lozenges, which leave an unpleasant taste when tobacco is subsequently smoked.

Some researchers have employed a combination of drugs and other treatments. Schwartz & Dubitzsky (1968*a*, *b*), for example, employed meprobamate with and without individual and group therapy. Their results suggest that the placebo was, if anything, more effective than the treatment.

Some success has been claimed through the use of acupuncture administered by insertion of a stainless steel stud in each ear (Choy, Purnell & Jaffe, 1978). Unfortunately the follow-up was insufficient to draw firm conclusions about this technique. However, one possible mechanism of acupuncture action is by opiate-like peptide release in the brain (Mayer & Watkins, 1981) and release of these peptides has been implicated as a possible reinforcer for smoking (see Chapter 2: Simple addiction models and Chapter 3: Reinforcing mechanisms of nicotine for smoking: The brain).

Individual counselling

Various procedures have been described in the literature. One such is the transactional analysis programme, in which smoking is viewed as a symptom of an underlying conflict. The goal of therapy is the identification and understanding of the conflict. Presumably, as the conflict abates, the need to smoke correspondingly diminishes. This technique is prototypic of a wide variety of individual therapeutic programmes.

The most common informal method of individual counselling is physician counselling, and this has been reviewed by Rose (1977b) and Lichtenstein & Danaher (1978). These reviews point to some rather surprising results. It appears that physicians have been discouraged from a counselling role, and that they are effective as counsellors only when dramatic symptoms are present. Even here, however, there is marked variation in success rates, which range from around 5% abstinence at six-month follow-up in a briefly counselled group (Porter & McCullough, 1972), to 38% for males and 11% for females at one-year follow-up (Handel, 1973), to 53% of males and 32% of females at one-year follow-up in patients presenting current respiratory symptoms (Burns, 1969). The carefully randomised trial reported by Russell, Wilson, Taylor & Baker (1979) reporting 10.3% and 19.1% of subjects quitting at one-year follow-up in control and maximal impact experimental groups, is also worth mentioning. In this general context, there are a good deal of data to show that ex-smokers themselves have linked increase in respiratory symptoms with smoking, and that this was a major precipitant for unaided quitting (Pechacek, 1979).

Clearly, this variability may in part be due to uncontrolled factors such as the nature and strength of the intervention (advice, pamphlets and so on) and individual physician style. Pincherle & Wright (1970) and Richmond (1977) both report a significant physician effect of this sort. Therefore, it seems that we have a fairly complex interaction between counselling style and the status of the smoker – whether, for example, he is a patient presenting respiratory symptoms, or not. This is clearly illustrated in some of the studies of cessation in patients hospitalised with first myocardial infarction. There are suggestions that from 30 to 50% of smokers in such groups stop smoking permanently, quitting rates being maintained for one or more years. When the initial routine advice is supplemented by more intensive counselling and active follow-up, the quitting rate appears to increase to around 60% (Burt et al., 1974).

In recent years, hypnotherapy has become a popular technique. However, while a number of claims have been made about the effectiveness of this procedure, it appears that such claims are extravagant. The early research led Johnston & Donoghue (1971) to conclude that 'there is almost no good research evidence attesting to the effectiveness of hypnosis in the elimination of smoking behaviour'. Data from more recent studies do nothing to refute this (Pederson, Scrimgedur & Lefcoe, 1975; Perry & Mullens, 1975; Barkley, Hastings & Jackson, 1977; Shewchuk et al., 1977).

Clearly, in all individual therapeutic programmes, the amount of time spent with the therapist and the relationship between the therapist and the client are important intervening variables. Supportive counselling of this sort, however, is a time-consuming and expensive procedure.

More broadly based intervention programmes

Group therapy procedures cover a wide range of techniques. They have the common characteristic, however, that clients are treated in relatively small groups, with the psychological factors involved in smoking and in smoking cessation generally being emphasised.

Some group therapy approaches are patterned after Alcoholics Anonymous. Treatment may consist of medical lectures, group discussions, instruction in habit change, and, for some subjects, drug (e.g., lobeline) treatment and/or the 'buddy' system, in which smokers, when motivated to have a cigarette, contact friends who dissuade them from smoking.

Of somewhat broader application are the Public Service Clinics, such as those of the American Cancer Society (ACS) and the Five-Day Plan, which have been perhaps the most actively promoted intervention strategy. Clinics of the Five-Day Plan, which use educational and fear-arousing communications, willpower, the buddy system, and a guide book of living instructions for the five days, employ total abstinence as the only success criterion.

However, only very limited outcome data of acceptable validity are available from these sources. For example, almost all the evaluations of the Five-Day Plan, showing good immediate abstinence rates of roughly 60–80%, with approximately 50% relapse by 1–3 months post-treatment, have been without controls. One of the few comparative studies of this treatment is that of Guilford (1972). He reports abstinence rates of 16–20% at one-year follow-up. These figures do not differ from those reported for unaided quitting (Pechacek, 1979).

A similar outcome is reported for ACS programmes which focus on insight development, group support and self-selected cessation techniques (Pyszka, Ruggels & Janowicz, 1973). Abstinence rates based on a random sample of participants in this programme were 41.7% post-treatment, 30% at six-month, 22% at one year and 18% at eighteen-month follow-up.

Other clinic programmes with similar or more elaborate formats, such as the Smoking Withdrawal Clinic Programmes, which are distinguished by an emphasis on educative and cognitive treatment aspects, and by treatment of large numbers of relatively unselected subjects, have reported similar outcome figures. These, however, are somewhat at variance with earlier data, such as those reported, for example, by the Ejrup (1963) Stockholm Clinic, which employed programmes consisting of 10 days of intensive educational, psychological and pharmacological (primarily lobeline) treatment. With 1021 subjects, an immediate quitting rate of 76% was reported, with the remaining subjects, who did not quit, reducing cigarette consumption by at least one-half.

By contrast, the Toronto Smoking Withdrawal Centre reports only 15–20% long-term abstinence amongst participants, a figure similar to that reported by the SmokeEnders (1971) Programme. In view of the generally accepted success rates for unaided control groups of around 16–19%, the impact of these programmes appears to be minimal, a fact which contradicts the earlier findings based on self-report. The placebo effect noted in control groups highlights the fact that many of the treatment effects in clinics remain undefined.

Other clinic programmes feature drugs, films, lectures, group discussions, with group meetings occurring at regular intervals. Examples are the Philadelphia Project, and the Smokers' Advisory Clinic of the British Ministry of Health.

One feature of most of these smoking clinic programmes is the high rates of attrition during the course of treatment. Nevertheless, the best of the clinics claim to produce results which are superior to those from the best of the behaviour modification studies in terms of *immediate* treatment effects.

Note that although the long-term figures reported may be little different from unaided quitting rates, it could be argued that participants are drawn from the remaining 75–80% who cannot quit unaided, so that treatment effects, despite the Guilford results, may still be occurring. This comment, of course, is relevant to all intervention procedures. A 20% quitting rate from a highly selected group of 'hard-core' smokers could be regarded as a significant treatment effect.

Treatment packages

A recent trend has been towards comprehensive programmes utilising combinations of techniques from both behavioural self-control and aversive control categories. Reviews of relevant studies (McAlister, 1975; Bernstein & McAlister, 1976; Lichtenstein & Danaher, 1976) report encouraging results. Initial success in treatment and maintained abstinence, up to one-year follow-up, has been reported by Pomerleau *et al.* (1978) and Brengelmann (1977). Best, Bass & Owen (1977) and Best, Owen & Trentadue (1978) using aversive smoking plus self-management techniques, report abstinence rates of 35–55% at six-month follow-up. Delahunt & Curran (1976) report that for female smokers a package (negative practice and self-control procedures) is superior to control procedures and to the individual components of the package. Data from six-month follow-up indicated that 56% of the combined treatment group were abstinent, while the figures for control and independent-component groups varied between 0 and 22%. Unfortunately, biological assay procedures were not available. Elliott (1977) reports roughly similar results. As Pechacek (1979) points out, however, these are the best of the available studies, others reporting much more limited success.

Again, it appears that the difficulties are great, and that success is to some extent a product of practical knowledge of the problems which guide the application of the treatment programme. Planned, extended contacts, plus adaptation of techniques to individual needs seem necessary for long-term success. To the extent that smoking typologies have validity, treatments need to be designed for the individual smoker. In addition, many of the studies are still bedevilled by some of the validation problems mentioned previously: the inconclusiveness of self-report, lack of supporting biological assay and inadequate follow-up. There is also the problem of the non-responder, a point well illustrated in the Brenglemann & Sedlmayr (1977) treatment-by-mail study. If we make the assumption that non-responders were still smoking, the success rate reported (47%) would in fact be reduced to 23%, which is not much different from that reported for non-treatment quitting. There is as yet little information on some very recent innovations in treatment, some of which involve media treatment, self-study books and so on. These techniques await controlled validation studies.

Thus, as far as the multi-component approach is concerned, recent data suggest that combinations of therapeutic procedures containing both motivational and skill-training components produce more favourable outcomes, although the increments are not striking (Delahunt & Curran, 1976; Lando, 1977; Elliott & Denney, 1978). Note, however, that at times combinations produce no significant gain over single therapies (Danaher, 1977) and, in some cases, may even decrease effectiveness (Lamontagne, Gagnon & Gaudette, 1978). For example, several studies have reported a decrease in the effectiveness of treatments when they are followed by phone calls or booster sessions to reinforce quitting (Best *et al.*, 1977; Elliott & Denney, 1978). It is obviously important to identify and deal with the range, frequency, periodicity and strength of the various controlling stimuli. If this is not done, the skills taught in the intervention programme may be only partly relevant to the smoker's problems and, indeed, may lure him into a false sense of security about his ability to control the habit. Where this occurs, the procedure may become counter-productive.

Maintenance of non-smoking

The limited success of most of the cessation techniques we have described, plus the fact that while treatment termination figures are quite encouraging, subsequent relapse rates are often dramatically high, has led many researchers to recognise that initial cessation is only one aspect of treatment. The novice ex-smoker therefore needs 'maintenance pro-gramming'. We have to build in the necessary, and sufficient, reinforcements not only to modify behaviour but also to maintain the change, and have to ensure that these reinforcers have a high probability of occurrence in the natural environment. Booster sessions and telephone support may be important. It may also be necessary to ensure a 'cognitive re-structuring' (i.e., change in attitudes, lifestyle and personal habits) of the successful quitter to maintain abstinence (Marlatt, 1979).

Generally speaking, maintenance programmes have not been very successful, although some isolated successes have been reported, for example that of Lando (1977), who employed a contingency contracting programme following an aversive procedure. Again, it seems that the effectiveness of post-termination maintenance programmes follows the same general pattern of single cessation techniques or combinations of techniques described earlier.

However, the spectrum of techniques available for non-smoking main-tenance is more circumscribed than is the case for smoking cessation. The directly suppressive (aversive) techniques, which focus on the smoking response, e.g., rapid smoking, which has been claimed to be one of the more effective techniques, are obviously irrelevant here. Maintenance strategies can therefore embrace only the self-monitoring, drug and counselling procedures.

One of the real problems of the maintenance of non-smoking is clearly the identification and elimination of the personal situational factors which support smoking, and which therefore may cause ex-smokers to relapse. In addition to this, of course, we have a complex interaction between individual personality characteristics and situational factors. For example, if nicotine is used to control anxiety, we would expect the more neurotic ex-smokers to be more susceptible to relapse. Attempts to utilise information about individual differences to maximise treatment effectiveness have not been very successful as yet (Pechacek, 1979), although it is fair comment that seldom has this factor been seriously considered in intervention programmes. There are good grounds for assuming that individual differences in personality characteristics have some effect on maintenance of non-smoking, as well as cessation, programmes.

We have already noted the fact that, as a group, high socioeconomic status (SES) smokers have been more successful in quitting the habit. In addition, there is some evidence that men are slightly more successful than women in quitting (Gritz, 1979). It is possible, of course, that this is a reflection of male/female personality differences, since there is evidence from smoking typologies that women tend to smoke more to relieve feelings of anxiety and anger (Russell *et al.*, 1974), this type of negative affect smoker being more 'addicted'. Given the important evidence from longitudinal studies that personality variables such as extraversion and emotional stability are predictive of greater success in quitting (Cherry & Kiernan, 1976), and that the personality norms of the general population clearly show that women score slightly lower both on extraversion and on emotional stability (Eysenck & Eysenck, 1975), we might expect women, on this basis, to be less successful in quitting.

Apart from SES and personality predictors, there is abundant evidence that the lighter smoker is more successful in quitting (Gordon, Kannel & McGee, 1974; Cherry & Kiernan, 1976). The finding that the successful quitter also consumes less coffee and alcohol (Friedman *et al.*, 1979) is consistent with the general finding of some correlations between cigarette, coffee, tea and alcohol consumption which provides empirical backing for a polydrug model of substance abuse (see Chapter 6).

Other important factors for maintenance of non-smoking are giving the smoker a positive attitude with regard to withdrawal symptoms, and his ability to deal with them, together with factors such as dismissal of fear (amongst women) that they will gain weight if they stop smoking. Clearly, specific plans should be formulated to aid the smoker to confront his or her predicted problem area.

As a final observation, we might note that the types of outcome usually reported for smoking cessation, i.e., good immediate cessation figures, but high relapse rates at six-month or one-year follow-up, parallel to a considerable degree outcome results from earlier studies, and from other drug abuse studies, although there are some obvious exceptions. Results from the most recent studies of substance abuse, as reviewed, for example, by Krasnegor (1980), do not differ substantially from those presented by Hunt & Matarazzo (1973) comparing relapse rates over time for heroin, smoking and alcohol. These data are presented in Fig. 18. Whether these figures reflect the inadequacy of intervention strategies vis-à-vis smoking in particular, or drug abuse in general, is a matter of conjecture. It is also uncertain whether the similarities in relapse rates imply that the dynamics underlying various modes of substance abuse are similar. This leads onto

Fig. 18. Relapse rates over time for heroin (filled circles), smoking (triangles) and alcohol (open circles). (From Hunt & Matarazzo, 1973. *Copyright (1973) by the American Psychological Association. Adapted by permission of the authors.* First published by Hunt, W. A., Barnett, L. W. & Branch, L. G., Oct. 1971, in *Journal of Clinical Psychology* by permission of Clinical Psychology Publishers, Co., Brandon, USA.)

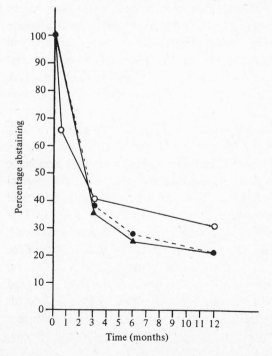

consideration of a polydrug model, which has considerable support from other studies (Cederlof *et al.*, 1977), and which we shall discuss in Chapter 6.

Summary

In view of the enormous amount of outcome research reported over the last twenty years, it is remarkable that relatively little success has been achieved in the area of smoking termination. It is estimated that 95% of the 29 million smokers who have quit in the USA since 1964 have done so of their own accord (National Cancer Institute, 1977). Survey data indicate that only a third or less of smokers motivated to quit are interested in formal programmes (Gallup Opinion Index, 1974) and that only a small minority of those who do express an interest actually attend programmes. Thus, the objective outcome data available are based on a small minority sample of the hard core of smokers.

As indicated in the Surgeon General's Report (1979) and in a number of reviews, it is abundantly clear that, while many of the behaviour modification and drug techniques which have been found to be successful in other areas of behaviour therapy have proved to be temporarily superior to control conditions in smoking cessation, the outcomes have not been maintained over any substantial follow-up period. Generally speaking, the percentages reported at one-year follow-up seldom differ from those reported for unaided quitting. On the other hand, some of the Public Health programmes report considerable success, particularly where smoking cessation is one aspect of, say, coronary prevention programmes. However, the results of these studies, in the main, are still confounded by weak designs and reliance on self-report. Acceptability of results is therefore questionable.

Whether or not the multi-component treatment approach will lead to a more promising outcome is a matter for debate. The same applies to the increasing focus on maintenance programming, where the multi-component approach might be expected to prove more successful. Here packages are aimed at giving the ex-smoker new skills needed to deal with, or adjust to his new non-smoking lifestyle.

If there is any validity in the smoking typologies we have previously described, it seems obvious that smoking cessation and non-smoking maintenance techniques, or combinations of techniques, have to be tailored to the individual smoker. His lifestyle, personality characteristics, tolerance of stress and so on may critically determine the extent to which various cessation and maintenance strategies are likely to be successful.

TERMINATION STRATEGIES: mass communication, health education and advertising

The specific and largely individualised intervention techniques discussed in the previous section seem to have met with limited success. As we have noted, it has been estimated that 95% of smokers who have quit in the USA since 1964 have done so as a result of their own efforts. The question arises as to the extent to which this so-called 'unaided quitting' has been influenced by public awareness of the health risks associated with smoking as a result of mass media coverage, public health programmes, increased no-smoking areas and so on.

General public health programmes

Under the rubric 'General Public Health Programmes' we should include the effects of specific 'one-off' events, such as the publication of reports by the US Surgeon General and the Royal College of Physicians in England, and the various media and public health campaigns mounted by agencies such as the Health Education Council.

The cumulative effect of such continuing publicity appears to have been a fairly substantial reduction in prevalence rates. In the period 1955–75, rates for males in the USA reduced from 52% to 39%, although for females there was an increase from 25% to 29%. Roughly similar figures are reported for the UK (see Introduction). Overall, prevalence rates have been reduced by 20–30% below the *predicted* 1975 level, although this is counterbalanced, to some extent, by a substantial increase in the consumption levels of the remaining smokers. During this period there has also been an almost complete shift to consumption of filter-tipped cigarettes (Surgeon General, 1979, Appendix A, p. 5), no doubt in part due to the belief that these are less hazardous. Also consistent with the view that publicity about the health risks of smoking has some effect on the smoker is the observation of temporary decline in total per capita consumption of cigarettes coinciding with periods of increased publicity, such as the times of publication of the various reports referred to above.

Of course, other factors might also be relevant to this overall reduction in smoking prevalence, e.g., a more positive attitude to physical health, which is reflected in jogging and healthier diet as well as in smoking and drinking levels. Interactions here may be very complex, so complex as to make it difficult to establish in any clear-cut fashion the exact role of anti-smoking programmes as such in smoking cessation. This is relevant to the O'Keefe (1971) observation that while television anti-smoking commercials may have produced changes in attitudes towards smoking,

they appear to have had minimal impact on smoking cessation. Only 1%
of ex-smokers credited the commercials with helping them to quit. Eiser,
Sutton & Wober (1978*a*, *b*) have also reported that commercials of this
sort have little effect on smoking cessation.

In general, most of the published reviews of the effects of media
anti-smoking campaigns suggest that the immediate effects are relatively
small (Eiser *et al.*, 1978*a*, *b*; Surgeon General, 1979). This may be due, in
part, to the fact that most of the anti-smoking and the more general health
programmes attach significance to repetition and to the 'threat' content
of the various messages. There seems to be an assumption in the literature
that sheer repetition of an anti-smoking message over multiple media will
attract attention, will change attitudes and change behaviour. This
expectation derives from the simple compliance model of Kelman (1958),
which is rather uncritically thought to apply to advertising in general. As
far as smoking cessation is concerned, however, this model seems to have
misdirected effort, making intervention even less effective than it might
otherwise have been.

A considerable amount of evidence from small-scale intervention studies
suggests that while the more vivid threat messages generate stronger
attitudes and intentions to quit immediately following the message, it is
equally clear that these do not persist, dissipating as the emotion associated
with the message weakens (Leventhal & Niles, 1965). Perhaps more
importantly, there is evidence that a strong fear message encourages
avoidance of threatening situations, e.g., not taking chest X-rays or not
exposing oneself to health information (Leventhal & Watts, 1966). Another
finding of interest is that a combination of messages which convey
information on personal vulnerability to damage and information on
threat, produces a smaller effect than either alone (Leventhal, 1970).
Leventhal (1974) comments that, although vivid threat messages arouse
more fear and stronger intentions to quit, in the absence of specific action
plans these do not lead to behaviour change. Conversely, specific action
plans themselves, without a fear message, seem to have little effect on
attitudes or behaviour.

Targetted programmes

A recent Finnish study investigating the effects of a series of
television counselling sessions which involved viewers to a greater extent
through organised 'self-help viewing groups', appears to be more promising
for smoking cessation (McAlister *et al.*, 1980). Unfortunately, in this case,
lack of control groups makes it difficult to evaluate the relative influence
of the television campaign as opposed to the specific group interventions.

This same situation applies in the case of directed community-wide programmes (Leventhal & Cleary, 1980). Fairly typical (of a programme with no control groups) is Ryan's (1973) report on the Cold Turkey Project in Greenfield, Iowa. At seven-month follow-up, only 3.9% of the active female smokers, and 14.2% of the active male smokers were abiding by their non-smoking pledges.

An interesting approach in this general area has been the employment of large-scale coronary prevention trials in which middle-aged men judged to be at risk for, but not exhibiting, coronary heart disease are exposed to anti-smoking counselling. This has been attempted in a number of countries, e.g., the US, Sweden, the UK and Finland. In these programmes, of course, smoking cessation is not the only target behaviour; attempts are also made, usually through nutritional counselling and other devices, to reduce serum cholesterol and blood pressure levels, both of which are considered to be critical factors in the aetiology of coronary heart disease.

Some of these programmes, such as the Coronary Prevention Evaluation Programme in Great Britain (Stamler, 1970a, b), the Multiple Risk Factor Intervention Trial (1977, 1979) in the USA, and a number of programmes in Sweden (Wilhelmsen, 1972) and the UK (Reid *et al.*, 1974), suggest quitting rates ranging from 30 to 50%. In most of these studies, however, biochemical assay techniques were unavailable, and it is difficult to accept the validity of the self-report data, especially when it is realised that, due to sample size, much follow-up was not face-to-face, which might be expected to encourage truthful reporting, but by telephone and post. There is also, of course, the question of the actual intensity of the intervention, which can range from routine advice to intensive personal counselling, and again this might be expected to have a marked effect on quitting rates.

A few studies have focused on total populations, and these are of especial interest. One such is that of the North Karelia Project (1976a, b), which was aimed at a reduction of cardiovascular disease in Eastern Finland. Smoking intervention as one aspect of the overall programme resulted in a reduction in the proportion of smokers from 53% to 43% in males aged 25–59 years. Female smoking rates, however, were relatively unchanged. Of interest also is the Stanford Heart Disease Prevention Programme (MacCoby, Farquhar, Wood & Alexander, 1977), which involved an extensive two-year mass media campaign and intensive counselling. Three years after the programme started the proportion of smokers had decreased by 3% in the control group, by 8% in the media-only treatment group, and by 24% in the media plus counselling community.

Of particular note is the Belgian study of Kornitzer, De Backer,

Dramaix & Thilly (1980). The impact of a health programme on smoking, blood pressure and serum cholesterol was examined on 16222 randomly selected male factory workers at high risk for heart disease, these being equally distributed between intervention and control groups. Of the intervention group, 18.7% reported quitting smoking as opposed to 12.2% of the control group. No differences between experimental and control groups were found for a random sample of non- high risk participants. The intervention material was media programmes, booklets and medical advice.

Advertising

The effect of a complementary strategy to targetted programmes, that of banning cigarette advertising, is difficult to evaluate. It has been suggested that the temporary drop in cigarette consumption in the UK for 1965 was due to the banning of cigarette advertising on television in that year (Atkinson & Skegg, 1974). Here, however, we should consider the possible effect of the preceding Report of the Royal College of Physicians (1962). It is possible that bans of this sort, together with media coverage of smoking risks, rather than causing an absolute downturn have prevented further increase in the consumption of tobacco (Surgeon General, 1979, Ch. 18, p. 22). The situation is further confused by the availability of alternative forms of advertising such as posters, shop displays and sport sponsorship into which the tobacco industry can divert its advertising resources. The cigarette industry has asserted that the major action of cigarette advertising is to shift brand preferences and to alter market shares between brands. This is perhaps true in countries where the market is relatively saturated and stable. However, cigarette advertising in a potentially expanding market (e.g., the so-called 'developing' world) may be a positive incentive to smokers, as opposed to merely shifting brand preferences. World production of cigarettes is still increasing, and is expected to reach a record 4,500 billion cigarettes per annum soon (ASH, 1981a). Some authors argue that cigarette advertising is critical in maintaining the social acceptability of smoking (Hoffman, 1979). The most important long-term consequence of this may be the indirect encouragement of the taking up of smoking by adolescents.

Price

Other factors, such as the price of cigarettes, appear to have a relatively minor influence on consumption, despite some earlier suggestions to the contrary. Tanner (1912), for example, in analysing the effects of duty increases on UK consumption of tobacco per capita for the years 1900–10, reported an upward trend in consumption during this period, which, however, was reversed at the three points of 'visitation' by the Chancellor of the Exchequer, in 1901, 1904 and 1909. Recovery followed after a year or so. Tanner was in no doubt about the effect of price on consumption, and commented 'In countries like Holland, where duties are very low, tobacco consumption runs to three times as much' (Tanner, 1912, p. 105).

More recent estimates are generally more conservative. Russell (1973), for example, estimates that for every 1% increase in price, consumption falls by 0.6%. Confounding factors are, of course, inflation, growth of real wages, shifts from unfiltered to filter-tipped cigarettes, changes in the age profile of the population and anti-cigarette campaigns themselves, including bans on television advertising (Surgeon General, 1979: Ch. 18, p. 23).

Differing emphases are given to these factors by different authors, partly due to the difference in socioeconometric models utilised. Thus, while most researchers acknowledge the effects of anti-smoking media campaigns, including bans on television advertising, some analyses give more emphasis to the 'real' (i.e., inflation-corrected) price of cigarettes (Russell, 1973; Peto, 1974) while others stress the relative importance of 'real' disposable income (Atkinson & Skegg, 1974).

There is some evidence, however, which suggests that the recent large price increases in the UK during the period 1980–1 may have reduced sales by up to 11% (ASH, 1981*b*). Here we are, of course, observing the combined effects of a large price increase and a levelling-off of real income in the years 1980–1, during which the UK experienced a recession, with over two million people unemployed. On more recent evidence (Business, 1982), an average of a 30% rise in UK cigarette prices over the period February 1981 to January 1982 has produced a decrease in the volume of sales of approximately 14%. Correction for inflation (conservatively estimated at 12%) over this time period produces a reduction in sales of 0.5% for every 1% increase in price. This is remarkably close to Russell's (1973) estimate. However, it is not known, as yet, whether this is a reflection of reduced prevalence or reduced consumption, or both.

Finally, we should re-emphasise that a general shift in attitudes towards a more 'healthy' lifestyle, in which increased exercise, better diet and reduced dependence on drugs of all kinds are important elements, makes it difficult to disentangle specific influences of the media or price on cigarette smoking. There does appear to be a smoking 'lifestyle', and it is entirely possible that reduced smoking prevalence is one aspect of a general change in this lifestyle. Possible consequences of such a change are discussed in Chapter 6.

School education/prevention

It is surely a truism that prevention is better than cure. Anti-smoking health education in schools attempts this goal. One of the earliest recorded examples of prevention of smoking in 'school', in this case an Oxbridge college, was an incident in which 'young Pupills, all Freshmen save one or two' were caught smoking by a master, and their pipes and tobacco confiscated and destroyed (Braithwait, 1617).

In the USA, during the later part of the nineteenth century, the Women's Christian Temperance Union mounted a campaign against alcohol and 'narcotics', especially tobacco. Particular emphasis was placed on morality and health education in schools, and this culminated in extensive legislation demanding school instruction on physiology and hygiene, including information about, and attitudes towards, alcohol and tobacco (Means, 1962). However, in spite of legislative success, this campaign has been criticised for being too moralising, for the preaching of zeal and negation, for frequent factual inaccuracy and for inappropriate matching of the factual materials to the age groups being taught (Surgeon General, 1979; Sect. 23–13).

At the beginning of the twentieth century, the 'International Anti-Cigarette League' (which, in spite of its title, was mainly based in the UK) had some success in curbing the sale of cigarettes to children. Indeed, this organisation, which numbered Winston Churchill and Baden-Powell on its board, seems to have been prototypic of many modern anti-smoking health education campaigns. It published its own gazette, inaugurated a vigorous system of education and 'pledges' in schools (similar to 'pledges' for alcohol abstinence by the nineteenth-century Temperance movements), and gained support in parliament (an Anti-Cigarette Bill was introduced into the House of Commons by Dr Macnamara in 1905). In addition, it attempted to curb cigarette advertising, promoted anti-smoking songs and disseminated literature and badges (see Fig. 19). Finally, it attempted some theorising about the actual rewards enjoyed by the smoker, as well as emphasising the costs in health, money, 'weak' attitudes (i.e., being slaves to a habit) and annoyance to non-smokers. However, at that time there was no definite proof of the association between cigarette smoking and disease, and the campaign appears to have petered out after accomplishing part of its major aim, that of preventing the sale to, and use of cigarettes by, minors. The year 1908 brought the prohibition to retailers supplying children under 16 years of age (Tanner, 1912). Unfortunately, as a recent survey has revealed, this law is extensively broken (ASH, 1981c).

More recent strategies for the prevention of cigarette smoking by

Fig. 19. Typical extracts from the pages of the *International Anti-Cigarette League Gazette* (1905).

.. THE ..

INTERNATIONAL AND ANTI-CIGARETTE LEAGUE

[FOUNDED - - - - MARCH, 1901]

GAZETTE.

ADVISORY BOARD :—

The Ven. Archdeacon SINCLAIR.
Rev. W. T. McCORMICK.
Major-General R. S. S. BADEN-POWELL, *Chairman.*
WINSTON L. S. CHURCHILL, Esq., M.P.

ROBERT FARQUHARSON, Esq., M.D., M.P.
Dr. T. J. MACNAMARA, M.P.
ANDREW MELROSE, Esq.
Dr. H. J. SPENSER.
Professor G. SIMS WOODHEAD, M.D., F.R.S.E.

Founder and Hon. Sec.—Rev. FRANK JOHNSON.

Headquarters: 57 & 59, LUDGATE HILL, LONDON.

No. 3.   *MAY and JUNE, 1905.*   MONTHLY, ONE HALFPENNY.

BETWEEN OURSELVES.

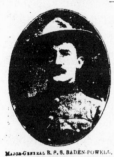

MAJOR-GENERAL R. S. S. BADEN-POWELL.

This month I have the pleasure of passing on a message from Major-General Baden-Powell, the famous defender of Mafeking. He is rendering us valuable assistance on the Advisory Board of the League, and though busy with important duties, yet finds time to assist every cause aiming at making the youth of the nation physically and mentally efficient.

Message from Major-General Baden-Powell.

War Office, Horse Guards, Whitehall, S.W.

I am glad to hear of the good progress which is being made by the I.A.-C.L. I believe that it has taken the evil in hand just in time to save the boys of England from becoming seriously injured by cigarette smoking. If every British boy will let cigarettes alone, we stand a good chance as a nation not only of holding our own, but of beating all competitors.

R. S. S. BADEN-POWELL.

The Anti-Cigarette Bill introduced into the House of Commons by Dr. Macnamara has made as yet no further progress. Resolutions in its favour have been passed at Bath, Glasgow, and other places, and newspapers like the *Sunday School Chronicle* and the *Schoolmaster* are doing much to keep the subject well before the public mind. In the former journal two interesting articles have appeared, the first giving the views of tobacconists on Dr. Macnamara's Bill, and the second the views of boy smokers themselves on the cigarette. From the former article it appears that some

---

SMOKERS' EARS.

THE effects of tobacco-smoking upon the ears, says a writer in the *Strand Magazine*, form the subject of interesting German anthropological investigations. Out of 1,000 persons examined, 760 were smokers. Of these, 696 were the children of smokers and about 356, or half of these, were stated to have been the grandchildren of habitual smokers. Of this latter number,

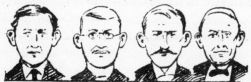

300 were distinguished by an adjustment of the ear more or less at right angles from the head, a peculiarity observable in only 7½ per cent. of the offspring of non-smokers and in 29 per cent. of the non-smokers. All this would seem to point to some action of nicotine upon the aural muscles, giving rise to the "smoker's ear."

adolescents may be conveniently divided into four main types: (a) those aiming to increase the knowledge of the harmful consequences of smoking on health; (b) those aiming to change attitudes towards the 'image' of the smoker, i.e., those emphasising the negative social aspects of smoking; (c) those demonstrating the immediate physiological effects of smoking and (d) those attempting to influence adolescent smoking through exemplars, whether these be classroom peers or adults such as teachers, parents and prominent youth culture 'idols'.

As in the case of the intervention strategies with adults, however, many of the programmes aimed at adolescents, although well meaning, lack adequate design, and have serious methodological flaws, such as failure to include control groups, inadequate follow-up and lack of objective assessments of smoking. This is clear from the major reviews of the large numbers of both formal and informal health education programmes in schools provided by Thompson (1978), Leventhal & Cleary (1980) and the Surgeon General (1979: Ch. 20). Given these reviews, we have not attempted to review all the studies reported but only give some examples, and detail those of special interest.

Increasing the knowledge about harmful consequences of smoking on health

This is the most basic approach to prevention possible, and it is underpinned by the assumption that if schoolchildren learn about the harmful consequences of smoking, they will act rationally and either stop smoking or be deterred from starting. Knowledge of health hazards is usually presented through lectures by teachers and/or visiting physicians, poster displays, simple smoking machine demonstrations of tar deposits from tobacco smoke, threat films, student participation in anti-smoking essays and group discussion. These programmes are generally successful in increasing knowledge about the harmful consequences of smoking and marginally increase positive attitudes in favour of not smoking, but apparently they do not produce substantial changes in actual behaviour (Leventhal & Cleary, 1980). For example, Briney (1967) found no relationship between knowledge of the effects of cigarette smoking and the practice of smoking amongst high school seniors in the USA. Similarly, in a large-scale Health Education Programme in the South East of England, Holland & Elliott (1968) found that in schools receiving a visit from a team of health educators, as opposed to control schools, there was no significant change in smoking habits. Anti-smoking propaganda, in this case, consisted of posters and discussions.

Some programmes have had slightly greater success. For example, Horn

(1960) reported roughly 10% less smoking in schools given messages about the potential future dangers of smoking. However, the results of this and similar programmes are generally so minimal that it has prompted concern that 'facts alone are not sufficient to deter teenagers from becoming smokers' (Surgeon General, 1979: Ch. 20, p. 6). This is perhaps unsurprising, given that the health hazards of smoking are so remote for the adolescent that they may be perceived as having little immediate personal relevance.

Changing attitudes towards smoking

A typical example of a programme which has attempted to change attitudes rather than simply increase the knowledge of health risks is the Maine Programme (Beckerman, 1963) in the USA. This programme used the original five communication messages of Horn, Courts, Taylor & Solomon (1959) in one package. These five messages were the remote effects of the health hazards of smoking, the current meaning of smoking, the two sides of the smoking issue, authoritative stands on the issue and assumption of an adult role with attempts to dissuade the parents from smoking. The package was presented in five educational exposures, spaced throughout the school year, including an audio-visual component, a discussion and pamphlets to take home and read. Questionnaire evaluation of the 26 experimental and 26 control schools revealed attitude changes by the end of the school year, and that changes in smoking behaviour emerged at the beginning of the next year. By then the original ninth grade group (15-year-olds) contained significantly fewer smokers in the experimental than in the control group. Unfortunately, although programmes of this nature produce significant changes in attitudes, and increased knowledge of the health hazards of smoking, changes in actual smoking behaviour are often small even though statistically significant (Thompson, 1978; Leventhal & Cleary, 1980).

Demonstration of the immediate physiological effects of smoking

For many adolescents, knowledge of the health hazards involved in smoking fails to have much impact because the threat appears to be far in the future. To increase the sense of immediacy and reality of the potential harmful effects of smoking for the adolescent, various programmes have been developed in the USA to demonstrate the more immediate physiological effects of cigarettes. These effects include an elevation in heart rate, a drop in skin temperature, increased hand tremor and a rise in exhaled CO (Evans et al., 1978). A similar programme is currently in the process of development by the Health Education Council in the UK.

Some success has been reported by Mitchell (1978). Thus, of the 249 students who were smokers before exposure to the programme, 24.5% had stopped smoking two months later and another 36% had decreased consumption considerably (Mitchell, 1978). However, insufficient control data have been reported to permit a clear evaluation. Nonetheless, the method is an interesting new departure, and may prove to be of some value.

Influences on adolescent smoking through exemplars

There is some evidence to suggest that social pressure exerted by peers and older siblings greatly encourages experimentation with cigarettes (Gorsuch & Butler, 1976). Smoking by family members, particularly parents, reduces barriers to peer pressure and increases opportunities for obtaining cigarettes for further experimentation (Borland & Rudolph, 1975). Other possible sources of negative exemplars are teachers who smoke, and high-status individuals, such as pop stars, television and film personalities, who smoke. It is difficult to quantify this effect, but given the tendency of children to learn by imitation, it is not unreasonable to suggest that these are potentially potent influences.

Most attempts to use non-smoking exemplars in smoking prevention programmes have involved some variation on peer teaching. There are two reasons for this. Firstly, there is the assumption that peer exemplars are more influential than adults. Secondly, it is difficult to persuade sufficient numbers of key adults (parents, teachers, 'pop stars') to set an example by giving up smoking themselves.

The clearest theoretical rationale for these methods is given by Evans (1976). Students are to be given small doses of the 'disease', peer pressure, so that they are 'innoculated' and later able to resist 'infection'. The innoculation is effected by use of illustrative films, discussion and role playing.

A number of smoking prevention programmes have utilised this strategy. A 'youth-to-youth' teaching element was incorporated in the San Diego Program (Surgeon General, 1979, Section 20–15). High school 'Key Club' members were encouraged to talk to 10- and 11-year-olds in schools serving as 'feeder' schools to their high schools. From 1971 to 1974, a total of 728 students, trained to conduct peer-training programmes, talked with 35445 students. Overall, the programme had mixed success. While a decrease in the proportion of boys smoking, by contrast with the nationwide trends, was reported, smoking among girls (aged 12–15 years) increased, in parallel to the nationwide trend of increased smoking amongst girls.

Evans and colleagues at the University of Houston (Evans *et al.*, 1978) report a study which they claim shows significant effects of a 'resisting peer pressure' programme in adolescents. Seven hundred and fifty male and female 12-year-olds were the target of either full treatment, partial treatment or no treatment control. The full treatment consisted of exposure to a series of videotapes demonstrating parental, advertising and peer pressures and ways to resist these pressures, together with 'giving knowledge of the immediate physiological effects of smoking'. The partial treatment consisted merely of feedback of the group's smoking behaviour results. A fake saliva-nicotine test was used to increase reliability of self-reported smoking rates. The smoking 'onset rate' was significantly lower for the treatment (approximately 10%) as opposed to the control (approximately 18%) groups. However, claims for success should be treated with reserve, since the partial treatment group achieved similar results (approximately 10% onset rate) to the full treatment group, in the absence of any 'resisting peer pressure' training.

A similar lack of success was reported by the Saskatoon smoking project in Canada. Eighth grade (13-year-old) student leaders from 32 schools attended a regional seminar on smoking and health, and then returned to their respective schools to plan and execute smoking programmes of their own. After two years there was no significant difference between the smoking habits of students who had been exposed to the student-directed education and students who had not (Thompson, 1978).

A more clear-cut study was the Stanford University peer teaching programme (Perry, Killen, Slinkard & McAlister, 1980). In this programme a team of 18 non-smoking and extraverted male and female high school students (aged 15–17) were specially selected and recruited to give a series of lectures to adjoining junior high schools. The target population was 289 pupils, 12 years of age from one school, together with the pupils in two adjoining schools (n = 400), acting as controls. Techniques included obtaining public commitments not to become smokers, identifying social pressures to smoke, and rehearsing and role-playing situations in which pressures to smoke were successfully resisted. Props included slides and videotapes to illustrate more vividly the social pressures involved. The programme also utilised exhaled CO measures to validate self-reports on smoking. Follow-ups at six months and one year indicated that the treatment population, as opposed to the control population, contained significantly fewer smokers, 8.1% of the treatment school pupils compared with 10.4% and 19.1% of the two control school pupils being smokers (as defined by smoking at least 1 cigarette per week). In assessing their results, the authors cautiously suggested that peer teaching might be a profitable avenue for further investigations.

Overall, the results of peer teaching have not been as great as originally hoped for. As Leventhal & Cleary (1980) suggest, the limited success of these programmes suggests that there is more to the initiation of smoking than social pressure. Children develop attitudes about smoking well before they try it. One study cited by Leventhal & McCleary (1980), that of Newman, Martin & Petersen (1978), suggested that intention to try cigarettes proved to be the best single predictor of later smoking. Evidence indicates that the young smoker is viewed by other children as tough, easy going, more often in trouble, careless and lazy (Bland, Bewley & Day, 1975; Bynner, 1970). This would appear to be a fairly accurate description (see the personality, behavioural and academic achievement characteristics of the very young smoker detailed in Chapter 4). Presumably this tough, rebellious and independent lifestyle is attractive to many potential smokers. Such individuals are extremely unlikely to be influenced by peer pressures, and thus are resistant to the youth-to-youth programmes. The youngsters who could be more susceptible to peer pressures may be those who feel anxious and inadequate, and use smoking as a means of gaining acceptance and identifying with the group.

An additional reason for the relative failure of these programmes could lie in the choice of the peer leader. Often this person is chosen on the basis of being confident, articulate and attractive. Whether such teenagers are likely to influence younger peers is not known. In fact, it has been observed that the 'hoods' who smoked the most did not want to emulate the 'popular' teenagers, who often emerge from a higher socioeconomic background (Surgeon General, 1979, Section 20-25; Newman, 1970).

On a more optimistic note, one final programme is worthy of mention. This is the programme fostered by the American Lung Association (Surgeon General, 1979, Ch. 20, p. 23), which is designed to begin as early as kindergarten age (< 5 years). Various health education units are tailored to meet the requirements of children from kindergarten age to eight years. These focus on increasing the individual's self-knowledge, both emotional and physiological, and on developing strategies for coping with the stresses and pressures of life. The outcome of this programme will not be known for several years, but it may offer hope of long-term success.

Conclusions

In the long term there is every reason to believe that anti-smoking efforts directed at schoolchildren will lead to continued declines in smoking. However, given the limited degree of success to date, this will be an extremely slow process. It is obvious that radical improvements are needed in the design and assessment of these campaigns. It is still true that many programmes suffer from design flaws which impede understanding of those elements of the programmes which are most crucial for success. In many cases there is inadequate follow-up. Few data are available on whether exposure of 10- to 11-year-olds to anti-smoking propaganda will affect their subsequent smoking behaviour at 15–17 years, even though this is clearly of crucial interest. There also needs to be greater acknowledgement of the differing motives for starting to smoke. For some adolescents smoking may be one aspect of rule-breaking and rebelliousness. Others may smoke to control anxiety, others again may simply be succumbing to social pressure to conform. These different motives clearly demand different intervention approaches.

SUMMARY: intervention and termination strategies

A wide variety of specific smoking cessation programmes, including behaviour therapy, drug therapy and individual and group counselling, has been developed. Assessment of the relative success of these programmes is made difficult by frequent use of poor designs, lack of extensive follow-up and lack of objective biological assays for verification of smoking cessation. Although widely varying initial smoking cessation rates have been reported, percentages abstinent at one-year follow-up seldom differ from those obtained for unaided quitting.

The majority of smokers who have quit have done so by their own efforts. Anti-smoking propaganda through the media, variations in the price of cigarettes and changes towards a more healthy lifestyle in general have no doubt prompted quitting and the shift to filter cigarettes. However, the relative importance of these factors is difficult to assess.

In the long term, anti-smoking efforts directed towards prevention in schoolchildren may offer a slower but more effective reduction in smoking prevalence. The evidence that factors such as socioeconomic status, sex and personality are important predictors for smoking recruitment and cessation suggests that more effort should be expended in tailoring smoking cessation and prevention programmes to meet varying individual needs.

6

Overview

In previous chapters, we have posed, and attempted to answer, what we regard as important and contentious issues in this field. At this stage, a brief recapitulation and evaluation seems timely.

In Part I we discussed the smoking/health debate and described theories of smoking recruitment and maintenance. Measured judgement about the viability of these theories, particularly those centring round lifestyle/genetic arguments, is difficult, for a variety of reasons. One problem is that many of the critical studies involve twin comparisons, and it is generally conceded that at times conventional twin methodology is not sufficiently robust to tease out important variables, especially where the parameters under study are highly complex. Even where significant differences are disclosed in comparisons between smoking and non-smoking Mz and Dz twins, it may be difficult to attribute these differences exclusively to genetical or to environmental influences.

Another problem is that most researchers have studied tobacco usage in isolation, neglecting the broader perspective of multiple drug use. Many studies, however, suggest that rather than a person who smokes tobacco, a truer picture is that of an individual who uses tobacco in conjunction with alcohol, tea, coffee and, to a lesser extent, tranquillisers. To take an example, the strength of the associations between the use of tobacco and the use of other psychoactive drugs is such that significant correlations can be demonstrated between coffee drinking and heart disease (Dawber, Kannel & Gordon, 1974; Surgeon General, 1979, Ch. 18, p. 14). It is highly unlikely that coffee is the guilty party, but it could be that smoking, which is associated with coffee drinking, is the culprit.

In the context of a multiple drug model, interactive effects may be of considerable importance, a point which is well illustrated in the Cederlof *et al.* (1977) study employing data from the Swedish Twin Registry. While hyper-mortality was clearly related to smoking in both Mz (45 to 31 deaths for highest to lowest smoking groups) and Dz (61 to 42 deaths) groups, when pairs with discordant drinking habits were excluded from the analysis, it was found that 25 deaths occurred in the highest smoking group compared with 25 in the lowest smoking group amongst 729 Dz twin pairs; corresponding figures for 640 Mz pairs were 21 and 20. This suggests an interactive effect of alcohol and tobacco on mortality rates. Perhaps the presence of both habits in individuals indicates a certain constitutional disposition.

This all being said, how do we interpret data revealing interrelationships between genetics, smoking, disease and personality? Let us first examine the conventional, usually medical assertion, the extreme environmentalist position, that smoking causes lung cancer and coronary heart disease. This claim is buttressed by considerable correlational data and toxicological studies of tobacco smoke itself. The counter-argument is that the association is to a degree artefactual, the link between smoking and disease occurring at the genetic dispositional level. While it must be admitted that the genetical data are somewhat inconclusive, we might comment that analysis of the links between marker genes which may be important for disease (e.g., that for Pi (alpha-1-antitrypsin) in the case of respiratory disease) and those genes which might determine smoking/general drug usage, is at a very early stage of enquiry (see Crumpacker *et al.*, 1979). At this point in time, it seems unwise to pre-judge the issue.

However, even if it can be argued that there is a genetical predisposition towards contracting diseases such as lung cancer, undoubtedly tar, a known carcinogen, substantially increases the risk. A similar situation is probably true for other lung diseases such as bronchitis. In other words, smokers who are genetically susceptible to the effects of cigarette smoke are most at risk. As far as heart disease is concerned, of course, the situation is much less clear-cut. A number of factors are involved, some genetic and some environmental, which, interactively, increase risk. As yet, there is no unequivocal evidence concerning the role of smoking as a primary causal factor in the aetiology of heart disease.

Perhaps the most cogent argument against the strict environmentalist position is that if we accept the direct smoking–disease causal relationship on the basis of correlational data alone, we would also have to assert that, in addition to lung cancer and heart disease, which have been the target areas for epidemiologists, smoking also 'causes' excessive drinking, increased suicides, backache, absenteeism, 'instability', and 'psychosocial discord', even in subjects as young as 15–17 years, some of whom smoke only one or two cigarettes a day. Clearly, causal links of this sort are extremely remote, and few would be prepared seriously to pursue this line of argument. Such a strict position is only tenable when laboratory evidence establishes a causal link between the offending agent in tobacco smoke and the relevant disease, and when other possible confounding variables (such as heredity, constitution and lifestyle) have either been excluded or taken into account, as is the case with tar and lung cancer, for example.

As far as the link between smoking and personality and their presumed genetic bases are concerned, it seems that while both personality and multiple drug use have been shown to have some genetic basis, it is very much a matter of conjecture as to how closely these aspects are linked at both genetic and phenotypic levels. Evidence for a particular smoking 'personality' is limited. It is more plausible to suggest that there are sub-groups of smokers who smoke for different reasons, an observation which has both theoretical and practical implications. For example, we can cite the impressive predictive power of the Cherry & Kiernan (1976) model of smoker sub-groups in which they demonstrated that, particularly for men, extraverted, stable, light smokers are much more likely to be successful in quitting smoking than introverted, neurotic, heavy smokers. This may have implications regarding the smoking/health debate in that certain putative smoking motives, e.g., emotional instability and 'anxiety', may themselves carry elevated mortality risks, even for non-smokers (Floderus, 1974).

On the basis of available evidence, we favour a model which suggests that smokers differ from non-smokers in regard to lifestyle, of which smoking is only one index amongst others such as alcohol drinking, drug use, eating habits and psychosocial discord. Some, perhaps all, are related to mortality, more so in interaction with smoking, so that we have a complex interaction of risk factors generating increased probabilities of increasing 'cause-specific' disease and raising overall morbidity and mortality rates. From the twin studies, it appears that on this lifestyle dimension, concordant smokers occupy one extreme position and concordant non-smokers occupy the other, with the discordant smokers at some uncertain value in the middle range. The fact that non-smokers in smoking-discordant pairs are still highly susceptible to certain cause-specific diseases is a vital piece of evidence. These individuals experience ill-health, both physical and mental, to a greater degree than concordant non-smokers. Whether this influence is primarily genetic or environmental is arguable. However, the fact that from the Swedish data Mz pairs fit the model better than Dz pairs (judging from the more pronounced lifestyle effects in the NET analyses), points to the stronger influence of genetic factors.

In Part II we examined in detail the action of a broad range of variables, primarily pharmacological, psychobiological and sociological, underlying recruitment to, and maintenance of, smoking. Generally speaking, it is apparent that major emphasis should be placed on pharmacological/psychobiological factors in relation to maintenance, and on psychosocial factors in relation to recruitment.

In describing the various theories of smoking maintenance in Part I, we briefly touched on evidence for the primacy of nicotine as a reinforcer for smoking behaviour. We expanded and elaborated this in the sections on nicotine pharmacokinetics and pharmacology. The former, in particular, provides some explanation as to why inhalation-type cigarette smoking is the most popular mode of tobacco usage, and why tobacco is never taken by swallowing. Inhalation is the fastest, most efficient and most easily controllable means of delivering nicotine to its postulated sites of action. Pharmacokinetics, in conjunction with conditioning theory, also offers an explanation of the so-called 'secondary reinforcing' aspects of cigarette smoking, in terms of the short latency between smoke inhalation and the arrival of nicotine at receptor sites in the CNS. As against this, pharmacokinetics poses searching questions for any simple addiction theory of smoking involving nicotine homeostasis. For the CNS in particular, there is compelling evidence that the most popular mode of tobacco use, and the one most difficult to give up, i.e., cigarette smoking, is the least effective means of maintaining *steady*, as opposed to rapidly *fluctuating* levels of nicotine at receptor sites.

However, merely looking at nicotine levels per se hardly advances our understanding of why nicotine should be so important in maintaining smoking. The critical observation involves the biphasic, i.e., the stimulant and depressant actions of nicotine, both peripherally and centrally. Clearly, the central action of nicotine is most important to the smoker, both stimulant and depressant effects (as measured by EEG, for example) being obtainable from smoking a cigarette. The type of effect will depend on a diversity of factors: the smoker's personality, the stimulating properties of the environment, the number of cigarettes habitually smoked and the amount of nicotine absorbed from the cigarette. This final factor is to an extent under the control of the smoker, who is able to obtain stimulant or depressant effects at will by varying the vigour with which a cigarette is smoked, and how much smoke is inhaled.

Thus the pharmacological evidence supports the assumption that one reinforcement for smoking is the role of nicotine as a psychological 'tool' to reduce tension or stress, or, conversely, to relieve monotony or fatigue, as the situation dictates. It could be claimed that nicotine from smoking induces 'pharmacological pleasure' in a manner analogous to that of electrical brain stimulation reward. On the other hand, the results of self-injection experiments with animals have not strongly supported this view. Persuading animals to self-inject nicotine or to smoke tobacco has proved an exceedingly difficult task.

As far as the effects of nicotine or smoking on performance are concerned, there are clearly some differences over interpretation of the available evidence. With some exceptions, it seems that the effects of smoking on vigilance, learning and memory are generally beneficial. Although we can make some conjectures about the mechanisms of nicotine action involved, there is the unresolved question of whether such enhancements are due to relief of withdrawal symptoms or are true increases in performance. So far, there is no compelling evidence one way or the other, although some studies of the effects of nicotine tablets/gum in non-smokers do indicate that true performance enhancement can occur. These are complemented by animal experiments concerning the effects of nicotine injections on maze learning, shuttle-box performance and bar-pressing, which demonstrate the beneficial effects of acute doses of nicotine in weighted equivalents to those obtained by human smokers. By contrast, there are some suggestions that with chronic nicotine administration the animal's performance becomes dependent on continued administration. This, of course, is more consistent with a physiological addiction than with an arousal modulation theory of smoking.

The current theoretical shift away from the earlier, rather crude addiction models of smoking maintenance parallels a similar movement in the recent drug addiction literature. Simple exposure models for drug abuse in general suggest that initial use of a drug (e.g., an opiate) engenders a powerful urge towards subsequent compulsive use. However, there is now an accumulation of evidence which cannot be accommodated within an exposure model: the fact that casual use of opiates is relatively widespread and that some heavily addicted groups, e.g., Vietnam veterans, show only moderate levels of recidivism following induction into civilian life. There is a growing body of opinion that metabolic theories, such as Goldstein's claim of a fundamental opiate avidity in mammals, or the recent claim that repeated exposure to opiates might create a long-term incapacity of the body to synthesise endorphins, their endogenous counterparts (Snyder, 1977), have proved not to be adequate. There have also been difficulties with conditioning explanations, the other influential theory of this genre, whether these employ a simple positive reinforcement or avoidance learning model, or more formally developed models such as opponent-process theory (Solomon, 1980), which integrates both elements.

As a consequence, there has been a pronounced swing towards adaptive theories (see Alexander & Hadaway, 1982), which view drug use as a coping strategy for handling stress of whatever origin, such strategies including, in addition to opiate use, smoking, drinking, over- and under-eating and the over-use of denial. According to theory, the particular mechanism employed is, to an extent, a function of the person's social experience and expectations, drug availability, cultural sanctions on drug use and so forth. The similarities between adaptive theories of opiate use and arousal modulation theories of smoking maintenance are indeed striking. Implicit also in both is a recognition of the possibility of drug migration or tradeoff, a point we shall return to later.

Turning now to recruitment, the evidence shows that psychosocial factors play a decisive role. Unfortunately, few definitive studies have been reported, presumably since the critical variables are difficult to manipulate using classic experimental designs. Exclusive reliance on correlational studies is hazardous, as we have already pointed out in our discussion of the smoking/health issue, although use of sophisticated designs and techniques of data analysis in some studies has avoided the most serious pitfalls. We can also make reasonable inferences from yoked research. For example, in the adolescent study reported, anxiety emerges as a critical variable with many of the smoking groups, although the exciting cause may differ between individuals and between groups. Complementary data have been reported showing that anxious subjects titrate themselves with nicotine, as do normal subjects placed in stressful situations.

Although the genetic factors identified in Part I no doubt exist, it is probable that they exert their influence through second-order variables represented in personality differences. Factors associated with taking up smoking are rebelliousness, risk-taking, stimulation-seeking and anxiety. These, in addition to sociocultural factors such as poor home relationships, sibling/peer smoking, and, to a lesser extent, parental smoking, can reasonably be regarded as causal. Other marker variables such as alcohol and other drug use may be associated with smoking in a non-causal fashion. The picture of the typical adolescent smoker, however, is blurred because young smokers do not form a homogeneous group even when subset by age and sex. Some smoke as a rule-breaking device, others are conforming to social pressures, others again find smoking a useful tranquilliser. A further confusing factor is the actual composition of the smoking group, which changes as new recruits join, while others quit. Nevertheless, the adolescent current smokers and ex-smokers share many of the psychosocial characteristics which distinguish the smoker from the non-smoker.

In Part III we described the successes and failures of various anti-smoking measures. Uncertainty about some of the factors underlying recruitment and maintenance has hindered the deployment of effective anti-smoking campaigns aimed at the adolescent and cessation programmes directed towards the committed smoker. There is no doubt that at this point in time such programmes have met with only limited success. This implies that, for the foreseeable future, there will probably be a substantial 'hard core' of smokers. The problem may be exaggerated in many underdeveloped countries, where recent figures suggest that cigarette consumption is increasing. Here we should also note the recent disclosure that smoking prevalence rates for females are escalating in many industrialised Western countries. It could be argued that, given these circumstances, efforts should be directed towards producing a 'safer' cigarette by removing toxic components such as CO and tar from cigarette smoke.

Two counter-arguments are relevant here. The first is that even if it were possible to construct such a 'safer' cigarette, the precise hazards of nicotine itself are unknown. Secondly, it could be argued that this strategy is misconceived, since it offers a 'bolt-hole' for the committed smoker who otherwise might be persuaded to stop smoking.

As far as intervention programmes with young children are concerned, special problems emerge. Perhaps the most crucial is that the known health hazards for the young child are remote, and can be easily displaced in his motivational hierarchy by more immediate and pressing needs. One interesting possibility which arises from the increasing knowledge about some genetic involvement in smoking and in smoking-related diseases is that of genetic screening for susceptibility to smoking risk. Clearly, those individuals who are genetically vulnerable on both counts face a double jeopardy, and preventive measures might be directed more particularly towards such individuals from an early age.

Another issue of some consequence is that of drug migration or 'tradeoff'. Throughout previous chapters, we have presented considerable evidence supporting a polydrug model. Rather than exhibiting the drug-specific cravings postulated by metabolic addiction theories, it is clear that many individuals are predisposed to multiple drug use, although the particular patterns of association may differ between age groups and social classes, and between cultures. Congruent with this is some evidence, admittedly patchy, that in certain professional and social class groups in which smoking has fallen significantly, other drug consumption has risen.

Does this imply that if the habitual user is denied his source of supply, for whatever reason (material in terms of price, psychological in terms of health threat), then he will migrate to other, more readily available drugs, a finding which has been reported with heroin users (Wishnie, 1977)? If so, what are the implications? If nothing else, it would presumably reshape our thinking about the overall strategy for attacking the problem of psychoactive drug abuse, since cessation programmes aimed at a single drug would be of dubious utility. A much broader approach would obviously be called for, in which attempts are made to encourage more positive, 'healthy' attitudes and activities, to meet what are clearly perceived by the individual as important and compelling needs.

Appendix

This appendix is not intended as a comprehensive or detailed guide to all the various techniques and concepts referred to in the text, but aims to be a quick reference guide for readers with different scientific backgrounds. Nor is any attempt made to include highly technical terms such as neurotransmitters, receptors and antagonists: the reader is referred to Chapter 3: Pharmacology of nicotine, or to the general references cited in the text, e.g., Cooper, Bloom & Roth (1978) for details.

Augmenting/reducing. This dichotomy refers to individual variations in the well-known positive relationship between stimulus intensity and evoked potential (EP) amplitude. Reducers respond with smaller than expected EP amplitudes, and augmenters with larger than expected EP amplitudes, with increasing stimulus intensity. The underlying dynamics of augmenting-reducing are unclear. However an analogy can be made with the concept of the 'inverted-U curve' relating performance efficiency with arousal. Presumably the augmenter is chronically under-aroused, and consequently the cortex performs more efficiently (i.e., expresses larger EP amplitude) with increased stimulus intensity. By contrast, the reducer has an optimal performance peak at lower arousal levels, consequently expressing larger EP amplitude at lower stimulus intensities. This notion is supported by data relating augmenting/reducing to other measures of physiological arousal, to sensory detection thresholds and to personality scales such as extraversion and sensation-seeking (see Mangan, 1982*b*).

Bolus (bolus injections, nicotine bolus). This refers to the method of rapid discrete injections or 'shots' of nicotine, to produce a series of nicotine-rich 'slugs' of blood travelling in the circulation, the so-called nicotine boli. This method is designed to mimic the nicotine blood bolus produced by inhalation of cigarette smoke. However, the nicotine blood bolus produced by rapid intravenous shots of nicotine is subject to mixing and dispersion as it is carried by the circulation through one side of the heart, through the lungs, and is then pumped through the other side of the heart to the brain and the rest of the body. By contrast, the nicotine blood bolus produced by inhalation of tobacco smoke has to travel only the latter part of this route. Consequently it is subject to less mixing and dispersion before reaching the brain. It will also reach the brain more rapidly than in the case of intravenous bolus injection.

Contingent negative variation (CNV). This is a slow negative potential shift recorded from the scalp. This negative potential occurs in the time interval between a warning stimulus (i.e., 'GET READY') and a subsequent imperative stimulus (i.e., 'GO!') signalling some motor activity such as pressing a button in a reaction time task. The CNV probably divides up into an initial orienting response component following the warning stimulus and a subsequent 'expectancy' wave or 'motor readiness' potential which occurs before the imperative stimulus. With relatively short time intervals between warning and imperative stimuli, these two components merge, but with longer intervals such as 10–20 s the individual components can be distinguished. The exact interpretation of the CNV is far from certain. However, increased CNV amplitude has been correlated with alertness and the degree of attention paid to the task. In appropriate doses, stimulant drugs usually increase, and depressant drugs usually decrease, the size of the CNV.

Critical flicker frequency (CFF). This is the frequency at which a flashing (strobe) light appears to the subject as having 'fused' into a steady continuous light, with no trace of flickering. In general, the CFF is raised with increased light flash intensity. Stimulant drugs usually increase, and depressant drugs usually decrease, CFF.

Electroencephalogram (EEG). The EEG is the electrical activity recorded normally from the surface of the scalp, but sometimes from electrodes inside the brain, mainly in animal experiments. The EEG is usually divided into different frequency bands: delta, 1–3 Hz; theta, 4–7 Hz; alpha, 8–12 Hz; beta, 13–30 + Hz. In general, the amount of low frequency, high amplitude delta activity decreases, and the amount of high frequency, low amplitude beta activity increases, in progressing from sleep to alertness. The notable exception to this rule is during the recurrent periods of 'paradoxical sleep' which occur during sleep. During these periods, the

EEG shows high frequency, low amplitude beta activity, which is associated with dreaming. Theta activity has been associated with the orienting response to a stimulus, and also in anticipation of motor activity. Alpha activity predominates during quiet wakefulness. Upon sensory stimulation, the alpha activity is replaced with beta activity, the so-called 'alpha-blocking' effect. Stimulant drugs usually increase the amount of high frequency activity (beta) and depressant drugs usually increase the amount of lower frequency activity (alpha and delta). However, some minor tranquillisers, such as valium, in appropriate doses, may produce 'mixed' effects, increasing delta *and* beta but decreasing alpha, thus indicating both depressant and stimulant (disinhibition?) actions. There is some evidence that depressant drugs in appropriate dosages increase theta activity whereas stimulant drugs decrease theta activity.

Evoked Potential (EP). This is sometimes called the evoked response (ER), and is labelled in terms of the modality of stimulation: e.g., visual evoked potential (VEP or VER) and auditory evoked potential (AEP or AER). The EP is the time-locked sequence of positive and negative waves in the EEG, which follows a stimulus such as a tone or light flash. In practice, many trials of stimuli are averaged in order to separate the EP from the random background EEG activity. Short latency, small-amplitude components, up to 10 ms post-stimulus, are produced by the brain stem. Longer latency components, up to 300 ms post-stimulus, of larger amplitude, reflect reticular system activation of the cortex. The later the EP component, the more 'cognitive' is thought to be the associated processing. The amplitude of components is usually increased by stronger stimuli, increased novelty of the stimulus and greater 'attention'. The latter effects are more characteristic of longer latency EP components. Stimulant drugs usually increase, and depressant drugs usually decrease, EP amplitude.

Extraversion. The common definition of extraversion (E) is in terms of sociability and impulsivity. However, the nature of the E scale in the EPQ (Eysenck & Eysenck, 1975) has been changed somewhat. This EPQ version of the E scale, which is now widely used, is largely composed of items measuring sociability. The impulsivity items, together with extra items of a similar nature and items measuring tendencies of a more psychotic nature, have been combined to form the P scale of the EPQ. There is some debate as to the validity of regarding the E scale of the EPQ as being equivalent to earlier versions of the E scale (Rocklin & Revelle, 1981). It appears likely that the 'new' version of the E scale in the EPQ is not very predictive of smoking, the reason being that the critical impulsivity items and closely related risk-taking and tough-mindedness items are now in the P scale. The P scale is predictive of smoking. Interested readers will find more details in Eysenck (1980), Rocklin & Revelle (1981) and Golding *et al.* (1983).

Inverted-U curve (or Yerkes–Dodson Law). This is a generalisation relating arousal to performance. The relationship between arousal and performance is curvilinear, with an optimum somewhere near the middle of the range. This means that as arousal increases so does performance, but that once the optimum has been passed, any further increase in arousal will produce a decrement in performance. The second part of this theory maintains that the optimum arousal level for any given task depends on the complexity of the task. The more complex and difficult a task, the lower the optimum arousal level, whereas the more straightforward the task, the higher the optimum arousal level for that particular task.

Monozygotic and dizygotic twins. Monozygotic (Mz) twins develop from a single fertilised egg-cell, the twin pair are genetically identical and usually identical in appearance. Dizygotic (Dz) twins develop from two concurrently fertilised egg-cells. From a genetic point of view, the partners in a Dz twin pair are similar to the same degree as are ordinary siblings (brothers and sisters). The statistical expectation as to the number of genes that they have in common is 0.5, the same as for ordinary siblings, and Dz twins may be of the same or opposite sex. However, Dz twins experience a much more similar environment both before and after birth than do ordinary siblings.

Paired Associate Learning. This refers to a learning task in which a cue stimulus is presented, and, within a few seconds, is replaced by the stimulus to be remembered. Recall is tested by the subject's correct response to the cue stimulus. For example, in verbal paired associate learning, 10 or 20 word pairs are presented sequentially over a number of successive trials until the subject has learnt the whole series perfectly. The number of trials taken to correctly anticipate the second word of each pair may be taken as an index of the speed of learning, or 'acquisition'. Retention of the material may be tested at some later time by repeating the process. High Interference material contains words with high natural associations, but in different pairs, e.g.:

Low Interference	shoe	book
	hide	pick
High Interference	miss	white
	black	take

Photic Driving. Photic driving occurs when repetitive flash stimuli entrain the EEG, producing EEG activity at the frequency of flash stimulation or some multiple of that frequency. In susceptible individuals photic driving may trigger EEG activity characteristic of epilepsy, and even epileptic attacks themselves. The efficiency of photic driving probably reflects the balance of cortical inhibitory and excitatory processes. However, interpretation is made difficult by the relative efficiency of driving at various frequencies, and large individual differences in response (see Mangan, 1982*b*).

Skin conductance (or electrodermal activity or Galvanic skin response, GSR). This refers to sweat gland activity, and is usually measured as the resistance or conductance between electrodes placed on areas of high sweat gland density such as the palm of the hand, finger tips or sole of the foot. It is dependent on autonomic nervous system activity, and changes with emotional state and with stimulation. In general, increased excitement, whether pleasurable or aversive, leads to an increased skin conductance level (SCL) and increased fluctuations in the SCL, so-called spontaneous fluctuations (SFs). A stimulus such as a tone will produce a rise in the SCL – a skin conductance response (SCR). Unless this stimulus signals some important event such as reward, or is itself noxious, the SCR will habituate, i.e., diminish in amplitude over successive stimulus presentations. The SCL, and especially SFs and the speed of SCR habituation, have commonly been used to measure autonomic excitation/inhibition balance. Depressant drugs usually decrease the number of SFs, diminish the SCR and speed habituation, and vice-versa for stimulants.

Stroop Test. In the Stroop Test the subject is required to name aloud the colour of the inks in which a series of colour names are printed. However, the colour names never correspond to the colour of the ink in which they are printed. Subjects find this incongruity very distracting and take longer to complete such a list than they take to name a list of colour blobs of equivalent length or, for that matter, a list in which the ink colour and the name of the colour are congruent. The extra difficulty found in completing the incongruous list, usually measured as a difference in time to completion, is called the Stroop Effect. Variants of this effect can be produced by utilising the sorting of cards with the colour words printed on them by ink colour as opposed to name of the colour word, or even using a numerical Stroop effect, e.g., reading such numbers as the number 1 composed as the pattern formed by many very small number 3s, and vice versa.

References

Abood, L. G., Lowy, K. & Booth, H. (1979). Acute and chronic effects of nicotine in rats and evidence for a noncholinergic site of action. *National Institute on Drug Abuse Research Monograph Series*, **23**, 136–49.

Abood, L. G., Reynolds, D. T., Booth, H. & Bidlack, J. M. (1981). Sites and mechanisms for nicotine's actions in the brain. *Neuroscience and Biobehavioural Reviews*, **5**, 479–86.

Agué, C. (1974). Cardiovascular variables, skin conductance and time estimation: changes after the administration of small doses of nicotine. *Psychopharmacologia*, **37**, 109–25.

Aiken, J. W. & Reit, E. (1968). Differential excitation of adrenergic and cholinergic sympathetic ganglion cells. *Pharmacologist*, **10**, 217.

Alexander, B. K. & Hadaway, P. F. (1982). Opiate Addiction: The case for an adaptive orientation. *Psychological Bulletin*, **92**, 367–81.

Alpern, H. I. & Jackson, S. J. (1978). Stimulants and depressants: Drug effects on memory. In *Psychopharmacology: A Generation of Progress*, ed. M. A. Lipton, A. DiMascio & K. F. Killam, pp. 663–75. New York: Raven Press.

Andersson, K. (1975). Effects of cigarette smoking on learning and retention. *Psychopharmacologia*, **41**, 1–5.

Andersson, K. & Hockey, G. R. J. (1977). Effects of cigarette smoking on incidental memory. *Psychopharmacology*, **52**, 223–6.

Ando, K. & Yanagita, T. (1981). Cigarette smoking in Rhesus monkeys. *Psychopharmacology*, **72**, 117–27.

Anon. (1674). *The Women's Petition Against Coffee*. London: By a Well-wisher. Reprinted in *Old English Coffee Houses* (1954). London: The Rodale Press.

Anton, F. (1978). *Art of the Maya*. Translated from the German by M. Whittall. London: Thames and Hudson Ltd.

Armitage, A. K. (1970). Tobacco Research Council Report. *Effects of Cigarette Smoking on Heart Rate*. London: Tobacco Research Council.

Armitage, A. K. (1978). The role of nicotine in the tobacco smoking habit. In *Smoking Behaviour: Physiological and Psychological Influences*, ed. R. E. Thornton, pp. 229–43. Edinburgh: Churchill Livingstone.

Armitage, A. K., Dollery, C. T., George, C. F., Houseman, T. H., Lewis, P. J. & Turner, D. M. (1975). Absorption and metabolism of nicotine from cigarettes. *British Medical Journal*, iv, 313–16.

Armitage, A. K., Dollery, C., Houseman, T., Kohner, E., Lewis, P. J. & Turner, D. (1978). Absorption of nicotine from small cigars. *Clinical Pharmacology and Therapeutics*, **23**, 143–51.

Armitage, A. K., Hall, G. H. & Morrison, C. F. (1968). Pharmacological basis for the tobacco smoking habit. *Nature*, **217**, 331–4.

Armitage, A. K., Hall, G. H. & Sellers, C. M. (1969). Effects of nicotine on electrocortical activity and acetylcholine release from the cat cerebral cortex. *British Journal of Pharmacology*, **35**, 152–60.

Armitage, A. K. & Turner, D. M. (1970). Absorption of nicotine in cigarette and cigar smoke through the oral mucosa. *Nature*, **226**, 1231–2.

ASH (Action on Smoking and Health) (1981a). World Production of Cigarettes. *ASH Information Bulletin*, No. 83, 3.

ASH (Action on Smoking and Health) (1981b). Effect of price increases on cigarette sales. *ASH Information Bulletin*, No. 83, 3.

ASH (Action on Smoking and Health) (1981c). ASH Survey: cigarette law ignored by tobacconists. *Times Health Supplement*, 13 Nov. 1981.

Ashton, H., Golding, J., Marsh, V. R., Millman, J. E. & Thompson, J. W. (1981). The seed and the soil: effect of dosage, personality and starting state on the response to delta-9-tetrahydrocannabinol in man. *British Journal of Clinical Pharmacology*, **10**, 579–89.

Ashton, H., Marsh, V. R., Millman, J. E., Rawlins, M. D., Telford, R. & Thompson, J. W. (1978). The use of event-related slow potentials of the brain as a means to analyse the effects of cigarette smoking and nicotine in humans. In *Smoking Behaviour: Physiological and Psychological Influences*, ed. R. E. Thornton, pp. 54–68. Edinburgh: Churchill Livingstone.

Ashton, H., Marsh, V. R., Millman, J. E., Rawlins, M. D., Telford, R. & Thompson, J. W. (1980). Biphasic dose-related responses of the CNV (contingent negative variation) to i.v. nicotine in man. *British Journal of Clinical Pharmacology*, **10**, 579–89.

Ashton, J., Millman, J. E., Telford, R. & Thompson, J. W. (1974). The effects of caffeine, nitrazepam and cigarette smoking on the contingent negative variation in man. *Electroencephalography and Clinical Neurophysiology*, **37**, 59–71.

Ashton, H., Stepney, R. & Thompson, J. W. (1979). Self-titration by cigarette smokers. *British Medical Journal*, *ii*, 357–360.

Ashton, H. & Watson, D. W. (1970). Puffing frequency and nicotine intake in cigarette smoking. *British Medical Journal*, *iii*, 679–81.

Atkins, S. H. (1936). Work for chimney-sweepers or a warning for tobacconists. *Shakespeare Association Facsimiles No. 11*. Oxford: Published for Shakespeare Association by Humphrey Milford, Oxford University Press.

Atkinson, A. B. & Skegg, J. L. (1974). Control of smoking and price of cigarettes – a comment. *British Journal of Preventive and Social Medicine*, **28**, 45–8.

Auerbach, D., Hammond, E. C. & Garfinkel, L. (1979). Changes in bronchial epithelium in relation to cigarette smoking. *New England Journal of Medicine*, **300**, 381–6.

Ax, A. F. (1953). The physiological differentiation between fear and anger in humans. *Psychosomatic Medicine*, **15**, 433–42.

Backhouse, C. I. & James, I. P. (1969). The relationship and prevalence of smoking, drinking and drug taking in delinquent adolescent boys. *British Journal of Addiction*, **64**, 75–9.

Balfour, D. J. K. & Benwell, M. E. M. (1981). The effects of chronic nicotine administration and withdrawal on 5-hydroxytryptamine synthesis and uptake by rat brain synaptosomes. *British Journal of Pharmacology Proceedings Supplement*, **72**, 490.

Barclays Bank (1961). *Tobacco*. London: Barclays Bank DCO.

Barkley, R. A., Hastings, J. E. & Jackson, T. L. (1977). The effects of rapid smoking and hypnosis in the treatment of smoking behaviour. *International Journal of Clinical and Experimental Hypnosis*, **25**, 7–17.

Barnes, G. & Fishlinsky, M. (1976). Stimulus intensity modulation, smoking and craving for cigarettes. *Addictive Diseases*, **2**, 479–84.

Barrell, J. J. & Price, D. D. (1977). Two experiential orientations towards a stressful situation and their related somatic and visceral responses. *Psychophysiology*, **14**, 517–21.

Bartol, C. (1975). Extraversion and neuroticism and nicotine, caffeine and drug intake. *Psychological Reports*, **36**, 1007–10.

Battig, K. (1970). The effect of pre- and post-trial application of nicotine on the 12 problems of the Hebb-Williams test in the rat. *Psychopharmacologia*, **18**, 68–76.

Beckerman, S. C. (1963). Report of an educational program regarding cigarette smoking among high school students. *Journal of the Maine Medical Association*, **54**, 60–3, 74.

Beckett, A. H., Gorrod, J. W. & Jenner, P. (1971*a*). The analysis of nicotine-1′-*N*-oxide in urine in the presence of nicotine and cotinine and its application to the study of in vivo nicotine metabolism in man. *Journal of Pharmacy and Pharmacology*, **23**, 55–61.

Beckett, A. H., Gorrod, J. W. & Jenner, P. (1971*b*). The effect of smoking on nicotine metabolism in vivo in Man. *Journal of Pharmacy and Pharmacology*, Supplement, **23**, 625–75.

Beckett, A. H. & Triggs, E. J. (1967). Buccal absorption of basic drugs and its application as an in vivo model of passive drug transfer through lipid membranes. *Journal of Pharmacy- and Pharmacology*, Supplement, **19**, 315–415.

Beese, D. H. (1972). Tobacco consumption in various countries. *Research Paper Number 6*, 3rd edn. London: Tobacco Research Council.

Ben-Meir, D. (1977). Fighting smoking habits in a country at war. In *Bibliography on Smoking and Health*, p. 262. Washington, DC: US Department of Health, Education and Welfare.

Berecz, J. M. (1976). Treatment of smoking with cognitive conditioning therapy: A self-administered aversion technique. *Behaviour Therapy*, **7**, 641–8.

Berggreen, S. (1981). Parental smoking at home and height of children. *British Medical Journal*, **283**, 1612.

Berkson, J. (1962). Smoking and lung cancer: another view. *Lancet*, **i**, 807–8.

Berlyne, D. E. (1960). *Conflict, Arousal and Curiosity*. New York: McGraw Hill.

Berlyne, D. E. (1971). *Aesthetics and Psychobiology*. New York: Appleton.

Berman, A. L. (1973). Smoking behaviour: How is it related to locus of control, death anxiety, and belief in afterlife? *Omega*, **4**, 149–55.

Bernstein, D. A. (1969). Modification of smoking behaviour: an evaluative review. *Psychological Bulletin*, **71**, 418–40.

Bernstein, D. A. & McAlister, A. (1976). The modification of smoking behaviour: Progress and problems. *Addictive Behaviours*, **1**, 89–102.

Berntson, G. G., Beattie, M. S. & J. M. Walker (1976). Effects of nicotine and muscarinic compounds on biting attack in the cat. *Pharmacology, Biochemistry and Behaviour*, **5**, 235–9.

Bertram, J. F. & Rogers, A. W. (1981). Recovery of bronchial epithelium on stopping smoking. *British Medical Journal*, **283**, 1567–9.

Best, J. A., Bass, F. & Owen, L. W. (1977). Mode of service delivery in a smoking cessation program for public health. *Canadian Journal of Public Health*, **68**, 469–73.

Best, J. A. & Hakstian, A. R. (1978). A situation-specific model for smoking behaviour. *Addictive Behaviors*, **3**, 79–92.

Best, J. A., Owen, L. E. & Trentadue, L. (1978). Comparison of satiation and rapid smoking in self-managed smoking cessation. *Addictive Behaviors*, **3**, 71–8.

Bevan, J. A. & Murray, J. F. (1963). Evidence for a ventilation modifying reflex from the pulmonary circulation in Man. *Proceedings of the Society for Experimental Biology and Medicine*, **114**, 393–6.

Bever, O. (1970). Why do plants produce drugs? Which is their function in the plants? *Quarterly Journal of Crude Drug Research*, **10**, 1541–9.

Bewley, B. R. & Bland, J. M. (1977). Academic performance and social factors related to cigarette smoking by schoolchildren. *British Journal of Preventive and Social Medicine*, **31**, 18–24.

Bewley, B. R., Bland, J. M. & Harris, R. (1974). Factors associated with the starting of cigarette smoking by primary school children. *British Journal of Preventive and Social Medicine*, **28**, 37–44.

Bewley, B. R., Day, I. & Ide, L. (1974). *Smoking by Children in Great Britain*. London: Social Science Research Council, Medical Research Council.

Bewley, B. R., Johnson, M. R. C., Bland, J. M. & Murray, M. (1980). Trends in children's smoking. *Community Medicine*, **2**, 186–9.

Bhagat, B. (1970). Influence of chronic administration of nicotine on the turnover and metabolism of noradrenaline in the rat brain. *Psychopharmacologia*, **18**, 325.

Bhattacharya, I. & Goldstein, L. (1970). Influence of acute and chronic nicotine administration on intra- and inter-structural relationships of the electrical activity in the rabbit brain. *Neuropharmacology*, **9**, 109–18.

Bianchini, F., Corbetta, F. & Pistola, M. (1977). *The Kindly Fruits*. London: Cassell.

Birchall, P. M. A. & Claridge, G. S. (1979). Augmenting–reducing of the visual evoked potential as a function of changes in skin conductance level. *Psychophysiology*, **16**, 482–90.

Bland, J. M., Bewley, B. R. & Day, I. (1975). Primary schoolboys: image of self and smoker. *British Journal of Preventive and Social Medicine*, **29**, 262–6.

BMJ Editorial (1978). Breathing other people's smoke. *British Medical Journal*, ii, 453–4.

Borland, B. L. & Rudolph, J. P. (1975). Relative effects of low socioeconomic status, parental smoking and poor scholastic performance on smoking among high school students. *Social Science and Medicine*, **9**, 27–30.

Bosse, R., Sparrow, D., Rose, C. L. & Weiss, S. T. (1981). Longitudinal effect of age and smoking cessation on pulmonary function. *American Review of Respiratory Disease*, **123**, 378–81.

Bovet-Nitti, F. (1969). Facilitation of simultaneous visual discrimination by nicotine in four inbred strains of mice. *Psychopharmacologia*, **14**, 193–9.

Braithwait, R. (1617). *The Smoaking Age or The Life and Death of Tobacco*. London: Oenozythopolis (Bodleian Library, Oxford).

Brawley, R. E. (1935). Studies of the pH of normal resting saliva: Diurnal variation. *Journal of Dental Research*, **15**, 79–86.

Brengelmann, J. C. (1975). Manual on smoking cessation therapy. Facts and suggestions for the treatment of smoking, 71 pp. Geneva: *International Journal of Health Education.*

Brengelmann, J. C. (1977). The organization of treatment for the cessation of smoking. In *Proceedings of the Third World Conference on Smoking and Health (Vol. II)*, ed. J. Steinfeld, W. Griffiths, K. Ball & R. M. Taylor, pp. 655–63. Washington, DC: US Department of Health, Education and Welfare.

Brengelmann, J. C. & Sedlmayr, E. (1977). Experiments in the reduction of smoking behaviour. In *Proceedings of the Third World Conference on Smoking and Health, N.Y. June 2–5 1975. Vol. II. Health Consequences, Education, Cessation Activities and Social Action*, ed. J. Steinfeld, W. Griffiths, K. Ball & R. M. Taylor, pp. 533–43. Washington, DC: US Department of Health, Education and Welfare, Public Service, National Institutes of Health, National Cancer Institute. DHEW Publication.

Brill, N. Q., Crumpton, E. & Grayson, H. M. (1971). Personality factors in Marihuana use. *Archives of General Psychiatry*, **24**, 163–5.

Briney, K. L. (1967). Relation of knowledge of effects of cigarette smoking to the practice of smoking among high school seniors. In *Studies and Issues in Smoking Behaviour*, ed. S. V. Zagona, pp. 53–5. Tucson, Arizona: University of Arizona Press.

Brooks, J. E. (1937). *Tobacco, its history illustrated by the books, manuscripts and engravings in the library of George Arents Junior*, 5 vol., last vol. published 1952. New York: Limited Edition (Bodleian Library, Oxford).

Brooks, J. E. (1953). *The Mighty Leaf: Tobacco Through the Centuries*. London: Alvin Redman.

Brown, B. B. (1973). Additional characteristic EEG differences between smokers and non-smokers. In *Smoking Behavior: Motives and Incentives*, ed. W. L. Dunn, Jr, pp. 67–81. Washington, DC: Winston and Sons.

Brown, D. A., Halliwell, J. V. & Scholfield, C. N. (1971). Uptake of nicotine and extracellular space markers by isolated rat ganglia in relation to receptor activation. *British Journal of Pharmacology*, **42**, 100–13.

Brown, D. A., Hoffmann, P. C. & Roth, L. J. (1969). 3H-nicotine in cat superior cervical and nodose ganglia after close-arterial injection in vivo. *British Journal of Pharmacology*, **35**, 406–17.

Brown, L. T., Ruder, V. G., Ruder, J. H. & Young, S. D. (1974). Stimulation seeking and the Change Seeker Index. *Journal of Consulting and Clinical Psychology*, **42**, 311.

Buchsbaum, M. (1971). Neural events and psychophysical law. *Science*, **172**, 502.

Burch, P. R. J. (1976). *The Biology of Cancer. A New Approach*. Lancaster: Medical and Technical Publishing.

Burgess, J. H. & Rapaport, E. (1968). Cardio-respiratory effects of nicotine injected into the human ascending aorta. *Canadian Medical Association Journal*, **98**, 110.

Burns, B. H. (1969). Chronic chest disease, personality, and success in stopping cigarette smoking. *British Journal of Preventive and Social Medicine*, **23**, 23–7.

Burt, A., Thornley, P., Illingsworth, D., White, P., Shaw, T. R. & Turner, R. (1974). Stopping smoking after myocardial infarction. *Lancet*, i, 304–6.

Business (1982). *20 Woodbines to cost £1*, by our Business Correspondent. London: *Daily Telegraph*, 9 Jan.

Buttes, H. (1599). *Dyets Dry Dinner: Consisting of Eight Severall Courses*. London: Tho. Creede for William Wood (Bodleian Library, Oxford).

Bynner, J. M. (1969). *The Young Smoker*. (Government Social Survey) London: HMSO.

Bynner, J. M. (1970). Behavioural research into children's smoking: some implications for anti-smoking strategy. *Royal Society of Health Journal*, **90**, 159–63.

Capell, P. J. (1978). Trends in cigarette smoking in the U.K. *Health Trends*, **10**, 49–54.

Carlyle, T. (1881). *Reminiscences*, vol. 1, ed. J. A. Froude. London: Longmans, Green and Co.

Carruthers, M. (1976). Modification of the noradrenaline related effects of smoking by beta-blockade. *Psychological Medicine*, **6**, 251–6.

Castelli, W. P., Garrison, R. J., Dawber, T. R., McNamara, P. M., Feinleib, M. & Kannel, W. B. (1981). The filter cigarette and coronary heart disease: The Framingham Study. *Lancet*, *ii*, 109–13.

Cattell, R. B. & Cattell, M. D. (1973). *Manual for the High School Personality Questionnaire, 'HSPQ'*. Windsor: National Foundation for Educational Research in England and Wales, Nelson Publishing Co.

Cattell, R. B. & Krug, S. (1976). Personality factor profile peculiar to the student smoker. *Journal of Counselling Psychology*, **14**, 116–21.

Cautela, J. R. (1970). Treatment of smoking by covert sensitization. *Psychological Reports*, **26**, 415–20.

Cederlof, R. (1966). The twin method in epidemiological studies on chronic disease. Dissertation of the Academy of the University of Stockholm. Cited in Cederlof, R., Friberg, L. & Lundman, T. (1977). The interactions of smoking, environment and heredity and their implications for disease etiology. A report of epidemiological studies on the Swedish twin registries. *Acta Medica Scandinavica, Supplement*, **612**.

Cederlof, R., Floderus, B. & Friberg, L. (1970). Cancer in Mz and Dz twins. *Acta Geneticae Medicae et Gemellologiae*, **19**, 69–74.

Cederlof, R., Friberg, L. & Lundman, T. (1977). The interactions of smoking, environment and heredity and their implications for disease etiology. A report of epidemiological studies on the Swedish twin registries. *Acta Medica Scandinavica, Supplement*, **612**.

CHD Report (1983). Prevention of coronary heart disease. Summary of a conference held at St. Thomas's Hospital, London, June 1982. *Journal of the Royal College of Physicians of London*, **17**, 66–73.

Cherek, D. R. (1981). Effects of smoking different doses of nicotine on human aggressive behavior. *Psychopharmacology*, **75**, 339–45.

Cherry, N. & Kiernan, K. (1976). Personality scores and smoking behaviour. A longitudinal study. *British Journal of Preventive and Social Medicine*, **30**, 123–31.

Cherry, N. & Kiernan, K. E. (1978). A longitudinal study of smoking and personality. In *Smoking Behaviour: Physiological and Psychological Influences*, ed. R. E. Thornton, pp. 12–18. Edinburgh: Churchill Livingstone.

Cheshire, P. J., Kellett, D. N. & Willey, G. L. (1973). Effects of nicotine and arousal on the monkey EEG. *Experientia*, **29**, 71–3.

Choy, D. S. J., Purnell, F. & Jaffe, R. (1978). Auricular acupuncture of smoking. In *Progress in Smoking Cessation*, ed. J. L. Schwartz, pp. 329–34. New York: American Cancer Society.

Clark, M. S. G. (1969). Self-administered nicotine solutions preferred to placebo by the rat. *British Journal of Pharmacology*, **35**, 367.

Clarke, R. V. G., Eyles, H. J. & Evans, M. (1972). The incidence and correlates of smoking among delinquent boys committed for Residential Training. *British Journal of Addiction*, **67**, 65–7.

Clausen, J. (1968). Adolescent antecedents of cigarette smoking: data from the Oakland growth study. *Social Science and Medicine*, **1**, 357–82.

Coan, R. W. (1973). Personality variables associated with cigarette smoking. *Journal of Personality and Social Psychology*, **26**, 86–104.

Colley, J. R. T. (1974). Respiratory symptoms in children and parental smoking and phlegm production. *British Medical Journal*, *ii*, 201–4.

Comer, A. K. & Creighton, D. E. (1978). The effect of experimental conditions on smoking behaviour. In *Smoking Behaviour: Physiological and Psychological Influences*, ed. R. E. Thornton, pp. 76–86. Edinburgh: Churchill Livingstone.

Conterio, F. & Chiarelli, B. (1962). Study of the inheritance of some daily life habits. *Heredity*, **17**, 347–59.

Cooper, J. R., Bloom, F. E. & Roth, R. H. (1978). *The Biochemical Basis of Neuropharmacology*, 3rd edn. New York: Oxford University Press.

Correspondence (1981). Correspondence concerning passive smoking. *British Medical Journal*, **283**, 914–17.

Corti, C. (1931). *A History of Smoking*. London: George G. Harrap and Co. Ltd.

Creighton, D. E. & Lewis, P. H. (1978). The effect of different cigarettes on human smoking patterns. The effect of smoking pattern on smoke deliveries. In *Smoking Behaviour: Physiological and Psychological Influences*, ed. R. E. Thornton, pp. 289–300. Edinburgh: Churchill Livingstone.

Crumpacker, P. W., Cederlof, R., Friberg, L., Kimberling, W. J., Sorenson, S., Vandenberg, S. G., Williams, J. S., McClean, G. E., Grever, B., Iyer, H., Krier, M. J., Pedersen, N. L., Price, R. A. & Roulette, I. (1979). A twin methodology for the study of genetic and environmental control of variation of human smoking behaviour. *Acta Geneticae Medicae et Gemellologiae*, **28**, 173–95.

Cryer, P. E., Haymond, M. W., Santiago, J. V. & Shah, S. D. (1976). Norepinephrine and epinephrine release and adrenergic mediation of smoking-associated hemodynamic and metabolic events. *New England Journal of Medicine*, **295**, 573–7.

C.T. (1615). *An Advice How To Plant Tobacco In England; With The Danger of the Spanish Tobacco*. London: Nicholas Okes (New York Public Library).

Cummins, R. O., Shaper, A. G., Walker, M. & Wale, C. J. (1981). Smoking and drinking by middle-aged British men: effects of social class and town of residence. *British Medical Journal*, *ii*, 1497–502.

Cynoweth, K. R., Ternai, B., Simeral, L. S. & Maciel, G. E. (1973). NMR studies of the conformation and electron distributions in nicotine and acetylcholine. *Molecular Pharmacology*, **9**, 144–51.

Danaher, B. G. (1977). Research on rapid smoking: interim summary and recommendations. *Addictive Behaviors*, **2**, 151–66.

Daroqui, M. R. & Orsingher, O. A. (1972). Effect of *alpha*-met-tyrosine pretreatment on the drug-induced increase of hippocampal RNA. *Pharmacology*, **7**, 366–70.

Darwin, C. (1871). *The Descent of Man and Selection in Relation to Sex*. New York: A. L. Burt Co.

Davison, G. C. & Rosen, R. L. (1972). Lobeline and reduction of cigarette smoking. *Psychological Reports*, **31**, 443–56.

Dawber, T. R., Kannel, W. B. & Gordon, T. (1974). Coffee and cardiovascular disease. Observations from the Framingham Study. *New England Journal of Medicine*, **291**, 871–4.

de Faire, U. (1974). Ischemic heart disease in death discordant twins. *Acta Medica Scandinavica, Supplement*, **568**.

De Good, D. E. & Valle, R. S. (1978). Self-reported alcohol and nicotine use and the ability to control occipital EEG in a bio-feedback situation. *Addictive Behaviors*, 3, 13.

De Quincey, T. (1821). *Confessions of an Opium Eater*. First published in London Magazine, 1821. Reprinted 1971. Harmondsworth, Middlesex: Penguin Books.

Delahunt, J. & Curran, J. P. (1976). Effectiveness of negative practice and self-control techniques in the reduction of smoking behaviour. *Journal of Consulting and Clinical Psychology*, 44, 1002–7.

Dember, W. N. & Earl, R. M. (1957). Analysis of exploratory, manipulatory and curiosity behaviours. *Psychological Review*, 64, 91–6.

Deneau, G. A. & Inoki, R. (1967). Nicotine self-administration in monkeys. *Annals of the New York Academy of Sciences*, 142, 277–9.

Dock, W. (1963). Ballistocardiographic patterns and nicotine. *Archives of Internal Medicine (Chicago)*, 112, 467–75.

Dohi, T., Kojima, S. & Tsujimojo, A. (1973). Comparative studies of hepatic nicotine metabolizing enzyme activities in monkeys and dogs. *Japanese Journal of Pharmacology*, 13, 748–51.

Doll, R. (1974). Smoking, lung cancer and Occam's razor. *New Scientist*, 61, 463–7.

Doll, R., Gray, R., Hafner, B. & Peto, R. (1980). Mortality in relation to smoking: 22 years' observations on female British doctors. *British Medical Journal*, 280, 967–71.

Doll, R. & Peto, R. (1976). Mortality in relation to smoking: 20 years' observations on male British doctors. *British Medical Journal*, ii, 1525–36.

Domino, E. F. (1965). Some behavioral actions of nicotine. In *Tobacco Alkaloids and Related Compounds*, ed. U. S. von Euler, pp. 145–62. New York: MacMillan.

Domino, E. F. (1967). Electroencephalographic and behavioural arousal effects of small doses of nicotine: A neuropsychopharmacological study. *Annals of the New York Academy of Sciences*, 142, 216–44.

Domino, E. F. (1973). Neuropsychopharmacology of nicotine and tobacco smoking. In *Smoking Behavior: Motives and Incentives*, ed. W. L. Dunn, Jr, pp. 5–31. Washington, DC: Winston and Sons.

Domino, E. F. (1979). Behavioural, electrophysiological, endocrine, and skeletal muscle actions of nicotine and tobacco smoking. In *Electrophysiological Effects of Nicotine, Proceedings of the International Symposium on the Electrophysiological Effects of Nicotine, Paris (France), 19–20 October, 1978*, ed. A. Rémond & C. Izard, pp. 133–46. Amsterdam: Elsevier/North-Holland Biomedical Press.

Domino, E. F. & von Baumgarten, A. M. (1969). Tobacco cigarette smoking and patellar reflex depression. *Clinical Pharmacology and Therapeutics*, 10, 72–9.

Drachman, D. A. (1978). Central cholinergic system and memory. In *Psychopharmacology: A Generation of Progress*, ed. M. A. Lipton, A. DiMascio & K. F. Killam, pp. 651–2. New York: Raven Press.

D'Souza, S. W., Black, P. & Richards, B. (1981). Smoking in pregnancy: associations with skinfold thickness, maternal weight gain and fetal size at birth. *British Medical Journal*, 282, 1661–3.

Duncan, R. (1951). *Tobacco Cultivation in England*. London: Falcon Press.

Dunlap, K. (1932). *Habits, Their Making and Unmaking*. New York: Liveright.

Dunn, A. J. (1980). Neurochemistry of learning and memory: An evaluation of recent data. *Annual Review of Psychology*, 31, 343–90.

Eaves, L. J. (1973). The structure of genotype and environmental covariation for personality measurements: an analysis of the PEN. *British Journal of Social and Clinical Psychology*, 12, 275–82.

Eaves, L. J. & Eysenck, H. J. (1975). The nature of extraversion: a general analysis. *Journal of Personality and Social Psychology*, **32**, 102–12.

Eaves, L. J. & Eysenck, H. J. (1976). A genetic model for psychoticism. *Behavior Genetics*, **6**, 359–62.

Eaves, L. J. & Eysenck, H. J. (1977). A genotype-environmental model of psychoticism. *Advances in Behaviour Research and Therapy*, **1**, 5–26.

Eaves, L. J. & Young, P. A. (1981). Genetic theory and personality differences. In *Dimensions of Personality*, ed. R. Lynn, pp. 130–79. Oxford: Pergamon.

Ebenezer, I. (1982). The effect of nicotine on the development of cortical slow potentials associated with discrimination in the rat. *British Journal of Pharmacology Proceedings Supplement*, **77**, 458.

Eiser, J. R., Sutton, S. R. & Wober, M. (1978a). Can television influence smoking? *British Journal of Addiction*, **73**, 215–19.

Eiser, J. R., Sutton, S. R. & Wober, M. (1978b). Can television influence smoking? Further evidence. *British Journal of Addiction*, **73**, 291–8.

Ejrup, B. (1963). A proposed medical regimen to stop smoking. The follow-up results. *Swedish Cancer Society. Yearbook 3*, 468–73.

Ek, S., Froberg, J., Kagan, A., Karlsson, C-G., Levi, L. & Palmblad, J. (1977). Cigarette smoking, nicotine content, cognitive factors and psychological stressors: an experimental study of physiological and psychological effects in smokers, non-smokers and abstainers. *Reports from the Laboratory for Clinical Stress Research*, no. **61**. Stockholm: Karolinska Institute.

Elgerot, A. (1976). Note on selective effects of short-term tobacco-abstinence on complex versus simple mental tasks. *Perceptual and Motor Skills*, **42**, 413–14.

Elliott, C. H. (1977). A multiple component treatment approach to smoking reduction. PhD Thesis, University of Kansas, 1976. *Dissertation Abstracts International*, **38**, 893-B–894-B.

Elliott, C. H. & Denney, D. R. (1978). A multiple-component treatment approach to smoking reduction. *Journal of Consulting and Clinical Psychology*, **46**, 1330–9.

Elliott, R. & Thysell, R. (1968). A note on smoking and heart rate. *Psychophysiology*, **5**, 280–3.

Elliott, R. & Tighe, T. (1968). Breaking the cigarette habit: Effects of a technique involving threatened loss of money. *Psychological Record*, **18**, 503–13.

Emboden, W. (1972). *Narcotic Plants*. London: Studio Vista.

Enstrom, J. E. (1979). Rising lung cancer mortality among non-smokers. *Journal of the National Cancer Institute*, **62**, 755–60.

Erwin, C. W. (1971). Cardiac rate responses to cigarette smoking. A study utilizing radiotelemetry. *Psychophysiology*, **8**, 75–81.

Essman, W. B. (1973). Nicotine-related neurochemical changes: some implication for motivational mechanisms and differences. *Smoking Behavior: Motives and Incentives*, ed. W. L. Dunn, Jr, pp. 51–65. Washington, DC: Winston and Sons.

Evangelista, A. M., Gattoni, R. C. & Izquierdo, I. (1970). Effect of amphetamine, nicotine and hexamethonium on performance of a conditioned response during acquisition and retention trials. *Pharmacology*, **3**, 91–6.

Evans, R. I. (1976). Smoking in children: developing a social psychological strategy of deterrence. *Preventive Medicine*, **5**, 122–7.

Evans, R. I., Rozelle, R. M., Mittelmark, M. B., Hansen, W. B., Bane, A. L. & Havis, J. (1978). Deterring the onset of smoking in children: knowledge of immediate physiological effects and coping with peer pressure, media pressure, and parent modelling. *Journal of Applied Social Psychology*, **8**, 126–35.

Eye and Ear Witness (1665). *The Character of a Coffee-House. Wherein is Contained a Description of the Persons Usually Frequenting It and Their Discourse and Humors.* London (Bodleian Library, Oxford).

Eysenck, H. J. (1953). *The Structure of Human Personality*. London: Methuen and Co. Ltd. New York: John Wiley and Sons.

Eysenck, H. J. (1957). *The Dynamics of Anxiety and Hysteria*. London: Routledge and Kegan Paul.

Eysenck, H. J. (Ed.) (1960). *Experiments in Personality, Vol. 1*. London: Routledge and Kegan Paul.

Eysenck, H. J. (1963). Smoking, personality and psychosomatic disorders. *Journal of Psychosomatic Research*, **7**, 107.

Eysenck, H. J. (1967). *The Biological Basis of Personality*. Springfield, Illinois: Charles C. Thomas.

Eysenck, H. J. (Ed.) (1968). *Handbook of Abnormal Psychology: An Experimental Approach*, (3rd printing). London: Pitman Medical Publishing Co.

Eysenck, H. J. (1973). Personality and the maintenance of the smoking habit. In *Smoking Behavior: Motives and Incentives*, ed. W. L. Dunn, Jr, pp. 113–46. Washington, DC: Winston and Sons.

Eysenck, H. J. (1977). *Crime and Personality*, revised edn. England: Granada Publishing Ltd.

Eysenck, H. J. (with contributions by L. J. Eaves) (1980). *The Causes and Effects of Smoking*. London: Maurice Temple Smith Ltd.

Eysenck, H. J. (1982). Schenk and the personality of the smokers. *Personality and Individual Differences*, **3**, 217–18.

Eysenck, H. J. & Eysenck, S. B. G. (1975). *Manual of the Eysenck Personality Questionnaire (Junior and Adult)*. London: Hodder and Stoughton.

Eysenck, H. J. & Eysenck, S. B. G. (1976). *Psychoticism as a Dimension of Personality*. London: Hodder and Stoughton Educational.

Eysenck, H. J. & Kamin, L. (1981). *Intelligence: the Battle For the Mind*. London and Sydney: Pan Books.

Eysenck, H. J. & O'Connor, J. (1979). Smoking, arousal and personality. In *Electrophysiological Effects of Nicotine. Proceedings of the International Symposium on the Electrophysiological Effects of Nicotine, Paris (France), 19–20 October, 1978*, ed. A. Rémond & C. Izard, pp. 147–57. Amsterdam: Elsevier/North Holland Biomedical Press.

Fagerstrom, K. O. & Gotestam, K. G. (1977). Increase in muscle tonus after tobacco smoking. *Addictive Behaviors*, **2**, 203–6.

Falkeborn, Y., Larsson, C. & Nordberg, A. (1981). Chronic nicotine exposure in the rat: a behavioural and biochemical study of tolerance. *Drug and Alcohol Dependence*, **8**, 51–60.

Feyerabend, C. T., Levitt, T. & Russell, M. A. H. (1975). A rapid gas-liquid chromatographic estimation of nicotine in biological fluids. *Journal of Pharmacy and Pharmacology*, **27**, 434–6.

Feyerabend, C. & Russell, M. A. H. (1978). Effect of urinary pH and nicotine excretion rate on plasma nicotine during cigarette smoking and chewing nicotine gum. *British Journal of Clinical Pharmacology*, **5**, 293–7.

Fisher, R. A. (1958a). Lung cancer and cigarettes. *Nature*, **182**, 108.

Fisher, R. A. (1958b). Cancer and smoking. *Nature*, **182**, 596.

Fisher, R. A. (1959). *Smoking. The Cancer Controversy*. Edinburgh and London: Oliver and Boyd.

Floderus, B. (1974). Psycho-social factors in relation to coronary heart disease and associated risk factors. *Nordisk Hygiensik Tidskrift*, Supplement **6**.

Flood, J. F., Bennet, E. L., Orme, A. E., Rosenzweig, M. R. & Jarvik, M. E. (1978). Memory: modification of anisomycin-induced amnesia by stimulants and depressants. *Science*, **199**, 324–6.

Foggitt, R. H. (1974). Personality and Delinquency. PhD Thesis, University of London.

Frankenhaeuser, M., Myrsten, A. L. & Post, B. (1970). Psychophysiological reactions to cigarette smoking. *Scandinavian Journal of Psychology*, **11**, 237–45.

Frankenhaeuser, M. A., Myrsten, A. L., Post, B. & Johansson, G. (1971). Behavioural and physiological effects of cigarette smoking in a monotonous situation. *Psychopharmacologia*, **22**, 1–7.

Frankenhaeuser, M., Myrsten, A. L., Waszak, M., Neri, A. & Post, B. (1968). Dosage and time effects of cigarette smoking. *Psychopharmacologia*, **13**, 311–19.

Frederiksen, L. W. (1976). Single-case designs in the modification of smoking. *Addictive Behaviors*, **1**, 311–19.

Frederiksen, L. W. & Frazier, M. (1977). Temporal distribution of smoking. *Addictive Behaviors*, **2**, 187–92.

Frederiksen, L. W., Miller, P. M. & Peterson, G. L. (1977). Topographical components of smoking behaviour. *Addictive Behaviors*, **2**, 55–61.

Frederiksen, L. W., Peterson, G. L. & Murphy, W. D. (1976). Controlled smoking: development and maintenance. *Addictive Behaviors*, **1**, 193–6.

Freud, S. (1901). Complete psychological works of Sigmund Freud. Translated from German by Strachey, J. (Ed.), *Infantile Sexuality II*, vol. VII (1901–1903), *Auto-Eroticism*, p. 182. London: Hogarth Press (1953 Edn).

Friberg, L., Cederlof, R., Lorich, U., Lundman, T. & de Faire, U. (1973). Mortality in twins in relation to smoking habits and alcohol problems. *Archives of Environmental Health*, **27**, 294–304.

Friberg, L., Kaij, L., Dencker, S. J. & Jonsson, E. (1959). Smoking habits in monozygotic and dizygotic twins. *British Medical Journal*, *i*, 1090.

Friedman, G. D., Siegelaub, A. B., Dales, L. G. & Seltzer, C. C. (1979). Characteristics predictive of coronary heart disease in ex-smokers before they stopped smoking: Comparison with persistent smokers and non-smokers. *Journal of Chronic Diseases*, **32**, 175–90.

Friedman, J., Goldberg, T., Horvarth, T. & Meares, R. (1974a). The effect of tobacco smoking on evoked potentials. *Clinical and Experimental Pharmacology and Physiology*, **1**, 249–58.

Friedman, J., Horvarth, T. & Meares, R. (1974b). Tobacco smoking and a 'stimulus barrier'. *Nature*, **248**, 455–6.

Frith, C. D. (1971a). The effect of varying the nicotine content of cigarettes on human smoking behaviour. *Psychopharmacologia*, **19**, 188–92.

Frith, C. D. (1971b). Smoking behaviour and its relationship to the smoker's immediate experience. *British Journal of Social and Clinical Psychology*, **10**, 73–8.

Funkenstein, D. H. (1955). The physiology of fear and anger. *Scientific American*, **192**, 74–80.

Gallup Opinion Index (1974). Public puffs on after ten years of warnings. *Gallup Opinion Index* (Report no. 108), 20–21.

Garg, M. (1969). The effect of nicotine on 2 different types of learning. *Psychopharmacologia*, **15**, 408–14.

Garg, M. & Holland, H. C. (1968). Consolidation and maze learning: A further study of post-trial injections of a stimulant drug (nicotine). *International Journal of Neuropharmacology*, **7**, 55–9.

Ginzel, K. H., Watanabe, S., Eldred, E. & Grover, F. (1968). Depression of gamma efferent activity by nicotine. *Federation Proceedings* (Federation of American Societies for Experimental Biology), **27**, 572.

Glasgow, R. E. (1978). Effects of a self-control manual, rapid smoking and amount of therapist contact on smoking reduction. *Journal of Consulting and Clinical Psychology*, **46**, 1439–47.

Goldfarb, T., Gritz, E. R., Jarvik, M. E. & Stolerman, I. P. (1976). Reactions to cigarettes as a function of nicotine and 'tar'. *Clinical Pharmacology and Therapeutics*, **19**, 767–72.

Goldfarb, T. L., Jarvik, M. E. & Glick, S. D. (1970). Cigarette nicotine content as a determinant of human smoking behaviour. *Psychopharmacologia*, **17**, 89–93.

Golding, J. F. (1980). Short Term Effects of Cigarette Smoking. D.Phil. University of Oxford.

Golding, J. F. & Mangan, G. L. (1982*a*). Arousing and de-arousing effects of cigarette smoking under conditions of stress and mild sensory isolation. *Psychophysiology*, **19**, 449–56.

Golding, J. F. & Mangan, G. L. (1982*b*). Effects of cigarette smoking on measures of arousal, response suppression and excitation/inhibition balance. *International Journal of the Addictions*, **17**, 793–804.

Golding, J. F., Harpur, T. & Brent-Smith, H. (1983). Personality, drinking and drug-taking correlates of cigarette smoking. *Personality and Individual Differences*, **4**, 703–6.

Goldsmith, J. R. & Landaw, S. A. (1968). Carbon monoxide and human health. *Science*, **162**, 1352–9.

Goodman, L. S. & Gilman, A. (1971). *Pharmacological Basis of Therapeutics*, 4th edn. New York: Macmillan.

Goodman Gilman, A., Goodman, L. S. & Gilman, A. (Eds.) (1980). *The Pharmacological Basis of Therapeutics*, 6th edn. New York: Macmillan.

Gordon, T., Kannel, W. B. & McGee, G. (1974). Death and coronary attacks in Man after giving up cigarette smoking. *Lancet*, *ii*, 1345–8.

Gori, G. B. (1977). Less hazardous cigarettes. In *Prevention and Detection of Cancer. Part I Prevention, Volume 1 Etiology*, ed. H. E. Nieburgs, pp. 791–804. New York: Marcel Dekker.

Gorrod, J. W. & Jenner, P. (1975). The metabolism of tobacco alkaloids. In *Essays in Toxicology*, ed. W. J. Hayes, Jr, vol. 6, pp. 35–78. New York: Academic Press.

Gorsuch, R. L. & Butler, M. C. (1976). Initial drug abuse: A review of predisposing social psychological factors. *Psychological Bulletin*, **83**, 120–37.

Gottesman, I. I. (1963). Heritability of personality: a demonstration. *Psychological Monographs*, **77**, 1–21.

Gottesman, I. I. (1968). Biogenetics of race and class. In *Social Class, Race, and Psychological Development*, ed. M. Deutsch, I. Katz & A. R. Jensen, pp. 11–51. New York: Holt, Rinehart and Winston.

Gottesman, I. I. & Shields, J. (1966a). Contributions of twin studies to perspectives in schizophrenia. In *Progress in Experimental Personality Research*, ed. B. A. Maher, pp. 1–80. New York: Academic Press.

Gottesman, I. I. & Shields, J. (1966b). Schizophrenia in twins. 16 years' consecutive admissions to a psychiatric clinic. *British Journal of Psychiatry*, 112, 809–18.

Grant, B. J. B. (1968). The nicotine habit. *Lancet*, i, 644.

Gray, J. A. (1971). *The Psychology of Fear and Stress*. London: Weidenfeld and Nicolson.

Griffiths, R. R., Bigelow, G. E. & Liebson, I. (1976). Facilitation of human tobacco self-administration by ethanol: A behavioural analysis. *Journal of Experimental Analysis of Behaviour*, 25, 279–92.

Gritz, E. R. (1979). Women and smoking: A realistic appraisal. In *Progress in Smoking Cessation*, ed. J. L. Schwartz, pp. 119–41. New York: American Cancer Society/WHO.

Gritz, E. R. & Siegel, R. K. (1979). Tobacco and smoking in animal and human behaviour. In *Modification of Pathological Behaviour*, ed. R. S. Davidson, pp. 419–76. New York: Gardner Press.

Guilford, J. S. (1972). Group treatment versus individual initiative in the cessation of smoking. *Journal of Applied Psychology*, 56, 162–7.

Guillerm, R. & Radziszewski, E. (1978). Analysis of smoking pattern including intake of carbon monoxide and influences of changes in cigarette design. In *Smoking Behaviour: Physiological and Psychological Influences*, ed. R. E. Thornton, pp. 361–70. Edinburgh: Churchill Livingstone.

Hall, G. H. (1970). Effects of nicotine and tobacco smoke on the electrical activity of the cerebral cortex and olfactory bulb. *British Journal of Pharmacology*, 38, 271–86.

Hall, G. H. & Morrison, C. F. (1973). New evidence for a relationship between tobacco smoking, nicotine dependence and stress. *Nature*, 243, 199–201.

Hall, G. H. & Turner, D. M. (1972). Effects of nicotine on the release of 3H-noradrenaline from the hypothalamus. *Biochemical Pharmacology*, 21, 1829–38.

Hall, R. A. M., Rappaport, H. K., Hopkins, H. K. & Griffin, R. (1973). Tobacco and evoked potential. *Science*, 180, 212–14.

Hancock, J. (1672). *Two Broad-Sides Against Tobacco. To Which is Added, Serious Cautions Against Excess in Drinking, Concluding with Two Poems Against Tobacco and Coffee*. London: Printed for John Hancock (Bodleian Library, Oxford).

Handel, S. (1973). Change in smoking habits in a general practice. *Postgraduate Medical Journal*, 49, 679–81.

Hankins, D., Drage, C., Zamel, N. & Kronenberg, R. (1982). Pulmonary functions in identical twins raised apart. *American Review of Respiratory Disease*, 125, 119–21.

Hanson, H. M., Ivester, C. A. & Morton, B. R. (1979). Nicotine self-administration in rats. *National Institute on Drug Abuse Research Monograph Series*, 23, 70–89.

Hare, R. D. (1975). Psychopathy. In *Research in Psychophysiology*, ed. P. Venables & M. Christie, pp. 325–48. New York: Wiley.

Harlow, H. F. & Harlow, M. K. (1962). Social deprivation in monkeys. *Scientific American*, 207, 137–46.

Harvald, B. & Hauge, M. (1965). Hereditary factors elucidated by twin studies. *Genetics and the Epidemiology of Chronic Diseases*, ed. J. V. Neel, M. W. Shaw & W. J. Schull, pp. 61–76. Washington DC: US Department of Health Education and Welfare.

Hauser, H., Schwarz, E., Roth, G. & Bickford, R. G. (1958). EEG changes related to smoking. *Electroencephalography and Clinical Neurophysiology*, 10, 576.

Hebb, D. O. (1949). *The Organisation of Behaviour: A Neuropsychological Theory*. New York: Wiley.

Heimstra, N. W. (1973). The effects of smoking on mood change. In *Smoking Behavior: Motives and Incentives*, ed. W. L. Dunn, Jr, pp. 197–207. Washington, DC: Winston and Sons.

Heimstra, N. W., Bancroft, N. R. & De Kock, A. R. (1967). Effects of smoking upon sustained performance in a simulated driving task. *Annals of the New York Academy of Sciences*, **142**, 295–307.

Herning, R. I., Jones, R. T., Bachman, J. & Mines, A. H. (1981). Puff volume increases when low-nicotine cigarettes are smoked. *British Medical Journal*, **283**, 187–9.

Herxheimer, A., Griffiths, R. L., Hamilton, B. & Wakefield, M. (1967). Circulatory effects of nicotine aerosol inhalation and cigarette smoking in man. *Lancet*, ii, 754–5.

Heston, L. L. (1966). Psychiatric disorders in foster home reared children of schizophrenic mothers. *British Journal of Psychiatry*, **112**, 819–25.

Hill, P. & Wynder, E. L. (1974). Smoking and cardiovascular disease: Effect of nicotine on the serum epinephrine and corticoids. *American Heart Journal*, **87**, 491–6.

Hirayama, T. (1981). Non-smoking wives of heavy smokers have a higher risk of lung-cancer: a study from Japan. *British Medical Journal*, **282**, 183–5.

Hjelle, L. A. & Clouser, R. (1970). Internal–external control of reinforcement in smoking behaviour. *Psychological Reports*, **26**, 562.

Hoffman, W. E. (1979). The impact of tobacco advertising and promotion on cigarette consumption. In *The Smoking Epidemic, a Matter of Worldwide Concern*, ed. L. M. Ramstrom, pp. 249–54. Stockholm: Almqvist and Wiksell International.

Holden, C. (1980). Identical twins reared apart. *Science*, **207**, 1323–8.

Holland, W. W. & Elliott, A. (1968). Cigarette smoking, respiratory symptoms, and anti-smoking propaganda. An experiment. *Lancet*, i, 41–3.

Holland, W. W., Halil, T., Bennett, A. E. & Elliott, A. (1969). Indications for measures to be taken in childhood to prevent chronic respiratory disease. *Millbank Memorial Quarterly*, **47**, no. 3, 215–27.

Homme, L. E. (1965). Perspectives in psychology. XXIV. Control of coverants, the operants of the mind. *Psychological Record*, **15**, 501–11.

Hopkins, J. M. & Evans, H. J. (1980). Cigarette smoke-induced DNA damage and lung cancer risk. *Nature*, **283**, 388–90.

Horn, D. (1960). Modifying smoking habits in high school students. *Children*, **7**, 63–5.

Horn, D. (1969). A scale to differentiate between types of smoker as related to the management of affect. *International Journal of the Addictions*, **4**, 649–59.

Horn, D., Courts, F. A., Taylor, R. M. & Solomon, E. S. (1959). Cigarette smoking among high school students. *American Journal of Public Health*, **49**, 1497–511.

Horn, J. M., Plomin, R. & Rosenman, R. (1976). Heritability of personality traits in adult male twins. *Behavior Genetics*, **6**, 17–30.

Hunt, W. A. & Matarazzo, J. D. (1973). Three years later: Recent developments in the experimental modification of smoking behaviour. *Journal of Abnormal Psychology*, **81**, 107–14.

Hutchinson, R. R. & Emley, G. S. (1973). Effects of nicotine on avoidance, conditioned suppression and aggression response measures in animals and man. In *Smoking Behavior: Motives and Incentives*, ed. W. L. Dunn, Jr, pp. 171–96. Washington, DC: Winston and Sons.

Ikard, F. F., Green, D. E. & Horn, D. A. (1969). A scale to differentiate between types of smoking as related to management of affect. *International Journal of Addictions*, **4**, 649–59.

International Anti-Cigarette League Gazette (1905). London: published monthly from 1901 to 1908 (Bodleian Library, Oxford).

Isaac, P. F. & Rand, M. J. (1969). Blood levels of nicotine and physiological effects after inhalation of tobacco smoke. *European Journal of Pharmacology*, **8**, 269–83.

Izard, C. (1978). Neuropsychology and Tobacco. In *Smoking Behaviour: Physiological and Psychological Influences*, ed. R. E. Thornton, pp. 44–53. Edinburgh: Churchill Livingstone.

Izard, C., Grob, R. & Rémond, A. (1979). Research into the electrophysiological effects of nicotine and their interpretation as arousal or sedation mechanisms. *Revue d'Electroencephalographie et de Neurophysiologie*, **9**, 348–65.

Jaffe, J. H. & Kanzler, M. (1979). Smoking as an addictive disorder. *National Institute on Drug Abuse Research Monograph Series*, **23**, 4–23.

James, Ist, King (1604). *A Counter-Blaste to Tobacco*. (Published under pseudonym 'R.B.' with Royal Coat of Arms) London: R.B. (Bodleian Library, Oxford).

Jarvik, M. E. (1967). Tobacco smoking in monkeys. *Annals of the New York Academy of Sciences*, **142**, 280–94.

Jarvik, M. E. (1970). The role of nicotine in the smoking habit. In *Learning Mechanisms and Smoking*, ed. W. A. Hunt, pp. 155–90. Chicago: Aldine.

Jarvik, M. E. (1973). Further observations on nicotine as the reinforcing agent in smoking. In *Smoking Behavior: Motives and Incentives*, ed. W. L. Dunn, Jr, pp. 33–50. Washington, DC: Winston and Sons.

Jarvik, M. E., Glick, S. D. & Nakamura, R. K. (1970). Inhibition of cigarette smoking by orally administered nicotine. *Clinical Pharmacology and Therapeutics*, **11**, 574–6.

Jarvis, M. J., Raw, M., Russell, M. A. H. & Feyerabend, C. (1982). Randomised controlled trial of nicotine chewing-gum. *British Medical Journal*, **285**, 537–40.

Jinks, J. L. & Fulker, D. W. (1970). Comparison of the biometric genetical MAVA and classical approaches to the analysis of human behaviour. *Psychological Bulletin*, **73**, 311–49.

Johnson, O. J. (1918). Effects of smoking on mental and motor efficiency. *The Psychological Clinic*, **12**, 132–40.

Johnston, D. M. (1965). Preliminary report on the effect of smoking on the size of visual fields. *Life Sciences*, **4**, 2215–21.

Johnston, D. M. (1966). Effect of smoking on visual search performance. *Perceptual and Motor Skills*, **22**, 619–22.

Johnston, E. & Donoghue, J. R. (1971). Hypnosis and smoking: A review of the literature. *American Journal of Clinical Hypnosis*, **13**, 265–71.

Johnston, L. M. (1942). Tobacco smoking and nicotine. *Lancet*, ii, 742.

Jones, M. C. (1924). A laboratory study of fear: The case of Peter. *Pedagogiai Szemle*, **31**, 308–15.

Jones, M. T., Hillhouse, E. W. & Cole, R. S. (1978). Role of GABA and other putative neurotransmitters in the regulation of corticotropin-releasing factor. In *Interactions between Putative Neurotransmitters*, ed. S. Garattini, J. F. Pujol & R. Samanin, pp. 245–61. New York: Raven Press.

Juel-Nielsen, N. (1960). 12 Mz pairs twins (1880–1934 born) brought up apart. Cited in Raaschou-Nielsen, E. (1960). Smoking habits in twins. *Danish Medical Bulletin*, **7**, 82–8.

Kales, J. D., Allen, C., Preston, T. A. & Tan, T-L. (1970). Changes in REM sleep and dreaming with cigarette smoking and following withdrawal. *Psychophysiology*, **7**, 347–8.

Karras, A. & Kane, J. M. (1980). Naloxone reduces cigarette smoking. *Life Sciences*, **27**, 1541–5.

Kelleher, R. T. & Morse, W. H. (1968). Determinants of the specificity of behavioural effects of drugs. *Ergebisse der Physiologie, Biologischen Chemie und Experimentellen Pharmakologie*, **60**, 1–56.

Kelman, H. C. (1958). Compliance, identification, and internalization: Three processes of attitude change. *Journal of Conflict Resolution*, **2**, 51–60.

Kershbaum, A., Pappajohn, D. J., Bellet, S., Hirabayashi, M. & Shafiiha, H. (1968). Effect of smoking and nicotine on adrenocortical secretion. *Journal of the American Medical Association*, **203**, 275–8.

Kier, L. B. (1968). A molecular orbital calculation of the preferred conformation of nicotine. *Molecular Pharmacology*, **4**, 70–6.

Kleinman, K. M., Vaughn, R. L. & Christ, T. S. (1973). Effects of cigarette smoking and smoking deprivation on paired-associate learning of high and low meaningful nonsense syllables. *Psychological Reports*, **32**, 963–6.

Knapp, P. H., Bliss, C. M. & Wells, H. (1963). Addictive aspects of heavy cigarette smoking. *American Journal of Psychiatry*, **119**, 966–72.

Knott, J. V. (1978). Smoking, EEG and input regulation in smokers and non-smokers. In *Smoking Behaviour: Physiological and Psychological Influences*, ed. R. E. Thornton, pp. 115–30. Edinburgh: Churchill Livingstone.

Knott, V. J. (1979a). Personality, arousal and individual differences in cigarette smoking. *Psychological Reports*, **45**, 423–8.

Knott, V. J. (1979b). Psychophysiological correlates of smokers and non-smokers: Studies on cortical, autonomic and behavioural responsivity. In *Electrophysiological Effects of Nicotine*, ed. A. Rémond & C. Izard, pp. 99–116. Amsterdam: Elsevier/North-Holland Biomedical Press.

Knott, V. J. & Venables, P. H. (1977). EEG alpha correlates of non-smokers, smokers, smoking and smoking deprivation. *Psychophysiology*, **14**, 150–6.

Knott, V. J. & Venables, P. H. (1978). Stimulus intensity control and cortical evoked response in smokers and non-smokers. *Psychophysiology*, **15**, 186–92.

Knudson, A. G. (1978). Retinoblastoma: A prototype hereditary neoplasm. *Seminars in Oncology*, **5**, 57–60.

Koenig, K. P. & Masters, J. (1965). Experimental treatment of habitual smoking. *Behaviour Research and Therapy*, **3**, 235–43.

Kornitzer, M., De Backer, G., Dramaix, M. & Thilly, C. (1980). The Belgian Heart Disease Prevention Project. *Circulation*, **61**, 18–25.

Kozlowski, L. T., Jarvik, M. E. & Gritz, E. R. (1975). Nicotine regulation and cigarette smoking. *Clinical Pharmacology and Therapeutics*, **17**, 93–7.

Krasnegor, N. A. (1980). Analysis and modification of substance abuse. *Behavior Modification*, **4**, 35–56.

Krutzer, C. S., Lichtenstein, E. & Mees, H. L. (1968). Modification of smoking behaviour: a review. *Psychological Bulletin*, **70**, 520–33.

Kumakura, K., Karoum, F., Guidotti, A. & Costa, E. (1980). Modulation of nicotinic receptors by opiate receptor agonists in cultured adrenal chromaffin cells. *Nature*, **283**, 489–92.

Kumar, R., Cooke, E. C., Lader, M. H. & Russell, M. A. H. (1978). Is tobacco smoking a form of nicotine dependence? In *Smoking Behaviour: Physiological and Psychological Influences*, ed. R. E. Thornton, pp. 244–58. Edinburgh: Churchill Livingstone.

Lacey, J. I. (1956). The evaluation of autonomic responses: toward a general solution. *Annals of the New York Academy of Sciences*, **67**, 123–64.

Lacey, J. I. (1967). Somatic response patterning and stress: Some revisions of activation theory. In *Psychological Stress: Issues in Research*, ed. M. H. Appley & R. Trumbull, pp. 14–42. New York: Appleton.

Lal, H., Miksic, S., Drawbaugh, R., Numan, R. & Smith, N. (1976). Alleviation of narcotic withdrawal syndrome by conditional stimuli. *Pavlovian Journal of Biological Science*, 11, 251–62.

Lamontagne, Y., Gagnon, M. A. & Gaudette, G. (1978). Thought-stopping, pocket timers and their combination in the modification of smoking behaviour. *British Journal of Addiction*, 73, 220–4.

Lancet (1979a). Smoking and intrauterine growth. *Lancet*, i, 536.

Lancet (1979b). Good memories or mere sieves? *Lancet*, i, 418–19.

Lando, H. A. (1977). Successful treatment of smokers with a broad spectrum behavioural approach. *Journal of Consulting and Clinical Psychology*, 45, 361–6.

Larson, P. S., Haag, H. B. & Silvette, H. (1961). *Tobacco: Experimental and Clinical Studies*. Baltimore, Maryland: Williams and Wilkins Co.

Larson, P. S. & Silvette, H. (1968). *Tobacco: Experimental and Clinical Studies. Supplement I*. Baltimore, Maryland: Williams and Wilkins Co.

Larson, P. S. & Silvette, H. (1971). *Tobacco: Experimental and Clinical Studies. Supplement II*. Baltimore, Maryland: Williams and Wilkins Co.

Laurence, D. R. (1973). *Clinical Pharmacology*, 4th edn. Edinburgh, London and New York: Churchill Livingstone.

Lebovits, B. & Ostfeld, A. (1971). Smoking and personality: A methodological analysis. *Journal of Chronic Diseases*, 23, 813–21.

Lee, P. N. (1976). Statistics of smoking in the United Kingdom. *Research Paper Number 1* (7th edn). London: Tobacco Research Council.

Lee, P. N. (1979). Has the mortality of male doctors improved with the reductions in their cigarette smoking? *British Medical Journal*, ii, 1538–40.

Lee, P. N. (1980). Correspondence: smoking and mortality of male doctors. *British Medical Journal*, 280, 562–3.

Leigh, G. (1982). The combined effects of alcohol consumption and cigarette smoking on critical flicker frequency. *Addictive Behaviors*, 7, 251–9.

Leventhal, H. (1970). Findings and theory in the study of fear communications. In *Advances in Experimental Social Psychology. Vol. 5*, ed. L. Berkowitz, pp. 119–86. New York: Academic Press.

Leventhal, H. (1974). Attitudes: Their nature, growth and change. In *Social Psychology: Classic and Contemporary Integrations*, ed. C. Nemeth, pp. 52–126. Chicago: Rand McNally.

Leventhal, H. & Cleary, P. D. (1980). The smoking problem: A review of the research and theory in behavioural risk modification. *Psychological Bulletin*, 88, 370–405.

Leventhal, H. & Niles, P. (1965). Persistence of influence for varying durations of exposure to threat stimuli. *Psychological Reports*, 16, 223–33.

Leventhal, H. & Watts, J. C. (1966). Sources of resistance to fear-arousing communications on smoking and lung cancer. *Journal of Personality*, 34, 155–75.

Levitt, E. E. & Edwards, J. A. (1970). A multivariate study of correlative factors in youthful cigarette smoking. *Developmental Psychology*, 1, 5–11.

Lewin, L. (1931). *Phantastica: Narcotic and Stimulating Drugs*. London: Kegan Paul, Trench, Trubner and Co.

Lichtenstein, E. & Danaher, B. G. (1976). Modification of smoking behaviour. A critical analysis of theory, research and practice. In *Progress in Behaviour Modification. Vol. 3*, ed. M. Hersen, R. M. Eisler & P. M. Miller, pp. 79–132. New York: Academic Press.

Lichtenstein, E. & Danaher, B. G. (1978). Role of the physician in smoking cessation. In *Chronic Obstructive Lung Disease: Clinical Treatment and Management*, ed. R. E. Brashear & M. L. Rhoades, pp. 227–41. St Louis, Missouri: C. V. Mosby.

Lichtenstein, E., Harris, E., Birchler, G. R., Wahl, J. M. & Schmahl, D. P. (1973). Comparison of rapid smoking, warm, smoky air, and attention placebo in the modification of smoking behaviour. *Journal of Consulting and Clinical Psychology*, **40**, 92–8.

Lilienfeld, A. M. (1959). Emotional and other selected characteristics of cigarette smokers and non-smokers as related to epidemiological studies of lung cancer and other diseases. *Journal of the National Cancer Institute*, **22**, 259.

Liljefors, I. (1970). Coronary heart disease in male twins. Hereditary and environmental factors in concordant and discordant pairs. *Acta Medica Scandinavica, Supplement*, **511**.

Liljefors, I. (1977). Coronary heart disease in male twins: 7-year follow-up of discordant pairs. 1st International Congress of Twin Studies, Rome, 1974. To be published in *Acta Geneticae Medicae et Gemellologiae*. Cited in Cederlof, R., Friberg, L. & Lundman, T. (1977). The interactions of smoking, environment and heredity and their implications for disease etiology. A report of epidemiological studies on the Swedish twin registries. *Acta Medica Scandinavica, Supplement*, **612**.

Lincoln (1969). Weight gain after cessation of smoking. *Journal of the American Medical Association*, **210**, 1765.

Loehlin, J. C. & Nichols, R. C. (1976). *Heredity, Environment and Personality*. Austin, Texas: University of Texas Press.

Lucchesi, B. R., Schuster, C. R. & Emley, G. S. (1967). The role of nicotine as a determinant of cigarette smoking frequency in man with observations of certain cardiovascular effects associated with the tobacco alkaloid. *Clinical Pharmacology and Therapeutics*, **8**, 789–96.

Lundman, T. (1966). Smoking in relation to coronary heart disease and lung function in twins. *Acta Medica Scandinavica, Supplement*, **455**.

McAlister, A. (1975). Helping people quit smoking: current progress. In *Applying Behavioural Science to Cardiovascular Risk*, ed. A. J. Enelow & J. B. Henderson, pp. 147–65. New York: American Heart Association.

McAlister, A., Puska, P., Koskela, K., Pallonen, U. & Maccoby, N. (1980). Mass communication and community organization for public health education. *American Psychologist*, **35**, 375–9.

McArthur, C., Waldron, E. & Dickinson, J. (1958). The psychology of smoking. *Journal of Abnormal and Social Psychology*, **56**, 267.

McCrae, R. R., Costa, P. T., Jr & Bosse, R. (1978). Anxiety, extraversion and smoking. *British Journal of Social and Clinical Psychology*, **17**, 269–73.

McKennell, A. C. (1970). Smoking motivation factors. *British Journal of Social and Clinical Psychology*, **9**, 8–22.

McKennell, A. C. (1973). A comparison of two smoking typologies. *Research Paper Number 12*. London: Tobacco Research Council.

MacCoby, N., Farquhar, J. W., Wood, P. D. & Alexander, J. (1977). Reducing the risk of cardiovascular disease: Effects of a community-based campaign on knowledge and behaviour. *Journal of Community Health*, **3**, 100–14.

Mandel, P., Mack, G., Kemf, E., Ebel, A. & Simler, S. (1978). Molecular aspects of a model of aggressive behaviour: neurotransmitter interactions. In *Interactions Between Putative Neurotransmitters in the Brain*, ed. S. Garattini, J. F. Pujol & R. Samanin, pp. 285–303. New York: Raven Press.

Mangan, G. L. (1982*a*). The effects of cigarette smoking on vigilance performance. *Journal of General Psychology*, **106**, 77–83.

Mangan, G. L. (1982*b*). *The Biology of Human Conduct*. Oxford: Pergamon.

Mangan, G. L. (1983). The effects of cigarette smoking on verbal learning and retention. *Journal of General Psychology*, **108**, 203–10.

Mangan, G. L. & Golding, J. (1978). An 'enhancement' model of smoking maintenance? In *Smoking Behaviour: Physiological and Psychological Influences*, ed. R. E. Thornton, pp. 87–114. Edinburgh: Churchill Livingstone.

Mangan, G. L. & Golding, J. F. (1983*a*). Factors underlining smoking recruitment and maintenance among adolescents. *Advances in Behaviour Research and Therapy*, **4**, 225–72.

Mangan, G. L. & Golding, J. F. (1983*b*). The effects of smoking on memory consolidation. *The Journal of Psychology*, **115**, 65–77.

Mangan, G. L. & Paisey, T. J. H. (1980). New perspectives in temperament/personality research: the 'behavioural' model of the Warsaw group. *Pavlovian Journal of Biological Science*, **15**, 159–70.

Manning, F. A. & Feyerabend, C. (1976). Cigarette smoking and foetal breathing movements. *British Journal of Obstetrics and Gynaecology*, **83**, 262–4.

Marais, E. (1936). *The Soul of the Ape*. New York: Atheneum.

Marlatt, E. (1979). Personal communication. Cited in Krasnegor, N. A. (1980). Analysis and modification of substance abuse. A behavioural overview. *Behaviour Modification*, **4**, 35–56.

Masironi, R. & Roy, L. (1982). *Cigarette Smoking in Young Age Groups. Geographic Prevalence*. Geneva: World Health Organization. Cited in Daily Telegraph (London), 27 March 1982.

Mason, S. T. (1979). Noradrenaline and behaviour. *Trends in NeuroSciences*, **2**, 82–4.

Matarazzo, J. D. & Saslow, G. (1960). Psychological and related characteristics of smokers and non-smokers. *Psychological Bulletin*, **57**, 493.

Mausner, B. & Platt, E. S. (1971). *Smoking: A Behavioural Analysis*. New York: Pergamon Press.

Mausner, J. S. (1970). Cigarette smoking among patients with respiratory disease. *American Review of Respiratory Diseases*, **102**, 704–13.

Mayer, D. J. & Watkins, L. R. (1981). Role of endorphins in endogenous pain control systems. In *Modern Problems of Pharmacopsychiatry*, **17**, ed. H. M. Emrich, pp. 68–96. Basel: S. Karger.

Maziere, M., Berger, G., Masse, R., Plummer, D. & Comar, D. (1979). The 'in vivo' distribution of carbon 11 labeled (−) nicotine in animals – a method suitable for use in man. In *Electrophysiological Effects of Nicotine*, ed. A. Rémond & C. Izard, pp. 31–47. Amsterdam: Elsevier/North-Holland Biomedical Press.

Means, R. K. (1962). *A History of Health Education in the United States*. London: Henry Kimpton.

Meylan, G. W. (1910). Meylan's results on smoking and scholarship. Appendix I in Hull, C. L. (1924). *The Influence of Tobacco Smoking on Mental and Motor Efficiency. Psychological Monographs*, **33**, 1–160.

Mitchell, V. (1978). Instant answers for students on what smoking does to the body. *American Lung Association Bulletin*, **10**, 6–9.

Mittler, P. (1971). *The Study of Twins*. Harmondsworth, Middlesex: Penguin Books Ltd.

Morley, S. G. (1947). *The Ancient Maya*. Stanford, California: Stanford University Press.

Morrison, C. F. (1967). Effects of nicotine on operant behaviour in rats. *International Journal of Neuropharmacology*, **6**, 229–40.

Morrison, C. F. (1968). The modification by physostigmine of some effects of nicotine on bar-pressing behaviour of rats. *British Journal of Pharmacology and Chemotherapy*, **32**, 28–33.

Morrison, C. F. & Stephenson, J. A. (1972). The occurrence of tolerance to a central depressant effect of nicotine. *British Journal of Pharmacology*, **46**, 151–6.

Munster, G. & Battig, K. (1975). Nicotine-induced hypophagia and hypodipsia in deprived and in hypothalamically stimulated rats. *Psychopharmacologia*, **41**, 211–17.

Murphree, H. B., Pfeiffer, C. C. & Price, L. M. (1967). EEG changes in man following smoking. *Annals of the New York Academy of Sciences*, **142**, 245–60.

Murphree, H. B. & Schultz, R. E. (1968). Abstinence effects in smokers. *Federation Proceedings* (Federation of American Societies for Experimental Biology), **27**, 220.

Murphy, G. (1970). Experiments in overcoming self-deception. *Psychophysiology*, **6**, 790–9.

Myrsten, A-L. & Andersson, K. (1975). Interaction between effects of alcohol intake and cigarette smoking. *Blutalkohol*, **12**, 253–65.

Myrsten, A-L. & Andersson, K. (1978). Effects of cigarette smoking on human performance. In *Smoking Behaviour: Physiological and Psychological Influences*, ed. R. E. Thornton, pp. 156–67. Edinburgh: Churchill Livingstone.

Myrsten, A-L., Andersson, K., Frankenhaeuser, M. & Elgerot, A. (1975). Immediate effects of cigarette smoking as related to different smoking habits. *Perceptual and Motor Skills*, **40**, 515–23.

Myrsten, A-L., Elgerot, A. & Edgren, B. (1977). Effects of abstinence from tobacco smoking on physiological arousal levels in habitual smokers. *Psychosomatic Medicine*, **39**, 25–38.

Myrsten, A-L., Post, B., Frankenhaeuser, M. & Johansson, G. (1972). Changes in behavioural and physiological activation induced by cigarette smoking in habitual smokers. *Psychopharmacologia*, **27**, 305–12.

Nathan, P. E. & Briddell, D. W. (1977). Behavioural assessment and treatment of alcoholism. In *Treatment and Rehabilitation of the Chronic Alcoholic*, ed. B. Kissin & M. Begleiter, pp. 301–49. New York: Plenum.

National Cancer Institute of the American Cancer Society (1977). *Cigarette Smoking Among Teenagers and Young Women*. Public Health Service, National Institutes of Health, National Cancer Institute, DHEW Publication No. (NIH) 77-1203. Washington, DC: US Department of Health, Education and Welfare.

Nauta, W. J. H. & Feirtag, M. (1979). The organization of the brain. *Scientific American*, **241**, 78–105.

Nelsen, J. M. & Goldstein, L. (1973). Chronic nicotine treatment in rats: Acquisition and performance of an attention task. *Research Communications in Chemical Pathology and Pharmacology*, **5**, 681–93.

Nelsen, J. M., Pelley, K. & Goldstein, L. (1973). Chronic nicotine treatment in rats: EEG amplitude and variability changes occurring within and between structures. *Research Communications in Chemical Pathology and Pharmacology*, **5**, 694–704.

Nelsen, J., Pelley, K. & Goldstein, L. (1975). Protection by nicotine from behavioural disruption caused by reticular formation stimulation in the rat. *Pharmacology, Biochemistry and Behaviour*, **3**, 749–54.

Nesbitt, P. D. (1973). Smoking, physiological arousal, and emotional response. *Journal of Personality and Social Psychology*, **25**, 137–45.

Newman, I. M. (1970). Peer pressure hypothesis for adolescent cigarette smoking. *School Health Reviews*, **1**, 15–19.

Newman, I. M., Martin, G. L. & Peterson, C. P. (1978). Attitudinal and normative factors associated with adolescent cigarette smoking. Paper presented at School Health Section Meeting, American Public Health Association, Los Angeles, October 1978. Cited in Leventhal, H. & Cleary, P. D. (1980). The smoking problem: A review of the research and theory in behavioural risk modification. *Psychological Bulletin*, **88**, 370–405.

Newman, L. M. (1972). Effects of cholinergic agonists and antagonists on self-stimulation behaviour in the rat. *Journal of Comparative Physiological Psychology*, **79**, 394–413.

North Karelia Project (1976a). In Puska, P., Koskela, K., Pakarinen, H., Puumalainen, P., Soirinen, V. & Tuomilehto, J. (1976). The North Karelia Project: A Programme for Community Control of Cardiovascular Diseases. *Scandinavian Journal of Social Medicine*, **4**, 57–60.

North Karelia Project (1976b). In Koskela, K., Puska, P. & Tuomilehto, J. (1976). The North Karelia Project: A First Evaluation. *International Journal of Health Education*, **19**, 59–66.

O'Brien, C. P., Testa, T., O'Brien, T. J., Brady, J. P. & Wells, B. (1977). Conditioned narcotic withdrawal in humans. *Science*, **195**, 1000–2.

O'Connell, D. L., Alexander, H. M., Dobson, A. J., Lloyd, D. M., Hardes, G. R., Springthorpe, H. J. & Leeder, S. R. (1981). Cigarette smoking and drug use in schoolchildren. II Factors associated with smoking. *International Journal of Epidemiology*, **10**, 223–31.

O'Connor, K. (1980). The contingent negative variation and individual differences in smoking behaviour. *Personality and Individual Differences*, **1**, 57–72.

O'Keefe, M. T. (1971). The anti-smoking commercials: A study of television's impact on behaviour. *Public Opinion Quarterly*, **35**, 242–8.

Ober, D. C. (1968). Modification of smoking behavior. *Journal of Consulting and Clinical Psychology*, **32**, 543–9.

Olds, M. E. & Domino, E. F. (1969). Comparison of muscarinic and nicotinic cholinergic agonists on self-stimulation behaviour. *Journal of Pharmacology and Experimental Therapeutics*, **166**, 189–204.

Orleans, C. T., Shipley, R. H., Williams, C. & Haac, L. A. (1981). Behavioural approaches to smoking cessation – I. A decade of research progress 1969–1979. II. Topical Bibliography 1969–1979. *Journal of Behavior Therapy and Experimental Psychiatry*, **12**, 125–44.

Orsingher, O. A. & Fulginiti, S. (1971). Effects of alpha-methyl-tyrosine and adrenergic blocking agents on the facilitating action of amphetamine and nicotine on learning in rats. *Psychopharmacologia*, **19**, 231–40.

Partanen, J., Bruun, K. & Markkanen, T. (1966). *Inheritance of drinking Behaviour. A Study on Intelligence, Personality, and Use of Alcohol of Adult Twins*. Stockholm: Almqvist and Wiksell.

Passmore, R. & Robson, J. S. (1976). *A Companion to Medical Studies. In Three Volumes. Volume 1: Anatomy, Biochemistry, Physiology and Related Subjects*. Oxford: Blackwell Scientific Publications.

Paton, W. D. M. & Perry, W. L. M. (1953). The relationship between depolarisation and block in the cat's superior cervical ganglion. *Journal of Physiology*, **119**, 43–7.

Paul, G. L. (1966). *Insight vs. Desensitization in Psychotherapy*. Stanford, California: Stanford University Press.

Payne, J. W. (1914). Payne's data: tabulated in Appendix A of Hull, C. L. (1924). *The Influence of Tobacco Smoking on Mental and Motor Efficiency. Psychological Monographs*, 33, 1–160.

Pechacek, T. F. (1979). Modification of smoking behaviour. Chapter 9. In *Smoking and Health: A report of the Surgeon General, U.S. Dept. of Health, Education & Welfare*, Publication No. (PHS) 79-50066. Washington, DC: US Government Printing Office.

Pederson, L. L., Scrimgedur, W. G. & Lefcoe, N. M. (1975). Comparison of hypnosis plus counselling, counselling alone and hypnosis alone in a community service smoking withdrawal program. *Journal of Consulting and Clinical Psychology*, 43, 920.

Perlman, H. H. & Dannenberg, A. M. (1942). The excretion of nicotine in breast milk and urine from cigarette smoking. *Journal of the American Medical Association*, 120, 1003–9.

Perry, C. L., Killen, J., Slinkard, L. A. & McAlister, A. L. (1980). Peer teaching and smoking prevention among junior high school students. *Adolescence*, 15, 277–81.

Perry, C. & Mullens, G. (1975). The effects of hypnotic susceptibility on reducing smoking behaviour treated by an hypnotic technique. *Journal of Clinical Psychology*, 31, 498–505.

Pertschuk, M. J., Pomerleau, O. F., Adkins, D. & Hirsh, C. (1979). Smoking cessation: The psychological costs. *Addictive Behaviors*, 4, 345–8.

Peto, J. (1974). Price and consumption of cigarettes: A case for intervention? *British Journal of Preventive and Social Medicine*, 28, 241–5.

Petrie, A. (1967). *Individuality in Pain and Suffering*. Chicago: Chicago University Press.

Pettigrew, J. D. (1978). The locus coeruleus and cortical plasticity. *Trends in NeuroSciences*, 1, 73–4.

Philaretus (1602). *Work for Chimney-sweepers: or A warning for Tabacconists*. Imprinted at London by T. Este, for Thomas Bushell (Bodleian Library, Oxford).

Philips, C. (1971). The EEG changes associated with smoking. *Psychophysiology*, 8, 64–74.

Phillis, J. & York, D. (1968). Nicotine, smoking and cortical inhibition. *Nature*, 219, 89–91.

Pickens, R. & Thompson, T. (1972). Simple schedules of drug self-administration in animals. In *Drug Addiction. Vol. 1. Experimental Pharmacology*, ed. J. M. Singh, L. H. Miller & H. Lal, pp. 107–20. Futura: Mount Kisco, New York.

Pikkarainen, J., Tukkunen, J. & Kulonen, E. (1966). Serum cholesterol in Finnish twins. *American Journal of Human Genetics*, 18, 115–26.

Pincherle, G. & Wright, H. B. (1970). Doctor variation in reducing cigarette consumption. *The Practitioner*, 205, 209–13.

Pomerleau, O. F. (1980). Why people smoke: current psychobiological models. In *Behavioral Medicine: Changing Health Life Styles*, ed. P. O. Davidson & S. M. Davidson, pp. 94–115. New York: Brunner-Mazel.

Pomerleau, O. F., Adkins, D. M. & Pertschuk, M. (1978). Predictors of outcome and recidivism in smoking-cessation treatment. *Addictive Behaviors*, 3, 65–70.

Pomerleau, O. F. & Pomerleau, C. S. (1977). *Break the Smoking Habit: A Behavioural Program for Giving Up Cigarettes*. Champaign, Illinois: Research Press.

Porter, A. M. & McCullough, D. M. (1972). Counselling against cigarette smoking. *The Practitioner*, 209, 686–9.

Pradhan, S. & Bowling, C. (1971). Effects of nicotine on self-stimulation in rats. *Journal of Pharmacology and Experimental Therapeutics*, **176**, 229–43.

Pradhan, S. & Guha, D. (1976). Studies on gross behaviour and electrocortical reactivity of the brain during various environmental and pharmacological states. *Research Communications in Psychology, Psychiatry and Behaviour*, **1**, 257–68.

Premack, D. (1959). Toward empirical behaviour laws. 1: positive reinforcement. *Psychological Review*, **66**, 219–33.

Pyke, S., Agnew, N. M. & Kopperud, J. (1966). Modification of an overlearned maladaptive response through a relearning program: A pilot study on smoking. *Behaviour Research and Therapy*, **4**, 197–203.

Pyszka, R. H., Ruggels, W. L. & Janowicz, L. M. (1973). *IR and D Report. Health Behaviour Change: Smoking Cessation*. Menlo Park, California: Stanford Research Institute.

Raaschou-Nielsen, E. (1960). Smoking habits in twins. *Danish Medical Bulletin*, **7**, 82–8.

Rachman, S. (1967). Systematic desensitization. *Psychological Bulletin*, **67**, 93–103.

Rae, G. (1975). Extraversion and neuroticism and attitudes. *British Journal of Social and Clinical Psychology*, **14**, 429–30.

Raw, M., Jarvis, M. J., Feyerabend, C. & Russell, M. A. H. (1980). Comparison of nicotine chewing gum and psychological treatments for dependent smokers. *British Medical Journal*, **281**, 481–4.

Rawbone, R. G., Murphy, K., Tate, M. E. & Kane, S. J. (1978). The analysis of smoking parameters: inhalation and absorption of tobacco smoke in studies of human smoking behaviour. In *Smoking Behaviour: Physiological and Psychological Influences*, ed. R. E. Thornton, pp. 171–94. Edinburgh: Churchill Livingstone.

Raymond, M. J. (1964). The treatment of addiction by aversion conditioning with apomorphine. *Behaviour Research and Therapy*, **1**, 287–91.

Razran, G. (1955). Partial reinforcement of salivary CRs in adult human subjects: preliminary study. *Psychological Reports*, **1**, 409–16.

Reich, W. (1949). *Character Analysis*. New York: Orgone Institute Press.

Reid, D. D., Brett, G. Z., Hamilton, P. J. S., Jarrett, R. J., Keen, H. & Rose, G. (1974). Cardiorespiratory disease and diabetes among middle-aged male civil servants. A study of screening and intervention. *Lancet*, *i*, 469–73.

Rémond, A., Martinerie, J. & Baillon, J-F. (1979). Nicotine intake compared with other psychophysiological situations through quantitative EEG analysis. In *Electrophysiological Effects of Nicotine. Proceedings of the International Symposium on the Electrophysiological Effects of Nicotine, Paris (France) 19–20 October 1978*, ed. A. Rémond & C. Izard, pp. 61–87. Amsterdam: Elsevier/North-Holland Biomedical Press.

Reynolds, C. & Nichols, R. (1976). Personality and behavioural correlates of cigarette smoking. One-year follow-up. *Psychological Reports*, **38**, 251–8.

Richmond, H. W. (1977). A fifteen-year prospective study of the incidence of coronary heart disease related to cigarette smoking habits in Cummins Engine Company management personnel with results of a vigorous anti-smoking education campaign. In *Proceedings of the Third World Conference on Smoking and Health. New York, June 2–5, 1975, Vol. II. Health Consequences, Education, Cessation Activities, and Social Action*, ed. J. Steinfeld, W. Griffiths, K. Ball & R. M. Taylor, pp. 275–81. US Department of Health, Education and Welfare, Public Health Service, National Institutes of Health, National Cancer Institute. DHEW Publication No. (NIH) 77–1413. Washington, DC: US Department of Health, Education and Welfare.

Rickles, W. H. (1972). Central nervous system substrates of some psychophysiological variables. In *Handbook of Psychophysiology*, ed. N. S. Greenfield & R. A. Sternbach, pp. 93–121. New York: Holt, Rinehart and Winston.

Risk Factor Intervention Trial (1977). Statistical design considerations in the National Heart and Lung Institute (NHLI) Multiple Risk Factor Intervention Trial (MRFIT). *Journal of Chronic Diseases*, **30**, 261–75.

Risk Factor Intervention Trial (1979). Multiple Risk Factor Intervention Trial (MRFIT): Smoking cessation procedures and cessation and recidivism patterns for a large cohort of MRFIT participants. In *Progress in Smoking Cessation: Proceedings of the International Conference on Smoking Cessation, June 21–23, 1978*, ed. J. L. Schwartz, pp. 183–98. New York: American Cancer Society.

Robins, L. N. (1966). *Deviant Children Grown Up*. Baltimore, Maryland: Williams and Wilkins.

Rocklin, T. & Revelle, W. (1981). The measurement of extraversion: A comparison of the Eysenck Personality Inventory and the Eysenck Personality Questionnaire. *British Journal of Social Psychology*, **20**, 279–84.

Rogot, E. (1974). *Smoking and general mortality among U.S. veterans, 1954–1969*. Department of Health, Education and Welfare Publication Number (NIH) 75–544. Bethesda, Maryland: National Institutes of Health.

Rogot, E. & Murray, J. L. (1980). Smoking and causes of death among U.S. veterans: 16 years of observation. *Public Health Reports*, **95**, 213–22.

Rolls, E. T. (1975). *The Brain and Reward*. Oxford: Pergamon Press.

Rose, G. (1977*a*). Ischaemic heart disease. *Journal of Medical Genetics*, **114**, 330–1.

Rose, G. (1977*b*). Physician counselling and personal intervention. In *Proceedings of the 3rd World Conference on Smoking and Health*, ed. J. Steinfeld, J. Griffiths, K. Ball & R. M. Taylor, pp. 515–23. US Department of Health, Education and Welfare (USDHEW) Publ. No. (NIH) 77–1413. Washington, DC: US Government Printing Office.

Rose, G. & Hamilton, P. J. S. (1978). A randomised controlled trial of the effect on middle-aged men of advice to stop smoking. *Journal of Epidemiology and Community Health*, **32**, 257.

Rosencrans, J. A. (1979). Nicotine as a discriminative stimulus to behaviour: Its characterisation and relevance to smoking behaviour. *National Institute on Drug Abuse Research Monograph Series*, **23**, 58–69.

Routtenberg, A. (1968). The 2-arousal hypothesis: Reticular formation and limbic system. *Psychological Review*, **75**, 51–80.

Royal College of Physicians (1962). *Smoking and Health*. London: Pitman.

Royal College of Physicians (1971). *Smoking and Health Now*. London: Pitman.

Royal College of Physicians (1977). *Smoking or Health*. London: Pitman.

Russell, M. A. H. (1971). Cigarette smoking: Natural history of a dependence disorder. *British Journal of Medical Psychology*, **44**, 1–16.

Russell, M. A. H. (1973). Changes in cigarette price and consumption by men in Britain, 1946–71: A preliminary analysis. *British Journal of Preventive and Social Medicine*, **27**, 1–7.

Russell, M. A. H. (1976). Tobacco smoking and nicotine dependence. In *Research Advances in Alcohol and Drug Problems. Vol. III*, ed. R. J. Gibbins, Y. Israel, H. Kalant, R. E. Popham, W. Schmidt & R. G. Smart, pp. 1–47. New York: Wiley and Sons.

Russell, M. A. H. (1979). Tobacco dependence: Is nicotine rewarding or aversive? *National Institute on Drug Abuse Research Monograph Series*, **23**, 100–22.

Russell, M. A. H. (1980). The case for medium-nicotine, low-tar, low-carbon monoxide cigarettes. In *Banbury Report 3: A Safe Cigarette? Proceedings of a meeting held at the Banbury Center, Cold Spring Harbor, N.H., October 14–16, 1979*, ed. G. B. Gori & F. G. Bock, pp. 297–310. New York: Cold Spring Harbor Laboratory.

Russell, M. A. H., Armstrong, E. & Patel, U. A. (1976). Temporal contiguity in electric aversion therapy for cigarette smoking. *Behaviour Research and Therapy*, **14**, 103–23.

Russell, M. A. H. & Feyerabend, C. (1978). Cigarette smoking: A dependence on high-nicotine boli. *Drug Metabolism Reviews*, **8**, 29–57.

Russell, M. A. H., Jarvis, M. J., Devitt, G. & Feyerabend, M. J. (1981). Nicotine intake by snuff users. *British Medical Journal*, **283**, 814–17.

Russell, M. A. H., Jarvis, M. J., Feyerabend, C. & Ferno, O. (1983). Nasal nicotine solution: a potential aid to giving up smoking? *British Medical Journal*, **286**, 683–4.

Russell, M. A. H., Peto, J. & Patel, V. A. (1974). The classification of smoking by factorial structure of motives. *Journal of the Royal Statistical Society (A)*, **137**, 313–46.

Russell, M. A. H., Wilson, C., Feyerabend, C. & Cole, P. V. (1976). Effect of nicotine chewing gum on smoking behaviour and as an aid to cigarette withdrawal. *British Medical Journal*, *ii*, 391–3.

Russell, M. A. H., Wilson, C., Taylor, C. & Baker, C. D. (1979). Effects of general practitioners' advice against smoking. *British Medical Journal*, *ii*, 231–5.

Ryan, F. J. (1973). Cold turkey in Greenfield, Iowa: A follow-up study. In *Smoking Behavior: Motives and Incentives*, ed. W. L. Dunn, Jr, pp. 231–41. Washington, DC: Winston and Sons.

Salber, E. J. (1964). Infant orality and smoking. *Journal of the American Medical Association*, **187**, 368–9.

Schachter, S. (1973). Nesbitt's paradox. In *Smoking Behavior: Motives and Incentives*, ed. W. L. Dunn, Jr, pp. 147–55. Washington, DC: Winston and Sons.

Schachter, S. (1975). Cited in 'Eat bicarbonates and smoke less'. *New Scientist*, **65**, 54.

Schachter, S. (1978). Pharmacological and psychological determinants of smoking. In *Smoking Behaviour: Physiological and Psychological Influences*, ed. R. E. Thornton, pp. 208–28. Edinburgh: Churchill Livingstone.

Schachter, S., Silverstein, B., Kozlowski, L. T., Perlick, D., Herman, C. P. & Liebling, B. (1977). Studies of the interaction of psychological and pharmacological determinants of smoking. *Journal of Experimental Psychology (General)*, **106**, 3–40.

Schechter, M. D. & Rand, M. J. (1974). Effect of acute deprivation of smoking on aggression and hostility. *Psychopharmacologia*, **35**, 19–28.

Schmahl, O. P., Lichtenstein, E. & Harris, D. E. (1972). Successful treatment of habitual smokers with warm, smoky air and rapid smoking. *Journal of Consulting and Clinical Psychology*, **38**, 105–11.

Schmiterlow, C. G., Hansson, E., Andersson, L. E., Applegren, L. E. & Hoffman, P. C. (1967). Distribution of nicotine in central nervous system. *Annals of the New York Academy of Sciences*, **142**, 2–14.

Schneider, N. G., Popek, P., Jarvik, M. E. & Gritz, E. R. (1977). The use of nicotine gum during cessation of smoking. *American Journal of Psychiatry*, **134**, 439–40.

Schulz, W. & Seehofer, F. (1978). Smoking behaviour in Germany – the analysis of cigarette butts (KIPA). *Smoking Behaviour: Physiological and Psychological Influences*, ed. R. E. Thornton, pp. 259–76. Edinburgh: Churchill Livingstone.

Schwartz, J. L. (1969). A critical review and evaluation of smoking control methods. *Public Health Reports*, **84**, 483–506.

Schwartz, J. L. & Dubitzky, M. (1968a). Requisites for success in smoking withdrawal. In *Smoking, Health and Behaviour*, ed. E. F. Borgatta & R. R. Evans, pp. 231–47. Chicago: Aldine.

Schwartz, J. L. & Dubitzky, M. (1968b). One-year follow-up results of a smoking cessation program. *Canadian Journal of Public Health*, **59**, 161–5.

Segal, M. (1978). The acetylcholine receptor in rat hippocampus; nicotinic, muscarinic or both? *Neuropharmacology*, **17**, 619–23.

Seltzer, C. C. (1980). Smoking and coronary heart disease: what are we to believe? *American Heart Journal*, **100**, 275–80.

Shekelle, R. B., Lepper, M., Liu, S., Maliza, C., Raynor, W. J., Jr, Rossof, A. H., Paul, O., Shryock, A. M. & Stamler, J. (1981). Dietary Vitamin A and risk of cancer in the Western Electric Study. *Lancet*, *ii*, 1185–90.

Shewchuk, L. A., Dubren, R., Burton, D., Forman, M., Clark, R. R. & Jaffin, A. R. (1977). Preliminary observations on an intervention program for heavy smokers. *International Journal of the Addictions*, **12**, 323–36.

Shields, J. (1962). *Monozygotic Twins Brought Up Apart and Brought Up Together*. London and New York: Oxford University Press.

Shields, J. (1973). Heredity and psychological abnormality. In *Handbook of Abnormal Psychology*, ed. H. J. Eysenck, pp. 540–603. London: Pitman Medical.

Shiffman, S. M. (1979). The tobacco withdrawal syndrome. *National Institute on Drug Abuse Research Monograph Series*, **23**, 158–84.

Siegel, S. (1978). A Pavlovian conditioning analysis of morphine tolerance. *National Institute on Drug Abuse Research Monograph Series*, **18**, 27–53.

Silverman, A. P. (1971). Behaviour of rats given a 'smoking dose' of nicotine. *Animal Behaviour*, **19**, 67–74.

Simeon, M. & Ariel, R. (1978). *Freud: The Psychoanalytic Adventure*. New York: Holt, Rinehart and Winston.

Smith, G. K. (1970). Personality and smoking: A review of the empirical literature. In *Learning Mechanisms in Smoking*, ed. W. A. Hunt, pp. 42–61. Chicago: Aldine.

SmokEnders (1971). Reported by Kanzler, M., Jaffe, J. H. & Zeidenberg, P. (1976). Long- and short-term effectiveness of a large-scale proprietary smoking cessation program – a four year follow-up of the SmokEnders participants. *Journal of Clinical Psychology*, **32**, 661–9.

Snyder, S. H. (1977). Opiate receptors and internal opiates. *Scientific American*, **236**, 44–56.

Sokolov, Y. N. (1963). *Perception and the Conditioned Reflex*. Oxford: Pergamon Press.

Solomon, R. L. (1977). An opponent-process theory of acquired motivation. In *Psychopathology: Experimental Models*, ed. J. D. Maser & M. E. P. Seligman, pp. 66–103. San Francisco: W. H. Freeman.

Solomon, R. L. (1980). The opponent-process theory of acquired motivation: The cost of pleasure and the benefits of pain. *American Psychologist*, **35**, 691–712.

Soskis, D. A. & Shagass, C. (1974). Evoked potential tests of augmenting–reducing. *Psychophysiology*, **11**, 175–90.

Stalhandske, T. (1970). Effects of increased liver metabolism of nicotine on its uptake, elimination and toxicity in mice. *Acta Physiologica Scandinavica*, **80**, 222–34.

Stamler, J. (1970a). Coronary risk factors and prevention of atherosclerotic coronary heart disease. *Chicago Medicine*, **73**, 509–18.

Stamler, J. (1970*b*). Acute myocardial infarction – progress in primary prevention. *British Heart Journal*, 33 (supplement), 145–64.

Stein, L. & Wise, C. D. (1967). Release of hypothalamic norepinephrine by rewarding electrical stimulation or amphetamine in the unanaesthetised rat. *Federation Proceedings* (Federation of American Societies for Experimental Biology), 26, 651.

Stepney, R. (1980). Consumption of cigarettes of reduced tar and nicotine delivery. *British Journal of Addiction*, 75, 81–8.

Stock, S. L. (1980). Risks the passive smoker runs. *Lancet*, ii, 1082.

Stolerman, I. P., Fink, R. & Jarvik, M. E. (1973*a*). Acute and chronic tolerance to nicotine measured by activity in rats. *Psychopharmacologia*, 30, 329–42.

Stolerman, I. P., Goldfarb, T., Fink, R. & Jarvik, M. E. (1973*b*). Influencing cigarette smoking with nicotine antagonists. *Psychopharmacologia*, 28, 247–59.

Straits, B. C. & Sechrest, L. (1963). Further support of some findings about the characteristics of smokers and non-smokers. *Journal of Consulting Psychology*, 27, 282.

Strickenberger, M. W. (1968). *Genetics*. New York: Macmillan.

Surgeon General (1964). *Smoking and Health: Report of the Advisory Committee to the Surgeon General of the Public Health Service*. Washington, DC: US Government Printing Office.

Surgeon General (1979). *Smoking and Health: A Report of the Surgeon General, U.S. Department of Health, Education and Welfare*. Washington, DC: US Government Printing Office.

Sutton, S. R., Russell, M. A. H., Feyerabend, C. & Saloojee, Y. (1978). Smokers' response to dilution of smoke by ventilated cigarette holders. In *Smoking Behaviour: Physiological and Psychological Influences*, ed. R. E. Thornton, pp. 330–5. Edinburgh: Churchill Livingstone.

Swain, T. (1974). Cold-blooded murder in the cretaceous. *Spectrum*, 120, 10–12.

Taggart, P. & Carruthers, M. (1972). Suppression by oxprenolol of adrenergic response to stress. *Lancet*, ii, 256–8.

Taha, A. & Ball, K. (1980). Smoking and Africa: the coming epidemic. *British Medical Journal*, 280, 991–3.

Tanner, A. G. (1912). *Tobacco: From the Grower to the Smoker. Pitman's Common Commodities and Industries*. London: Sir Isaac Pitman and Sons Ltd.

Tarriere, C. & Hartemann, F. (1964). Investigation into the effects of tobacco smoke on a visual vigilance task. In *Proceedings of the Second International Congress of Ergonomics, Dortmund*. Supplement to *Ergonomics*, 525–30.

Thomas, C. B. (1960). Characteristics of smokers compared with nonsmokers in a population of healthy, young adults, including observations on family history, blood pressure, heart rate, body weight, cholesterol and certain psychologic traits. *Annals of Internal Medicine*, 53, 697.

Thomas, C. B. (1973). The relationship of smoking and habits of nervous tension. In *Smoking Behavior: Motives and Incentives*, ed. W. L. Dunn, Jr, pp. 157–69. Washington, DC: Winston and Sons.

Thomas, C. B. & Cohen, B. H. (1955). The familial occurrence of hypertension and coronary disease, with observations concerning obesity and diabetes. *Annals of Internal Medicine*, 42, 90–5.

Thomas, C. B., Fargo, R. & Enslein, K. (1970). Personality characteristics of medical students as reflected by the Strong vocational interest test with special reference to smoking habits. *Johns Hopkins Medical Journal*, 127, 323.

Thomas, C. B. & Ross, D. C. (1968). Precursors of hypertension and coronary disease among healthy medical students: Discriminant analysis function IV. Using certain habits of daily life (sleeping, eating, drinking, studying and exercise) as the criteria. *Johns Hopkins Medical Journal*, **122**, 196.

Thompson, E. L. (1978). Smoking education programs. 1960–1976. *American Journal of Public Health*, **68**, 250–7.

Thoracic Society (1983). Comparison of four methods of smoking withdrawal in patients with smoking related diseases: Report by a subcommittee of the Research Committee of the British Thoracic Society. *British Medical Journal*, **286**, 595–7.

Tobin, K. J., Jenouri, G. & Sackner, M. A. (1982). Effect of naloxone on change in breathing pattern with smoking. A hypothesis on the addictive nature of smoking. *Chest*, **82**, 530–7.

Todd, G. F. (1978). Cigarette consumption per adult of each sex in various countries. *Journal of Epidemiology and Community Health*, **32**, 289–93.

Todd, G. F. & Mason, J. I. (1959). Concordance of smoking habits in monozygotic and dizygotic twins. *Heredity*, **13**, 417–44.

Tokuhata, G. K. (1963). Smoking habits in lung-cancer proband families and comparable control families. *Journal of the National Cancer Institute*, **31**, 1153–71.

Tokuhata, G. K. (1964). Familial factors in human lung cancer and smoking. *American Journal of Public Health*, **54**, 24–32.

Tokuhata, G. K. & Lilienfeld, A. M. (1963a). Familial aggregation of lung cancer in humans. *Journal of the National Cancer Institute*, **30**, 289–312.

Tokuhata, G. K. & Lilienfeld, A. M. (1963b). Familial aggregation of lung cancer among hospital patients. *Public Health Reports*, **78**, 277–83.

Tomkins, S. S. (1966). Psychological model for smoking behaviour. *American Journal of Public Health and Nation's Health*, **56**, 17–20.

Tomkins, S. S. (1968). A modified model of smoking behaviour. In *Smoking, Health and Behaviour*, ed. E. Borgatta & R. Evans, pp. 165–86. Chicago: Aldine.

Tooley, J. T. & Pratt, S. (1967). An experimental procedure for the extinction of smoking behaviour. *Psychological Record*, **17**, 209–18.

Toronto Smoking Withdrawal Study Centre (1973). In Delarue, N. C. (1973). A study in smoking withdrawal. The Toronto smoking withdrawal study centre – description of activities. *Canadian Journal of Public Health, Smoking and Health Supplement*, **64**, S5–19.

Travell, J. (1960). Absorption of nicotine from various sites. *Annals of the New York Academy of Sciences*, **90**, 13–30.

Trends in Neurosciences (1978). Mechanisms of action of benzodiazepines. *Trends in NeuroSciences*, **1**, 5.

Trevelyan, G. M. (1945). *English Social History*, 3rd impression. London: Longmans.

Tsujimoto, A., Nakashima, T., Tamino, S., Dohi, T. & Kurogochi, Y. (1975). Tissues distribution of [^{3}H]nicotine in dogs and rhesus monkeys. *Toxicology and Applied Pharmacology*, **32**, 21–31.

Tucci, J. R. & Sode, J. (1972). Chronic cigarette smoking. Effect on adrenocortical and sympathoadrenomedullary activity in man. *Journal of the American Medical Association*, **221**, 282–5.

Turner, D. M. (1969). The metabolism of [^{14}C]nicotine in the cat. *Biochemical Journal*, **115**, 889–96.

Turner, D. M. (1971). Metabolism of small multiple doses of (^{14}C) nicotine in the cat. *British Journal of Pharmacology and Chemotherapy*, **41**, 521–9.

Turner, D. M., Armitage, A. K., Briant, R. H. & Dollery, C. T. (1975). Metabolism of nicotine by the isolated perfused dog lung. *Xenobiotica*, **5**, 539–51.

Turner, J. A. M., Sillett, R. W. & Ball, K. P. (1974). Some effects of changing to low-tar and low-nicotine cigarettes. *Lancet*, *ii*, 737–9.

Turner, J. A. M., Sillett, R. W. & McNichol, M. W. (1977). Effect of cigar smoking on carboxyhaemoglobin and plasma nicotine concentrations in primary pipe and cigar smokers and ex-cigarette smokers. *British Medical Journal*, *ii*, 1387–9.

Turner, P., Granville-Grossman, K. L. & Smart, J. V. (1965). Effect of adrenergic receptor blockade on the tachycardia of thyrotoxicosis and anxiety state. *Lancet*, *ii*, 1316–19.

Ulett, J. A. & Itil, T. M. (1969). Quantitative electroencephalogram in smoking and smoking deprivation. *Science*, **164**, 969–70.

Ullmann, L. P. & Krasner, L. (1969). *A Psychological Approach to Abnormal Behaviour*. Englewood Cliffs, New Jersey: Prentice Hall.

Vagg, P. R. & Hammond, S. B. (1976). The number and kind of invariant personality (Q) factors: a partial replication of Eysenck and Eysenck. *British Journal of Social and Clinical Psychology*, **15**, 121–9.

Van Laer, E. K. & Jarvik, M. E. (1963). Smoking behaviour in monkeys. *The Pharmacologist*, **5**, 240.

Vandenberg, S. G. (1967). Hereditary factors in normal personality traits (as measured by inventories). In *Recent Advances in Biological Psychiatry*, vol. 9, ed. J. Wartis, pp. 65–104. New York: Plenum Press.

Vasquez, A. & Toman, J. (1967). Some interactions of nicotine with other drugs upon central nervous system function. *Annals of the New York Academy of Sciences*, **142**, 201–15.

Venables, P. H. & Martin, I. (1967). *A Manual of Psychophysiological Methods*. Amsterdam: North Holland Publishing Co.

Vogel, W., Broverman, D. & Klaiber, E. L. (1977). Electroencephalographic responses to photic stimulation in habitual smokers and non-smokers. *Journal of Comparative and Physiological Psychology*, **91**, 418–22.

Vogt, T., Selvin, S., Widdowson, G. & Hulley, S. (1977). Expired air carbon monoxide and serum thiocyanate as objective measures of cigarette exposure. *American Journal of Public Health*, **67**, 545–9.

Wachtel, P. L. (1967). Conceptions of broad and narrow attention. *Psychological Bulletin*, **68**, 417–29.

Wald, N. J. (1978). Smoking as a cause of disease. In *Recent Advances in Community Medicine*, ed. A. E. Bennett, pp. 73–96. Edinburgh, London and New York: Churchill Livingstone.

Wald, N., Doll, R. & Copeland, G. (1981). Trends in tar, nicotine, and carbon monoxide yields of U.K. cigarettes manufactured since 1934. *British Medical Journal*, **282**, 763–5.

Wald, N., Idle, M. & Boreham, J. (1981). Serum cotinine levels in pipe smokers: evidence against nicotine as a cause of coronary heart disease. *Lancet*, *ii*, 775–7.

Walker, R. E., Nicolay, R. C., Kluczny, R. & Rudel, R. G. (1969). Psychological correlates of smoking. *Journal of Clinical Psychology*, **25**, 42.

Warburton, D. M. & Wesnes, K. (1978). Individual differences in smoking and attentional performance. In *Smoking Behaviour: Physiological and Psychological Influences*, ed. R. E. Thornton, pp. 19–43. Edinburgh: Churchill Livingstone.

Warwick, K. M. & Eysenck, H. J. (1963). The effects of smoking on the CFF threshold. *Life Sciences*, **4**, 219–25.

Waters, W. E. (1971). Smoking and neuroticism. *British Journal of Medicine*, **25**, 162–4.

Watt, J. M. & Breyer-Brandwijk, M. G. (1962). *The Medicinal and Poisonous Plants of Southern and Eastern Africa*. London: E. and S. Livingston Ltd.

Weatherley, D. (1965). Some personality correlates of the ability to stop smoking cigarettes. *Journal of Consulting Psychology*, **29**, 483–5.

Webster, D. D. (1964). The dynamic quantitation of spasticity with automated integrals of passive motion resistance. *Clinical Pharmacology and Therapeutics*, **5**, 900–8.

Weeks, D. J. (1979). Do chronic cigarette smokers forget people's names? *British Medical Journal*, *ii*, 1627.

Wennmalm, A. (1982). Effect of cigarette smoking on basal and carbon dioxide stimulated cerebral blood flow in man. *Clinical Physiology*, **2**, 529–35.

Wesnes, K. & Warburton, D. M. (1978). The effects of cigarette smoking and nicotine tablets upon human attention. In *Smoking Behaviour: Physiological and Psychological Influences*, ed. R. E. Thornton, pp. 131–47. Edinburgh: Churchill Livingstone.

Wilde, G. J. S. (1964). Behaviour therapy for addicted cigarette smokers: A preliminary investigation. *Behaviour Research and Therapy*, **2**, 107–9.

Wilhelmsen, L. (1972). A smoking cessation program in a field trial. In *Preventive Cardiology. Proceedings of an International Symposium, Skovde, Sweden, August 21st*, ed. G. Tibblin, A. Keys & L. Werko, pp. 97–102. New York: John Wiley and Sons.

Williams, D. G. (1980). Effects of cigarette smoking on immediate memory and performance in different kinds of smoker. *British Journal of Psychology*, **71**, 83–90.

Winett, R. A. (1973). Parameters of deposit contracts in the modification of smoking. *Psychological Record*, **23**, 49–60.

Wishnie, H. (1977). *The Impulsive Personality*. New York: Plenum.

Wolpe, J. (1958). *Psychotherapy by Reciprocal Inhibition*. Stanford, California: Stanford University Press.

Wundt, W. M. (1874). *Grubdzuge der Physiologischen Psychologie*. Leipzig: Englemann.

Yanagita, T. (1977). Brief review on the use of self-administration techniques for predicting drug dependence potential. In *Predicting Dependence Liability of Stimulant and Depressant Drugs*, ed. T. Thompson & K. R. Unna, pp. 231–60. Baltimore, Maryland: University Park Press.

Yates, A. (1958). The application of learning theory to the treatment of tics. *Journal of Abnormal and Social Psychology*, **56**, 175–82.

Yoshida, K., Kato, Y. & Imuro, H. (1980). Nicotine-induced release of noradrenaline from hypothalamic synaptosomes. *Brain Research*, **182**, 361–8.

Zuckerman, M. (1979). *Sensation Seeking: Beyond the Optimal Level of Arousal*. New Jersey: Lawrence Erlbaum Associates.

Zuckerman, M., Bone, R. N., Neary, R., Mangelsdorff, D. & Brustman, B. (1972). What is the sensation-seeker? Personality trait and experience correlates of the sensation seeking scale. *Journal of Consulting and Clinical Psychology*, **39**, 308–21.

Zuckerman, M., Neary, R. S. & Brustman, B. A. (1970). Sensation-seeking scale correlates in experience (smoking, drugs, alcohol, 'hallucinations' and sex) and preference for complexity (designs). *Proceedings of the 78th Annual Convention, American Psychological Association*, pp. 317–18.

Index